Analytic Neurology: Examining the Evidence for Clinical Practice

Analytic Neurology: Examining the Evidence for Clinical Practice

Michael Benatar, M.B.ChB., D.Phil.

Clinical Fellow in Neurology, Harvard Medical School
and Beth Israel Deaconess Medical Center, Boston

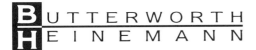

BUTTERWORTH
HEINEMANN

An imprint of Elsevier Science
Amsterdam Boston London New York Oxford Paris
San Diego San Francisco Singapore Sydney Tokyo

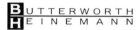
An imprint of Elsevier Science

200 Wheeler Road
Burlington, MA 01803

Library of Congress Cataloging-in-Publication Data

Benatar, Michael.
    Analytic Neurology: Examining the Evidence for Clinical Practice / Michael Benatar
      p. cm.
    Includes index.
    ISBN 0-7506-7440-7
     1. Neurology—Research. 2. Nervous system—Pathophysiology. I. Title.

    RC337 .B46 2003
    616.8'007'2—dc21

2002026155

Publisher: Susan F. Pioli
Editorial Assistant: Joan Ryan

SSC/MVY

Printed in the United States of America.

9 8 7 6 5 4 3 2 1

To my parents

Contents

Acknowledgments

I am indebted to my friends and teachers who have unselfishly given of their time, energy, and expertise to read and comment critically on sections of this book—Louis Caplan, Michael Ronthal, Clifford Saper, Roland Eastman, John Newsom-Davis, Seward Rutkove, Tim Vartanian, Frank Drislane, Daniel Tarsy, Daniel Press, Jonathan Edlow, and Sean Savitz.

I am particularly grateful to Roland Eastman, who first introduced me to neurology, encouraged me to turn to the literature for answers to clinical questions, and to read this literature as critically as possible.

I would like to thank my editor at Butterworth–Heinemann, Susan Pioli, for the enthusiasm with which she received the proposal for this project and for the energetic and efficient manner in which she helped bring this book to publication.

Finally, I would like to acknowledge my parents and brothers for their encouragement. I am grateful to them for this and for so much more.

Introduction

The everyday practice of clinical neurology does not require an extensive knowledge of the medical literature. In fact, very competent practicing clinicians may lack such knowledge. The reasons for this are manifold and relate to the fact that physicians very often know what should be done, even if they lack an understanding of the reasons why. In part, this state of affairs is a function of the nature of postgraduate medical education. Residents often work excessively long hours with substantial implicit learning from exposure to the way in which more senior colleagues practice. Residents, therefore, may learn more from day-to-day clinical experience than they do by poring over the medical literature. And when they do read, the focus may be on textbooks rather than on the primary data. Residency programs compensate by providing an education through didactic lectures, but these often amount to broad overviews that focus on *what* to do rather than on *why* we do what we do. The study of the primary literature that forms the basis for clinical practice is often neglected. The result is that physicians may pass through their postgraduate medical education without ever acquiring a real understanding of the foundations for clinical practice. Having not developed the curiosity and motivation to explore the primary literature as residents, physicians may be unlikely to acquire these traits in their later careers. It may often be the case that practice in fact is based on anecdote and lore rather than on hard evidence, but there is value in knowing that the evidence is lacking rather than simply being ignorant of whether or not it is present.

Some might take issue with the claim that practicing neurologists lack a detailed knowledge of the available literature. Those who do should, for example, ask whether they have ever heard the concern raised that patients who have migraine with aura might harbor an arteriovenous malformation (AVM) that is responsible for their symptoms. Is there any published literature on the subject other than a few isolated case reports? Are there any epidemiologic data that inform on this matter? What is the prevalence of AVMs in the general population, and how does this compare to the incidence in the population of patients who have migraine with aura? Are there any data supporting the claim that migraine that always affects the same side of the head or body should raise suspicion of an underlying AVM? As it turns out, there is very little in the literature to inform on the matter. The available data, in fact, suggest that the prevalence of AVMs may even be higher in the general population than amongst migraineurs. One could very easily deal with this concern in everyday clinical practice by obtaining a brain magnetic resonance image to exclude an underlying AVM. In this instance, ignorance of the literature results in safe practice, but this may not be the case in a different clinical circumstance. Although safe, such practice is not necessarily rational. I would venture that rationality dictates that we try to practice in the realm of the probable rather than the possible.

This background illustrates the motivation for this book, the aim of which is to ask these sorts of fundamental (and sometimes annoying) questions and, where possible, to offer answers. This book offers an exploration of the literature and an examination of the evidence that supports current practice in clinical neurology. As explained below, the approach adopted is not that used by the evidence-based medicine (EBM) discipline, and it also differs from the formal systematic review, such as that produced by the Cochrane Collaboration.

The dominant theme running through this book is the notion that clinical practice should be based on knowledge of the evidence that is outlined in the available literature. The idea that medical practice should be *evidence based* is well known and widely accepted. This has been the underpinning and *raison d'être* for the discipline of EBM that has been founded on the virtues of the randomized controlled trial (RCT). Although recognizing the utility of the RCT for its formal demonstration of the efficacy of a therapeutic measure in a well-defined study population, such trials are not without limitations. For example, the smaller the benefit to be gained from a therapeutic intervention, the larger the sample size needed. To obtain the statistical power necessary to demonstrate the relatively small benefit of a particular treatment modality, the organizers of RCTs must often recruit very large numbers of patients. A practical consequence of the need to recruit such large numbers of patients is the requirement for broad inclusion criteria. For example, many studies of therapeutic interventions in stroke have included all patients with ischemic stroke irrespective of whether the underlying pathophysiology is that of cardioembolism, large-artery atherosclerosis, or lacunar disease. The benefits of anticoagulation may outweigh the risks for certain stroke types but not for others. Although *lumping* may provide the numbers required for statistical power, this approach has at least two regrettable consequences. The first is that the efficacy of an intervention in a select group of patients may be diluted out and lost by including a different group of patients. The second problem is that broad inclusion criteria may limit the applicability of the results of the study to the individual patient. Therefore, for an RCT to yield a statistically meaningful result, a balance must be achieved between the need for a large sample size and the criteria used to define the study population. Such a balance often may not be obtained. The solution, however, does not lie in the abandonment of the clinical trial as a means of gathering clinical information. Instead, it is necessary to recognize the limitations of the available studies, to work toward the design of trials with more appropriate inclusion and exclusion criteria, and to exercise caution in the extrapolation of study results to individual patients. And when data from RCTs are not available, it is necessary to rely on the best available data. The goal of this book is to present the data as they exist and to try to describe both their value and limitations.

Problems in clinical neurology are approached by asking questions and then seeking the answers. The style of this book is predicated on this approach. Within each chapter, a series of questions is posed and the answers sought through a critical appraisal of the relevant literature. The aim has been to gather the best available evidence, even if this constitutes poor-quality data by EBM standards. Where relevant and available, RCTs have been cited. However, when such data are lacking, I have resorted to citing data that range in quality from prospective uncontrolled trials to retrospective case series. The point is that even in the absence of good-quality data from RTCs, it still makes sense to base practice on knowledge of the available data. After all, the published literature does represent the collective neurologic experience and, as such, offers insights that exceed the capability of individual neurologists. The use of steroids in the treatment of myasthenia gravis is a good example. Although there have been no large prospective randomized, placebo-controlled trials of steroids in myasthenia gravis, the available data support their use as first-line immunosuppressive therapy. Controversy persists, however, regarding the optimal dose and schedule for the initiation of therapy. Knowing the limits of the available data helps to engender a sense of humility in the conviction with which a particular practice is held.

A careful reading of the literature is perhaps more easily said than done. In part, this is because of its magnitude and the wide variation in its quality. More important, however, is the observation that much, if not most, of the published literature does not seem to have been written with the general neurologist reader in mind. Although it is clearly necessary for publications to include a detailed account of the study methodology, authors (and editors) seem to have forgotten that most readers require assistance in discerning the strengths and weaknesses of what often constitute highly technical reports. Most will be familiar with the practice of reading the *introduction* and *discussion* sections of a paper and skimming over or skipping the *methods* and perhaps even the *results* sections because of their daunting technicality. Readers often, therefore, place their trust in the investigators responsible for the trial and in the reviewers and editors who have seen fit to publish the study in question. It is not uncommon, however, for authors to present their results in a biased fashion and to fail to provide an adequate discussion of the validity and possible alternative interpretations of their data. Moreover, the review and publication process encourages this sort of approach in the sense that negative studies and studies with more equivocal results are less likely to become published in prominent journals, if at all. Publication bias thus limits the prominence with which negative studies are published. The Fraxiparine in Ischemic Stroke (FISS) and FISS-bis studies provide excellent examples. FISS was a randomized, double-blind, placebo-controlled trial of low-molecular-weight heparin (Fraxiparine) in the treatment of 308 patients with acute ischemic stroke. The conclusion from this study was that the use of heparin was associated with a 31% reduction in the relative risk of death or dependency at 6 months. The study was published in the prominent *New England Journal of Medicine*. The follow-up FISS-bis study was designed as a replication study with a larger sample. The conclusion from this study was that heparin did not confer any advantage in terms of the primary endpoint of death or Barthel Index (see Appendix 3 [Barthel Index]) score of less than 85. Notwithstanding the importance of these results, this study was published only in abstract form in the more obscure and less available journal *Cerebrovascular Disease*.

It has not been possible to cover all of clinical neurology in this book. The choice of subject material, therefore, is of necessity somewhat idiosyncratic. The first eight chapters of this book are devoted to various aspects of cerebrovascular disease, mostly concerning the outcome and management of ischemic stroke but also including chapters on intracerebral hemorrhage and subarachnoid hemorrhage. The first chapter on the risk of stroke recurrence has been included because this knowledge provides the necessary background and perspective for evaluating the relative benefits of the various therapeutic interventions that are discussed in the individual chapters on antiplatelet therapy, anticoagulant therapy, thrombolysis, carotid stenosis, and atrial septal aneurysms. The chapter on the antiphospholipid syndrome deals largely with the relationship between antiphospholipid antibodies and stroke in the young. The next three chapters focus on the demyelinating disorders, including optic neuritis, acute disseminated encephalomyelitis, and multiple sclerosis. Then follow chapters on neuromuscular and spinal cord disease, including Guillain-Barré syndrome, chronic inflammatory demyelinating polyradiculoneuropathy, myasthenia gravis and Bell's palsy, motor neuron disease, and cervical spondylosis as well as spinal cord trauma and compression. Individual chapters are devoted to Parkinson's disease, headache, and the treatment of dementia and seizures. A series of appendices includes all of the scales and scoring systems that are referred to in the studies discussed in this book. These have been included because insight into the nature of these scales is helpful in reading and understanding the literature.

A number of factors have influenced the choice of subjects. Chief amongst these has been the frequency with which particular issues have been raised in the course of my clinical practice, which has been characterized by an emphasis on inpatient neurology. The practice of stroke neurology, for example, which dominates in-hospital practice, has increasingly become influenced by the results of large prospective controlled trials. Furthermore, the morbidity and mortality of stroke are significant, and the treatments used often carry the risk of significant morbidity. The need, therefore, for a rational evidence-based practice is especially acute. For this reason, a significant number of chapters have been devoted to various aspects of stroke neurology.

Another important factor that has influenced the selection of subject material has been the disparity I have observed between the quality of the data on the one hand and the strength of conviction behind a particular practice held by some neurologists on the other. The place and timing of thymectomy in myasthenia gravis provide an excellent example. Is early thymectomy appropriate in patients with newly diagnosed myasthenia who have presented in crisis? Some advocate the aggressive use of plasma exchange or intravenous immunoglobulin followed by early thymectomy once the crisis has been averted. Others might object to this practice based on the questionable utility of thymectomy and the belief that the risks of surgery exceed the potential benefits at a stage in the disease when adequate immunosuppression has not yet been achieved. The truth is that these two approaches have not been compared head-to-head in a prospective fashion. However, a careful review of the data tends more to support than to undermine the position that thymectomy is of questionable benefit. Certainly, there is no evidence to support the contention that thymectomy should be performed acutely or in the very early stages of the disease. The literature on myasthenia gravis is characterized by a particular paucity of large prospective randomized, placebo-controlled trials, and, as such, practice is very often based more on lore than on evidence. Knowing that this is the case should serve to cultivate a sense of humility and open-mindedness to the possibility that the lore of a particular practice may not be appropriate.

As explained previously, one aim of this book is to make the reader aware of the evidence that supports clinical practice. Certain topics, therefore, have been included primarily because there are important landmark papers that have changed or profoundly affected the way in which we practice. The use of plasma exchange and intravenous immunoglobulin in the treatment of Guillain-Barré syndrome and chronic inflammatory demyelinating polyradiculoneuropathy is a prime example. Other subjects, such as the treatment of Bell's palsy, have been chosen because there appears to be little controversy surrounding the use of steroids and acyclovir, and yet the data supporting this practice are not unequivocal. It is useful to be aware of the limitations of these data even if such an awareness will not lead to an immediate change in practice.

For each of the neurologic diseases addressed, many others have been neglected, including lumbar spondylosis, carpal tunnel syndrome, brain tumors, and many more. Failure to include discussions of these disorders reflects the necessity of choice rather than any underestimation of their importance. This choice has been made on the basis of the factors outlined above. Although lumbar spondylosis, for example, is an important cause of morbidity and accounts for a significant number of outpatient neurology consultations, its management remains unsatisfactory, and the literature is not very informative in terms of selecting or prioritizing treatment strategies. There are no major studies that impact significantly on common practice, and the approach to treatment of this common condition is not based on adequate evidence.

Even within each chapter, it has been necessary to be selective with regard to the range of questions asked. It has been possible to cover the stroke literature more extensively, as many more chapters have been devoted to these issues. There has had to be greater selectivity in material covered in other chapters. In large part, the particular questions have been selected because of the frequency with which they have emerged in my clinical experience, but such selection has also been strongly influenced by the availability of studies that have bearing on the issues at stake.

It might be asked whether a book of this sort is really necessary given that there is little that is controversial or novel in the preceding comments. However, there are very few (if any) books that have been based on the premises outlined above. Moreover, it is surprising just how much of clinical neurology is practiced in a vacuum isolated from knowledge of the relevant literature. Ultimately, there can be no substitute for a careful reading of the literature oneself. The hope is that this book will serve as second best, introducing the reader to the literature that is relevant to a range of clinical issues and helping to provide some insights into the strengths and limitations of this literature. At times, some of the details provided in describing many of the studies will seem tiresome, but these details are included precisely because they give a sense of how a particular study was performed. This helps the reader to recognize the strengths and shortcomings of the trial in question.

Concern might also be raised about the ability of a book such as this to provide current information. It is true that new studies are continually being published, and our understanding and knowledge of neurologic disease are in ever-evolving states. Nevertheless, the present literature will always form the basis for the design and implementation of future trials, and knowing where the gaps lie in the current literature provides the necessary perspective for reading and understanding newer studies. It is also hoped that this book will provide not just a review of the available literature but that it will also stimulate and cultivate the approach that has been advocated.

M.B.

CHAPTER 1

Risk of Ischemic Stroke Recurrence

Introduction

There are many reasons why it would be useful to be able to estimate the risk of stroke after a transient ischemic attack (TIA) or stroke. Patients and their families want to know the likelihood of their having a stroke in the future. Also, if we are to evaluate the efficacy of secondary prevention treatment strategies, it is crucial to have an idea of the natural history of the disease in question. What are the chances of a recurrent stroke? Does this risk depend on whether the index event was a TIA or a stroke? Is the risk greatest in the immediate period after the index event? What are the factors that predict the risk of stroke recurrence? The answers to these questions have practical implications. For example, should patients with TIAs be admitted for urgent investigation, or can this be accomplished in the ambulatory setting?

However, the literature on stroke recurrence is extensive and difficult to encapsulate. The questions about stroke recurrence have been addressed by many studies, each with its own limitations, and there really is no single key study that has best addressed the issue. One problem is that the studies have varied in so many respects. Some have been retrospective and others prospective. The population under investigation has differed, being predominantly community or hospital based. The proportion of patients who were treated with antiplatelet agents or anticoagulants has varied, and this may impact upon the risk of recurrent stroke. The inclusion and exclusion criteria have not been uniform, and some studies, for example, have excluded patients who developed a stroke as a complication of cerebral angiography or carotid endarterectomy.

Another major issue that has plagued the literature on stroke recurrence relates to the fact that stroke is not a homogeneous condition, with the primary distinction being between hemorrhagic and ischemic stroke. The heterogeneity is significant even amongst ischemic stroke patients. Intuitively, it might be expected that stroke recurrence would differ for cardioembolism, large-artery atherosclerosis, small vessel ischemia, and lacunar stroke.

Nevertheless, we are constrained by the available literature. What follows is an attempt to wade through a number of the more recent studies, recognize their limitations, and yet also try to use the evidence they present to inform on the question of the risk of stroke recurrence.

Does the Risk of Stroke Recurrence Depend on Whether the Index Event Was a Transient Ischemic Attack or a Stroke?

Traditionally, a distinction has been made between neurologic deficits that resolve within 24 hours (TIA) and those that are persistent beyond this time period (stroke). Increasingly, however, especially with the use of sophisticated magnetic resonance imaging, it is becoming apparent that this is an artificial distinction. Diffusion-weighted imaging may show areas of tissue infarction when symptoms last less than 24 hours, and yet diffusion-weighted imaging may be negative in patients whose deficits persist for longer. These observations complicate any effort to answer the question posed above, but because the available studies examining the risk of stroke recurrence have employed clinical (not magnetic resonance imaging) criteria to distinguish TIA and stroke, it is the clinical definition of TIA that is used in the following discussion.

Given the varying risk of stroke recurrence reported in the literature depending on the nature of the study and population under investigation, it is difficult to use different studies to compare the relative risks of recurrent stroke after first TIA or stroke. Fortunately, there are reports of the risk of recurrent stroke after TIA or stroke in the same population.[1,2]

The Oxfordshire Community Stroke Project (OCSP) was a prospective community-based study of over 100,000 people that identified 184 patients with a TIA during the study period.[1] The mean age of the patient population was 69.4 years with 56% men. One hundred five patients (57%) received regular aspirin, 15 (8%) were treated with warfarin, and six (3%) underwent carotid endarterectomy. There were 45 first-ever strokes, and all but one were likely ischemic in nature. Sixteen (36%) were minor strokes and caused no long-term disability, and there were 15 (8%) stroke-related deaths. The risk of stroke was 4.4% during the first month, 8.8% during the first 6 months, 11.6% during the first year, and 29.3% over 5 years (Table 1-1). No analysis is provided to demonstrate whether treatment had any effect on the risk of stroke recurrence.

The OCSP also identified 675 patients with a first stroke.[2] The mean age of this patient population was 72 years (47% men). Cerebral infarction accounted for 545 (81%) of these strokes, the remainder being due to primary intracerebral hemorrhage, subarachnoid hemorrhage, or an unidentified process. Few of these patients received either antiplatelet therapy (6%) or anticoagulant therapy (1%), and the risks of stroke recurrence, therefore, are likely to be a reliable reflection of the natural history following stroke. There were 135 first recurrent strokes during the follow-up period

TABLE 1-1
Risk of Ischemic Stroke Recurrence

Index Event	Risk of Stroke at Indicated Time Interval			
	1 Mo (%)	*6 Mos (%)*	*1 Yr (%)*	*5 Yrs (%)*
Transient ischemic attack	4.4	8.8	11.6	29.3
Stroke	—	8.6	13.2	29.5

(although the type of stroke was only recorded in 42% of cases). Thirty-two (24%) of these were minor with no residual deficit, and 52 (39%) were severe. The risk of stroke was 8.6% at 6 months, 13.2% at 1 year, and 29.5% at 5 years (see Table 1-1).

These findings suggest that the risk of recurrent stroke is similar irrespective of whether the index event is a TIA or a stroke.

Is the Risk of Stroke Recurrence Greatest in the Short Term after the Index Event?

The importance of establishing whether the risk of recurrent stroke is greatest in the time period immediately after a TIA or stroke is that it has implications for the timing of investigation and initiation of secondary prevention strategies.

Aggregate (predominantly retrospective) data, summarized by the Cerebral Embolism Task Force,[3] suggest that the risk of recurrent embolic stroke is approximately 12% within the first 2 weeks (almost 1% per day) after an index cardioembolic stroke. These data are not entirely consistent with more recent prospective studies that have suggested that the risk of recurrence of cardioembolic stroke is approximately 12% per year (see following section). However, they do suggest that the risk appears to be greatest shortly after the index event.

Similarly, the Stroke Data Bank study found that the cumulative risk for recurrent stroke was 2% at 14 days, 3.3% at 30 days,[4] and 14.1% at 2 years,[5] and the OCSP found that the risk of stroke after TIA was 4.4% during the first month, 8.8% during the first 6 months, 11.6% during the first year, and 29.3% over 5 years.[1]

In a more recent (2000) retrospective study, Johnston et al.[6] examined the risk of stroke after the diagnosis of TIA by an emergency department (ED) physician. Patients seen in the ED who were diagnosed as having had a TIA were identified for inclusion in this study. TIA was defined on the basis of the World Health Organization criteria of rapidly developed clinical signs of focal or global disturbance of cerebral function lasting less than 24 hours, with no apparent nonvascular cause. In general, the diagnosis was made by an ED physician, but patient records were reviewed by a neurologist. The diagnosis of TIA was thought improbable by a neurologist in 96 patients (5.6%). The primary outcome was stroke occurring within 90 days of TIA presentation. The diagnosis of stroke required confirmation by two neurologists. The study included 1,707 patients, 99% of whom were evaluated within 1 day of the onset of symptoms. Mean age was 72 years, and mean symptom duration was 207 minutes. Strokes occurred in 180 patients (10.5%) within 90 days, 91 (approximately 50%) of which occurred during the first 2 days. Age older than 60 years, diabetes mellitus, duration of the episode greater than 10 minutes, signs or symptoms of weakness, or speech impairment during the episode were identified as independent risk factors for stroke within the 90-day study period. The 5.3% 2-day risk and 10.5% 90-day risk of stroke occurrence observed in this study are substantially greater than the risks reported by the OCSP. One reason for this may be that in the OCSP, patients were enrolled a median of 3 days after the index TIA, which implies that the early (2-day) risk of stroke was not captured by this study. On the other hand, the study by Johnston et al. is also subject to criticism. The study was retrospective, the diagnosis of TIA was made by an ED physician (with approval by a neurologist), and the mean duration of TIAs was unusually long, raising further concern about the veracity of the diagnosis.

Notwithstanding its limitations, the available data suggest that the risk of recurrent stroke is greatest shortly after the index event.

Does the Risk of Stroke Recurrence Depend on the Stroke Subtype of the Index Event?

Ischemic stroke is not a single disease but rather a broad term that is used to encompass a range of pathogenetic processes that includes cardioembolism, large vessel disease with artery-to-artery embolism, and small vessel disease (lacunar) stroke. It is not surprising that the risk of recurrent stroke might vary depending on the nature of the pathophysiologic mechanism of the first (index) stroke. Although many studies that have examined stroke recurrence have not differentiated between these various sorts of strokes, a number of studies have focused on this very important issue.

The European Atrial Fibrillation Trial was a prospective study of secondary prevention in nonrheumatic atrial fibrillation after TIA or stroke. These investigators found the risk of recurrent stroke in untreated patients with nonrheumatic atrial fibrillation to be 12% within the first year.[7] Of note is that this annual risk is very similar to the 11.6–13.2% reported for all stroke types in the OCSP.[1,2]

The Stroke Data Bank was a prospective observational study of patients hospitalized with acute stroke.[4,5] Ischemic stroke type was classified on the basis of causal mechanism into infarction due to large-artery atherosclerosis, lacunar stroke, cardioembolism, and stroke of undetermined cause. Data were available for 1,273 patients with ischemic stroke. In the study of early stroke recurrence,[4] there were 40 recurrent noniatrogenic strokes, iatrogenic strokes (e.g., stroke that resulted from cerebral angiography or carotid endarterectomy) having been excluded from the analysis. Thirty-one (77.5%) of these 40 strokes were of the same subtype as the index stroke. For all ischemic strokes, the cumulative risk of recurrence within the first month was 3.3% (similar to the 4.4% reported in the OCSP[1]). Analysis by stroke subtype, however, demonstrated that the risk was lowest (2.2%) for lacunar stroke, intermediate (4.3%) for cardioembolism, and highest (7.9%) for large-artery atherosclerotic stroke (Table 1-2).

The Stroke Data Bank population was then examined at 2 years to determine the risk of late stroke recurrence.[5] The estimated 2-year cumulative recurrence rate for all patients was 14.1%. When analyzed by stroke subtype, the cumulative 2-year recurrence was 14.6% for lacunar stroke, 14.7% for embolic stroke, 21.9% for large-vessel atherosclerotic stroke, and 10.5% for infarction of unknown cause (see Table 1-2).

Moroney et al. prospectively examined 297 patients who were hospitalized with an ischemic stroke and determined the risk of recurrent stroke within 3 months. The overall cumulative risk of stroke recurrence was 7.4%. When analyzed by stroke subtype, the risk of recurrent stroke was 13.1% in patients with large vessel atherothrombotic stroke, 11.3% in the cardioembolic group, and 1.2% in patients with lacunar stroke[8] (see Table 1-2).

The Dutch TIA Trial Study Group enrolled patients with TIA and nondisabling stroke. Events were classified as being due to small or large vessel disease, with approximately 1,200 patients in each group. All patients were treated with aspirin (either 30 mg or 283 mg per day). The overall stroke recurrence rate for each group was 3.6% per year. Patients with a large vessel disease index event were more likely to have a recurrent large vessel ischemic stroke. In contrast, recurrent strokes in patients with a small vessel index event were equally likely to have recurrent small and large vessel strokes.[9]

TABLE 1-2
Risk of Ischemic Stroke Subtype Recurrence

Stroke Subtype	Risk of Recurrent Stroke at Specified Time Interval from the Index Event			
	1 Mo (%)	*3 Mos (%)*	*1 Yr (%)*	*2 Yrs (%)*
All strokes	3.3[4]–4.4[1]	7.4[8]	13.2[2]	14.1[5]
Cardioembolic	4.3[4]	11.3[8]	12.0[7]	14.7[5]
Lacunar	2.2[4]	1.2[8]	—	14.6[5]
Atherothrombotic	7.9[4]	13.1[8]	—	21.9[5]

In summary, the risk of both early and late recurrence does vary for different types of ischemic strokes. The overall impression is that the risk of recurrent stroke is lowest for lacunar stroke, intermediate for cardioembolic stroke, and greatest for large-artery atherothrombotic stroke.

Are Recurrent Strokes of the Same Subtype as the Index Event?

Identification of the underlying mechanism of recurrent stroke is the key to effective secondary prevention. Early studies suggested that recurrent stroke is usually of the same type as the first stroke, but a significant proportion of strokes were classified as being of unknown etiology.[5] In a more recent (1998) retrospective study of 121 episodes of recurrent stroke in 102 patients admitted to the stroke center at Lausanne University Hospital, the authors similarly found that recurrent stroke was most often the same type as the first stroke. The recurrence rate of same-type stroke was 77% for cardioembolic stroke, 65% for large-artery atherosclerosis, and only 48% for lacunar stroke.[10] However, on average, the recurrent stroke was often (38%) not of the same type as the first, and this was particularly true for lacunar infarction (52%).

A recent (2000) study examined the mechanism of recurrent stroke in patients whose index event had been a carotid TIA or stroke. These investigators included patients from the North American Symptomatic Carotid Endarterectomy Trial and reported the mechanism of subsequent stroke on the side ipsilateral to the asymptomatic carotid artery. They found that the combined risk of cardioembolic and lacunar stroke was almost equal to that of large-artery stroke.[11] Given the nature of this study, it is not possible to establish precisely how many recurrent strokes are of a different subtype. However, these results do indicate that the mechanism of recurrent stroke is very often different from the initial event in patients with an initial carotid artery TIA or stroke.

In summary, the available evidence suggests that recurrent strokes are frequently of the same type as the initial stroke but that a different mechanism underlies a significant proportion of recurrent strokes. The implication is probably that patients with a first stroke require aggressive investigation to determine not only the likely etiology of the index event, but also whether there are any other coexisting risk factors that might predispose to recurrent stroke of a different type.

What Are the Risk Factors for Stroke Recurrence?

Data on the risk factors for recurrent stroke are inconsistent and relatively meager compared to the data available on risk factors for initial stroke. For example, hypertension was identified as a risk factor in some studies[4,12] but not others.[5,8] Similarly, diabetes was found to increase the risk of recurrent stroke in some studies[4,5] but not others.[12] In part, this is because of the retrospective nature of some of these studies and their failure to perform multivariate analysis of putative risk factors. The Lehigh Valley Recurrent Stroke Study was a prospective study that examined the importance of potential risk factors (hypertension, diabetes, myocardial ischemia, atrial fibrillation, and other arrhythmias) to the risk of stroke recurrence. Investigators followed 621 patients with an initial ischemic stroke and detected 77 recurrent strokes over an average follow-up of 2 years. They found that only hypertension and atrial fibrillation were independently associated with an increase of recurrent stroke.[13] In the study of recurrent stroke in patients from the North American Symptomatic Carotid Endarterectomy Trial, it was apparent that the risk factors varied for the different types of recurrent strokes. For example, diabetes was a risk factor for large-artery and lacunar stroke, hypertension was also a risk factor for lacunar stroke, and a history of myocardial ischemia and atrial fibrillation increased the risk of recurrent cardioembolic stroke.[12]

In summary, the risk factors for recurrent stroke are likely to differ for various stroke subtypes and have not yet been clearly established. It is, nevertheless, sensible to attend to risk factors like hypertension, diabetes, and atrial fibrillation that are clearly associated with increased general morbidity and mortality, even in the absence of evidence that these are clearly risk factors for recurrent stroke.

Summary

- The risk of recurrent stroke is similar irrespective of whether the index event is a TIA or a stroke.
- The risk of recurrent stroke is greatest in the short term after a TIA or stroke, approximating 4% in the first month, 9% in the first 6 months, and 12% during the first year.
- There are insufficient data to be confident of the very short-term (i.e., within days) risk of stroke after a TIA. This knowledge would be very helpful in making a decision about the acuity with which investigations should be performed and management instituted.
- The risk of recurrence is lowest for lacunar stroke, intermediate for cardioembolic stroke, and greatest for large-artery atherothrombotic stroke.
- Most recurrent strokes are of the same type as the initial stroke, but a significant minority are of a different type.
- The risk factors for stroke recurrence have not been clearly established but likely include hypertension, diabetes, and atrial fibrillation.

References

1. Dennis M, Bamford J, Sandercock P, Warlow C. Prognosis of transient ischemic attacks in the Oxfordshire Community Stroke Project. *Stroke* 1990;21:848–853.
2. Burn J, Dennis M, Bamford J, et al. Long-term risk of recurrent stroke after a first-ever stroke. The Oxfordshire Community Stroke Project. *Stroke* 1994;25:333–337.
3. Cardiogenic brain embolism. Cerebral Embolism Task Force. *Arch Neurol* 1986;43:71–84.
4. Sacco RL, Foulkes MA, Mohr JP, et al. Determinants of early recurrence of cerebral infarction. The Stroke Data Bank. *Stroke* 1989;20:983–989.
5. Hier DB, Foulkes MA, Swiontoniowski M, et al. Stroke recurrence within 2 years after ischemic infarction. *Stroke* 1991;22:155–161.
6. Johnston SC, Gress DR, Browner WS, Sidney S. Short-term prognosis after emergency department diagnosis of TIA. *JAMA* 2000;284:2901–2906.
7. Secondary prevention in non-rheumatic atrial fibrillation after transient ischaemic attack or minor stroke. EAFT (European Atrial Fibrillation Trial) Study Group. *Lancet* 1993;342:1255–1262.
8. Moroney JT, Bagiella E, Paik MC, et al. Risk factors for early recurrence after ischemic stroke: the role of stroke syndrome and subtype. *Stroke* 1998;29:2118–2124.
9. Kappelle LJ, van Latum JC, van Swieten JC, et al. Recurrent stroke after transient ischaemic attack or minor ischaemic stroke: does the distinction between small and large vessel disease remain true to type? Dutch TIA Trial Study group. *J Neurol Neurosurg Psychiatry* 1995;59:127–131.
10. Yamamoto H, Bogousslavsky J. Mechanisms of second and further strokes. *J Neurol Neurosurg Psychiatry* 1998;64:771–776.
11. Inzitari D, Eliasziw M, Gates P, et al. The causes and risk of stroke in patients with asymptomatic internal-carotid-artery stenosis. North American Symptomatic Carotid Endarterectomy Trial Collaborators. *N Engl J Med* 2000;342:1693–1700.
12. Prencipe M, Culasso F, Rasura M, et al. Long-term prognosis after a minor stroke: 10-year mortality and major stroke recurrence rates in a hospital-based cohort. *Stroke* 1998;29:126–132.
13. Lai SM, Alter M, Friday G, et al. A multifactorial analysis of risk factors for recurrence of ischemic stroke. *Stroke* 1994;25:958–962.

CHAPTER 2

Antiplatelet Therapy and Ischemic Stroke

Introduction

The rationale for antiplatelet therapy in the treatment and prevention of stroke is based on the knowledge that platelets play an active role in the pathogenesis of atherosclerotic lesions and thrombosis. More specifically, endothelial injury results in platelet adhesion and activation, with release of both vasoactive substances and mitogenic factors. These platelet-derived factors promote progression of the atherosclerotic lesion towards rupture and thrombosis. Each of the antiplatelet agents in common use exhibits different mechanisms of action. The antithrombotic effect of aspirin results from its ability to inhibit the production of thromboxane A_2, a prostaglandin that induces platelet aggregation and vasoconstriction. Dipyridamole elevates cyclic adenosine monophosphate that results in inhibition of thromboxane A_2 with consequent vasodilation and inhibition of platelet aggregation. Ticlopidine also inhibits the adenosine phosphate pathway of platelet aggregation, and clopidogrel inhibits platelet binding to fibrinogen.

Most of the trials of antiplatelet therapy in the prevention of stroke have used ischemic stroke as their endpoint, without attention to whether the stroke was the result of cardioembolism, large-artery atherosclerosis, or lacunar stroke. In fact, many of the studies have employed the endpoint of vascular event (myocardial infarction, stroke, or vascular death). The result is that there are limited data regarding the efficacy of antiplatelet therapy in the prevention of specific stroke types.

Nevertheless, we are bound to work within the framework of the available evidence. Occasionally, decisions about the use of antiplatelet therapy in specific circumstances are based in part on the presumed mechanism of the stroke. For example, it may be argued that antiplatelet therapy is appropriate in circumstances where endothelial injury and platelet activation are thought to be the primary mechanisms responsible for the stroke. It should be realized, however, that these are theoretical arguments and usually not founded on specific evidence. The aim of this chapter is to explore the evidence that supports the use of aspirin and other antiplatelet agents in the treatment and prevention of ischemic stroke.

Is Aspirin Beneficial in the Prevention of Stroke?

Although aspirin has been shown to be beneficial in the primary prevention of myocardial infarction, such an effect has not been demonstrated for the primary prevention of stroke, except in the context of atrial fibrillation (see the section Is Aspirin Effective for the Prevention of Stroke Due to Atrial Fibrillation?). However, there is ample evidence for the salutary effect of aspirin in secondary stroke prevention. The evidence from randomized trials published before 1990 is summarized in the most recent systematic review performed by the Antiplatelet Trialists' (APT) Collaboration. Aspirin was the most common antiplatelet agent used in the trials summarized in this review that included 18 studies in which stroke or transient ischemic attack (TIA) was the index event. Recurrent nonfatal stroke occurred in 8.2% of patients treated with an antiplatelet agent and 10.2% of controls, yielding a (statistically significant) relative risk reduction of 19.6% and an absolute risk reduction of 2.0%.[1] Similarly, the second European Stroke Prevention Study of over 6,000 patients with TIA or stroke found that the risk of stroke recurrence over the 2-year follow-up period was 12.9% in patients treated with aspirin (50 mg per day) and 15.8% in the placebo group.[2] Relative to placebo, this translates into a relative risk reduction of 18.4% and an absolute risk reduction of 2.9% for aspirin (Table 2-1).

These results indicate that although aspirin is unequivocally protective against recurrent stroke, the magnitude of this effect is small (absolute risk reduction of 2–3%), hence the efforts to establish whether a different dose of aspirin might have an even greater beneficial effect or whether the substitution or addition of another antiplatelet agent might result in a greater reduction in the risk of subsequent stroke. These two issues are discussed in the sections that follow.

What Is the Optimal Dose of Aspirin for Long-Term Secondary Stroke Prevention?

The optimal dose of aspirin for long-term secondary stroke prevention has been the subject of considerable debate over the years. The APT systematic review published in 1994 included trials that employed aspirin dosages that varied from 75 mg to 1,500 mg per day. This review included trials in which the effects of aspirin were studied in patients with a variety of atherosclerotic diseases. For the combined endpoint of stroke, myocardial infarction, or vascular death, the odds reductions for low- (75–160 mg), medium- (160–325 mg), and high-dose (500–1,500 mg) aspirin compared to controls were 26%, 28%, and 21%, respectively.[1] Algra and colleagues selected 10 of the trials that had been included in the APT systematic review. These were the controlled trials (all but one of which were placebo controlled) that had examined the effect of aspirin alone on the combined risk of stroke, myocardial infarction, or vascular death only in patients whose initial event had been a

TABLE 2-1
Effect of Aspirin on Stroke Recurrence

	Treatment	Risk of Stroke (%)	Absolute Risk Reduction (%)	Relative Risk Reduction (%)
Antiplatelet Trial- ists' Group[a]	Antiplatelet	8.2	2.0	19.6
	Control	10.2	—	—
The Second Euro- pean Stroke Pre- vention Study-2[b]	Aspirin	12.9	2.9	18.4
	Placebo	15.8	—	—

[a]The time period during which these risks of stroke were observed is not clear.
[b]Data shown are for the 2-year risk of stroke.

stroke or TIA (rather than any atherosclerotic disease). They found the over-all risk reduction to be 13% in the low-dose (less than 100 mg) trials, and 14% in the medium- to high-dose trials. The confidence intervals of these estimates overlapped almost completely, and this allowed an overall esti-mate to be made. Combining all of these trials, they found the overall rela-tive risk reduction to be 13% with a corresponding odds reduction of 16%.[3]

In summary, low- to medium-dose (75–325 mg) aspirin has been stud-ied most frequently and shown repeatedly to be protective against stroke, myocardial infarction, and death. Higher and lower dosages have not been shown to be either more or less protective.

Is the Combination of Aspirin and Dipyridamole Superior to Aspirin Alone for the Secondary Prevention of Stroke?

The first European Stroke Prevention Study compared the combination of 990 mg aspirin (330 mg three times per day) and 225 mg dipyridamole (75 mg three times per day) to placebo in the secondary prevention of stroke. Approx-imately 1,800 patients were followed prospectively for 2 years, with stroke and death (from any cause) being the primary endpoints of the study. The combination treatment conferred a 38% reduction over placebo in the relative risk of secondary stroke.[4] This reduction was substantially higher than that reported in the studies that had used aspirin alone. The second European Stroke Prevention Study was designed, therefore, to directly compare aspirin and dipyridamole individually as well as the combination to placebo. Over 6,000 patients with TIA or stroke were randomized to receive aspirin (25 mg twice per day), extended-release dipyridamole (200 mg twice per day), the combination of aspirin and dipyridamole, or placebo. The risk of stroke recur-rence over the 2-year follow-up period[2] is summarized in Table 2-2. These

TABLE 2-2
Effect of Aspirin and Dipyridamole on the Risk of Stroke Recurrence: The Second
European Stroke Prevention Study

Treatment	Two-Year Risk of Stroke (%)	Absolute Risk Reduction (%)	Relative Risk Reduction (%)
Aspirin	12.9	2.9	18.4
Dipyridamole	13.2	2.6	16.5
Both	9.9	5.9	37.3
Placebo	15.8	—	—

Note: Aspirin dose 25 mg twice daily; dipyridamole dose 200 mg twice daily.

results suggest that the combination of aspirin and dipyridamole is superior to
either individual agent in the secondary prevention of stroke.

What Are the Relative Benefits of Aspirin and Clopidogrel (Plavix) in Secondary Stroke Prevention?

The Clopidogrel versus Aspirin in Patients at Risk of Ischemic Events
(CAPRIE) trial is the key study that illuminates the question of the benefits
of clopidogrel and aspirin in secondary stroke prevention. It should be realized, however, that the study population included patients with ischemic
stroke, myocardial infarction, or atherosclerotic peripheral artery disease,
and similar to the APT review, the primary outcome measure in this study
was the combined risk of ischemic stroke, myocardial infarction, and vascular disease. Almost 20,000 patients were randomized to receive either
aspirin (325 mg per day) or clopidogrel (75 mg per day), with a mean follow-
up period of 1.9 years. An intention-to-treat analysis of the primary outcome cluster revealed an overall relative risk reduction of 8.7% in favor of
clopidogrel. It is instructive to consider that this conclusion is based on
annual event rates of 5.32% in the clopidogrel group and 5.83% in the aspirin group (an absolute risk reduction of 0.51%) (Table 2-3). In absolute numbers, clopidogrel would be expected to prevent about 24 outcome events
(ischemic stroke, myocardial infarction, or limb amputation) in 1 year,
compared to 19 per 1,000 patients treated with aspirin.[5]

What Are the Relative Benefits of Aspirin and Ticlopidine in Secondary Stroke Prevention?

The question of the relative benefits of aspirin and ticlopidine in the secondary prevention of stroke was the subject of the Ticlopidine Aspirin Stroke

TABLE 2-3
Effect of Clopidogrel on the Risk of Stroke Recurrence: Clopidogrel versus Aspirin
in Patients at Risk of Ischemic Events

Treatment	Stroke Risk (%)	Absolute Risk Reduction (%)	Relative Risk Reduction (%)
Clopidogrel	5.32	0.51	8.70
Aspirin	5.83	—	—

Study.[6] This was a randomized controlled trial that was designed to determine whether ticlopidine was more effective than aspirin in the secondary prevention of stroke. Patients with a history of amaurosis fugax, TIA, or minor stroke within the preceding 3 months were eligible for inclusion in the study. Those with cardioembolic disease were excluded. A total of 3,069 patients were randomized to receive either ticlopidine 250 mg twice daily (n = 1,529) or aspirin 650 mg twice daily (n = 1,540). Twelve patients (nine in the aspirin group and three in the ticlopidine group) were subsequently excluded. There were no significant baseline differences between the two treatment groups, and compliance with treatment was generally good. The primary endpoint of the study was defined as the composite of nonfatal stroke or death from all causes. The occurrence of stroke (composite of fatal and nonfatal) was defined as a secondary endpoint. During the follow-up period, the primary endpoint (death from any cause or nonfatal stroke) occurred in 306 patients receiving ticlopidine and 349 patients who were treated with aspirin. There were 172 strokes amongst the ticlopidine group and 212 in the aspirin group. Kaplan-Meier analysis of the primary endpoint showed a significant cumulative benefit of ticlopidine therapy. At 3 years, the combined risk of death or nonfatal stroke was 17% for the ticlopidine group and 19% for the aspirin group, representing a relative risk reduction of 12%. The stroke rates and risk reductions at 3 years are summarized in Table 2-4.

   These differences, although statistically significant, are small and of questionable clinical significance. The potential benefits of ticlopi-

TABLE 2-4
Effect of Ticlopidine on the Risk of Stroke Recurrence: Ticlopidine Aspirin
Stroke Study

Treatment	Stroke Risk (%)	Absolute Risk Reduction (%)	Relative Risk Reduction (%)
Aspirin	13	3	23
Ticlopidine	10	—	—

dine might also be outweighed by the small, but real, incidence of severe neutropenia.

Is Aspirin Beneficial in the Treatment of Acute Ischemic Stroke?

The aforementioned studies all examined the effects of aspirin (and other antiplatelet agents) started within a number of months of the index TIA or stroke. The question being asked here is whether there is any advantage to the use of aspirin in the context of an acute ischemic stroke. This issue has been addressed by two large, prospective placebo-controlled trials.

The International Stroke Trial (IST) enrolled approximately 20,000 patients within 48 hours of the onset of ischemic stroke. Patients were randomized to receive subcutaneous heparin, 300 mg aspirin, both, or neither. Half of the patients were randomized to receive heparin (half of whom in turn each received one of two doses of heparin) and the other half to avoid heparin. Using a factorial design, half of the patients were then randomized to receive aspirin and half to avoid aspirin. The result was that there were multiple treatment groups:

Aspirin + heparin 12,500 IU
Aspirin + heparin 5,000 IU
Aspirin + no heparin
No aspirin + heparin 12,500 IU
No aspirin + heparin 5,000 IU
No aspirin + no heparin

Relevant to this discussion of the potential benefit of aspirin in the acute treatment of ischemic stroke is the analysis reported in terms of "aspirin" versus "avoid aspirin" irrespective of whether patients received heparin. Notwithstanding this unusual method of analysis, those who received aspirin had significantly fewer recurrent ischemic strokes within 14 days compared to those who did not receive aspirin (2.8% vs. 3.9%) (Table 2-5). This

TABLE 2-5
Use of Aspirin in the Acute Management of Ischemic Stroke: International Stroke Trial Study

Treatment	Stroke Risk (%)	Absolute Risk Reduction (%)	Relative Risk Reduction (%)
Aspirin	2.8	1.1	28.2
No aspirin	3.9	—	—

study demonstrated that the use of aspirin is associated with a significant reduction of 11 per 1,000 deaths or nonfatal stroke at 14 days.[7]

The Chinese Acute Stroke Trial (CAST) also enrolled approximately 20,000 patients within 48 hours of the onset of ischemic stroke. Patients were randomized to receive 160 mg aspirin or placebo. This study demonstrated a significant reduction of 5.4 per 1,000 deaths at 4 months (the primary endpoint), a significant reduction of 6.8 per 1,000 deaths or nonfatal stroke at 4 months, and a nonsignificant trend towards reduced likelihood of death or dependency at the time of hospital discharge.[8] There was also a nonsignificant trend towards a reduction in the endpoint of fatal and nonfatal recurrent stroke among aspirin-treated patients. This study has been criticized because a computerized tomographic scan was not required (either before or after randomization). However, there was no excess of hemorrhagic complications in the aspirin-treated group, suggesting that there was no significant misclassification of strokes as ischemic by relying purely on clinical criteria.

The Cochrane collaboration performed a systematic review of antiplatelet therapy for acute ischemic stroke. They included the IST and CAST studies as well as six other smaller randomized controlled trials of antiplatelet therapy started within 14 days of acute ischemic stroke. They found that treatment was associated with a significant increase of 13 per 1,000 patients who were alive and independent at the end of the designated follow-up period. In addition, an increase of 10 per 1,000 treated patients made a complete recovery from their stroke.[9]

The overall impression is that medium-dose aspirin (160–300 mg per day) is a safe and effective therapy for acute ischemic stroke. There are insufficient data to indicate whether alternative antiplatelet regimens are as effective. Although aspirin is associated with a small increase in symptomatic intracranial (and extracranial) hemorrhage, this is offset by the reduction in the rate of recurrence of ischemic stroke. Subgroup analyses in the IST and CAST studies indicated that the beneficial effects of aspirin are not dependent on age, gender, or stroke type, suggesting that aspirin is beneficial across the spectrum of patients with acute ischemic stroke.

Is Aspirin Effective for the Prevention of Stroke Due to Atrial Fibrillation?

This issue of whether aspirin is effective for the prevention of stroke due to atrial fibrillation has been addressed in both primary and secondary prevention trials. In the Stroke Prevention in Atrial Fibrillation trial, 703 patients with nonrheumatic atrial fibrillation were randomized in a double-blind fashion to receive aspirin (325 mg per day) or placebo. Patients were followed for a mean of 1.3 years for the primary endpoint of ischemic stroke or

TABLE 2-6
Effect of Aspirin on Stroke Recurrence in Atrial Fibrillation: Stroke Prevention Atrial Fibrillation Study

Treatment	Event Risk (%)	Absolute Risk Reduction (%)	Relative Risk Reduction (%)
Aspirin	3.6	2.7	42.0
Placebo	6.3	—	—

systemic embolism. Although a small percentage of patients had a history of TIA or stroke more than 2 years before enrollment, the Stroke Prevention in Atrial Fibrillation was essentially a primary prevention trial. The annual event (stroke and systemic embolism) rates and risk reductions are summarized in Table 2-6. The absolute risk reduction of 2.7% translates into 27 fewer ischemic strokes or episodes of systemic embolism per 1,000 patients treated.[10]

The European Atrial Fibrillation Trial was a prospective study of secondary prevention in nonrheumatic atrial fibrillation after TIA or stroke. In one part of this study, patients with a TIA or stroke within the preceding 3 months were randomized to receive aspirin (300 mg per day) or placebo. The risk of recurrent stroke within the first year was 12% in the placebo group and 10% in the aspirin-treated patients.[11] This difference was not statistically significant.

In summary, aspirin is effective in the primary prevention of stroke in patients with nonrheumatic atrial fibrillation. However, although there is a trend towards aspirin also being effective in the secondary prevention of stroke in this patient population, these results did not reach statistical significance. The relative utility of anticoagulants for primary and secondary prevention of stroke in nonrheumatic atrial fibrillation is discussed in the next chapter.

Summary

- Antiplatelet therapy reduces the risk of vascular events (myocardial infarction, stroke, or vascular death) in patients with a previous TIA or stroke (APT).
- Most of the evidence supports the use of medium-dose aspirin (75–325 mg per day) for the secondary prevention of stroke (APT).
- Aspirin is a safe and effective therapy for acute ischemic stroke, and its use within 48 hours of an ischemic stroke reduces the short-term risk of recurrent stroke (IST and CAST).

TABLE 2-7
Summary of the Effects of Antiplatelet Therapy on the Risk of Stroke Recurrence

Study	Treatment	Risk of Stroke (%)	Absolute Risk Reduction (%) (Relative to Control)	Relative Risk Reduction (%) (Relative to Control)
Antiplatelet Trialists' Group	Antiplatelet therapy	8.2	2.00	19.6
	Control	10.2	—	—
The Second European Stroke Prevention Study	Aspirin (50 mg)	12.9	2.90	18.4
	Dipyridamole (400 mg)	13.2	2.60	16.5
	Aspirin + dipyridamole	9.9	5.90	37.3
	Control (placebo)	15.8	—	—
Clopidogrel versus Aspirin in Patients at Risk of Ischemic Events	Clopidogrel	5.32	0.51	8.7
	Aspirin	5.83	—	—
Ticlopidine Aspirin Stroke Study	Aspirin	13.0	3.00	23.0
	Ticlopidine	10.0	—	—
Stroke Prevention Atrial Fibrillation Study	Aspirin	3.6	2.70	42.0
	Placebo	6.3	—	—
Canadian Cooperative Study Group	Aspirin	15.9	7.20	31.2
	No aspirin	23.1	—	—

- There is reasonable evidence that the combination of aspirin and dipyridamole is more effective than aspirin alone in the secondary prevention of stroke (the first European Stroke Prevention Study and the second European Stroke Prevention Study).
- Clopidogrel is slightly more effective than aspirin in the secondary prevention of vascular events (myocardial infarction, stroke, amputation, or vascular death) (CAPRIE).
- Ticlopidine is slightly more effective than aspirin in reducing the composite risk of death or nonfatal stroke, as well as the combined endpoint of fatal and nonfatal stroke (Ticlopidine Aspirin Stroke Study).
- Aspirin is beneficial for the primary prevention of stroke secondary to atrial fibrillation (Stroke Prevention in Atrial Fibrillation).
- The results of these studies of the effects of antiplatelet therapy in reducing the risk of stroke are summarized in Table 2-7. Note that the stroke rates cited for the different studies relate to follow-up peri-

ods of varying duration and are not, therefore, directly comparable. Comparisons may be drawn from the calculated risk reductions.

References

1. Collaborative overview of randomised trials of antiplatelet therapy—I: prevention of death, myocardial infarction, and stroke by prolonged antiplatelet therapy in various categories of patients. Antiplatelet Trialists' Collaboration. *BMJ* 1994;308:81–106.
2. Diener HC, Cunha L, Forbes C, et al. European Stroke Prevention Study 2. Dipyridamole and acetylsalicylic acid in the secondary prevention of stroke. *J Neurol Sci* 1996;143:1–13.
3. Algra A, van Gijn J. Aspirin at any dose above 30mg offers only modest protection after cerebral ischaemia. *J Neurol Neurosurg Psychiatry* 1996;60:197–199.
4. The European Stroke Prevention Study (ESPS). Principal end-points. The ESPS Group. *Lancet* 1987;2:1351–1354.
5. A randomised, blinded, trial of clopidogrel versus aspirin in patients at risk of ischaemic events (CAPRIE). CAPRIE Steering Committee. *Lancet* 1996;348: 1329–1339.
6. Hass WK, Easton JD, Adams HP, et al. A randomized trial comparing ticlopidine hydrochloride with aspirin for the prevention of stroke in high-risk patients. Ticlopidine Aspirin Stroke Study Group. *N Engl J Med* 1989;321: 501–507.
7. The International Stroke Trial (IST): a randomized trial of aspirin, subcutaneous heparin, both, or neither among 19,435 patients with acute ischaemic stroke. International Stroke Trial Collaborative Group. *Lancet* 1997;349:1569–1581.
8. CAST: randomised placebo-controlled trial of early aspirin use in 20,000 patients with acute ischaemic stroke. CAST (Chinese Acute Stroke Trial) Collaborative Group. *Lancet* 1997;349:1641–1649.
9. Gubitz G, Sandercock P, Counsell C. Antiplatelet therapy for acute ischaemic stroke. *Cochrane Database Syst Rev* 2000;2:CD000029.
10. Stroke Prevention in Atrial Fibrillation Study. Final results. *Circulation* 1991;84:527–539.
11. Secondary prevention in non-rheumatic atrial fibrillation after transient ischaemic attack or minor stroke. EAFT (European Atrial Fibrillation Trial) Study Group. *Lancet* 1993;342:1255–1262.

CHAPTER 3

Anticoagulants in the Treatment of Ischemic Stroke

Introduction

In considering the role of anticoagulants in the management of patients with stroke, it is useful to make a distinction between the use of heparin in the treatment of acute stroke and the use of warfarin for the prevention of recurrent stroke.

The use of heparin in the management of acute ischemic stroke remains controversial, and practice varies substantially from one academic center to another. This is perhaps surprising given that repeated studies of both unfractionated and low-molecular-weight heparin, administered either subcutaneously or intravenously, have failed to demonstrate a beneficial effect. Those who favor the use of heparin (correctly) argue that stroke is not a homogeneous disorder and that heparin is likely to be beneficial only under circumstances in which the formation of red clot is important in the pathogenesis of stroke. Examples might include thrombus formation in an enlarged left atrium or thrombosis that occurs over an ulcerated atherosclerotic plaque in a large artery. To include these patients in a study of those with lacunar stroke, in whom (based on pathophysiology) heparin is less likely to be beneficial, has the effect of diluting the beneficial effect in the former group. It is true that most studies have lumped together patients with all forms of ischemic strokes, and in those studies in which stroke subtypes are recognized, there is some evidence for a differential effect of heparin. One difficulty, however, at least in the past, has been that the pathophysiologic mechanism of acute stroke may not be immediately apparent. The argument, therefore, has been that for the purposes of a study of an acute therapy, it is necessary to treat all patients with ischemic stroke in a similar manner. With the advent of modern imaging techniques, however, it should now be possible to delineate the likely underlying pathophysiology within minutes to hours. What is needed, therefore, are studies of the use of heparin in the treatment of acute stroke that is likely (based on underlying pathophysiology) to benefit from anticoagulation (e.g., large-artery occlusions and severe stenoses).

Similarly, in studies of the prevention of recurrent stroke, it is appropriate to consider separately those with different underlying mechanisms of the index stroke. It should also be recognized, however, that the mechanism of recurrent stroke often differs from that of the initial event (see Chapter 1).

What is the role of heparin in the management of acute ischemic stroke? Does it matter whether heparin is administered subcutaneously or intravenously? Is heparin indicated only for stroke of a particular pathophysiology? Does long-term anticoagulation with warfarin reduce the risk of recurrent stroke, irrespective of the underlying pathophysiology? Or is warfarin only effective in the prevention of cardioembolic stroke in patients with atrial fibrillation? These questions are the focus of this chapter.

Should Heparin Be Used in the Management of Acute Ischemic Stroke?

The use of heparin in the management of acute ischemic stroke has been the subject of many randomized trials that have varied in quality and size. Although the results of these trials, in general, have shown that heparin is not beneficial in the treatment of acute ischemic stroke, a fairly widespread use of heparin persists. To date, there has been only one prospective randomized placebo-controlled trial of intravenous unfractionated heparin.[1] This study included 225 patients and found no significant difference between the two groups with regard to functional status at 1 week, 3 months, and 1 year after the stroke.

Subsequent trials have studied either low-molecular-weight heparin (administered either intravenously or subcutaneously) or subcutaneous (s.c.) unfractionated heparin. The International Stroke Trial was an open trial in which approximately 20,000 patients with acute ischemic stroke were randomized to receive aspirin, heparin, both, or neither.[2] The heparin used was unfractionated and administered subcutaneously in 1 of 2 doses, 5,000 IU twice a day (low dose) or 12,500 IU twice a day (medium dose). The primary endpoints were death at 14 days and death or dependency at 6 months. Compared to those randomized to "avoid heparin," the use of heparin (either low or medium dose) was not associated with a significant reduction in either of the primary outcome measures (Table 3-1). Although heparin was associated with a reduction in the incidence of recurrent ischemic stroke, this benefit was offset by a similar-sized increase in the risk of hemorrhagic stroke. Of interest is that subgroup analysis revealed that low-dose heparin was associated with a significant reduction in early death or stroke, with only a slight (nonsignificant) excess of major extracranial hemorrhage. Two criticisms of this study are the awkward nature of the analysis performed (i.e., heparin vs. "avoid heparin," irrespective of concurrent aspirin therapy) and the failure to monitor the international normalized ratio (INR) and adjust the dose of heparin accordingly.

TABLE 3-1
Heparin Trials

Study	Treatment	Analysis	Primary Endpoint(s)	Results
International Stroke Trial[2]	Unfractionated heparin s.c. (12,500 IU vs. 5,000 IU twice daily)	Heparin vs. no heparin	Death at 14 days Death or dependency at 6 mos	No effect
Fraxiparine in Stroke Study[3]	Low-molecular-weight heparin s.c.	Heparin vs. placebo	Death or dependency at 6 mos	RR reduction of 31% in favor of heparin
Fraxiparine in Stroke Study–bis[4] (replication study with larger sample size)	Low-molecular-weight heparin s.c.	Heparin vs. placebo	Death; Barthel Index <85	No effect
Trial of ORG 10172 in Acute Stroke Treatment[5]	Low-molecular-weight heparin i.v.	Heparin vs. placebo	3-month favorable outcome on Barthel or Glasgow Outcome Scale	RR reduction of 20% in the large-artery atherosclerotic group
Heparin in Acute Embolic Stroke Trial[7]	Low-molecular-weight heparin s.c.	Heparin vs. aspirin	Recurrent ischemic stroke within 14 days	No effect

RR = relative risk.

The Fraxiparine in Stroke Study was a randomized, double-blind, placebo-controlled study of low-molecular-weight heparin (Fraxiparine) in the treatment of acute ischemic stroke.[3] Three hundred eight patients were randomized to receive placebo, high-dose (4,100 anti–factor Xa IU twice daily) Fraxiparine, or low-dose (4,100 anti–factor Xa IU daily) Fraxiparine, administered subcutaneously for 10 days. The primary endpoint was death or dependency at 6 months. The use of high-dose heparin was associated with a (significant) 31% reduction in the relative risk of death or dependency at 6 months. This beneficial effect was not accompanied by an increased risk of hemorrhagic or other complications. When Fraxiparine

TABLE 3-2
Trial of ORG 10172 in Acute Stroke Treatment Study Results

	ORG 10172 (%)	Placebo (%)	p Value
Favorable outcome at 3 mos (all stroke subtypes combined)[a]	75.2	73.7	0.49
Favorable outcome at 3 mos (large-artery atherosclerotic stroke)[a]	68.1	54.7	0.04
Very favorable outcome at 3 mos (large-artery atherosclerotic stroke)[b]	43.4	29.1	0.02

[a]*Favorable outcome* defined as Glasgow Outcome Scale score of I or II and modified Barthel Index score of 12–20.
[b]Glasgow Outcome Scale score of I and modified Barthel Index score of 19–20.

was re-examined in a larger cohort of 767 patients in a study with similar design, the beneficial effect, however, was no longer demonstrable[4] (see Table 3-1).

The Trial of ORG 10172 in Acute Stroke Treatment was a prospective double-blind, placebo-controlled trial of heparin in acute ischemic stroke.[5] Patients presenting within 24 hours of onset of an acute ischemic stroke were randomized to receive either low-molecular-weight heparin administered intravenously for 7 days (initial bolus followed by a continuous infusion, with the rate of infusion adjusted to maintain anti–factor Xa activity in a therapeutic range) or placebo. The study included 1,281 patients, and the primary endpoint was a favorable outcome (determined by Glasgow Outcome Scale and Barthel Index) at 3 months (see Appendix 3 [Barthel Index] and Appendix 10 [Glasgow Outcome Scale]). Overall, there was no significant difference in the outcome between the two groups (Table 3-2). However, for strokes due to large-artery atherosclerosis, the rate of favorable outcome was significantly higher in the low-molecular-weight heparin group (see Tables 3-1 and 3-2). Hemorrhagic complications were also more frequent in this group.

The Cochrane Collaboration conducted a systematic review of these and other randomized trials of anticoagulants for the treatment of acute ischemic stroke.[6] They concluded that immediate anticoagulant therapy in patients with acute ischemic stroke is not associated with net short- or long-term benefit and that the data from their review do not support the routine use of any type of anticoagulant in acute ischemic stroke.

The available data, therefore, do not support the indiscriminate use of unfractionated or low-molecular-weight heparin (administered either intravenously or subcutaneously) in the treatment of acute ischemic stroke. For the most part, all of these studies lumped together patients with ischemic stroke of any cause. At least in theory, it may be that patients with specific subtypes of ischemic strokes, or those with the greatest risk of short-term stroke recurrence, may benefit from treatment with heparin. In this regard, it is of interest that subgroup analysis in the Trial of ORG 10172 in Acute Stroke Treatment did indicate a more favorable outcome in patients with large-artery atherosclerotic stroke. It may be no coincidence that these are the patients with the highest risk of recurrent stroke (see Chapter 1). The utility of heparin has also been examined in patients with embolic stroke and atrial fibrillation. In a subgroup analysis of patients with atrial fibrillation, the International Stroke Trial (which compared s.c. unfractionated heparin with aspirin and placebo) found that the reduction in the risk of recurrent ischemic stroke was offset by the increased risk of intracerebral hemorrhage.[2] Similarly, the Heparin in Acute Embolic Stroke Trial (which compared the use of s.c. low-molecular-weight heparin to aspirin in the treatment of acute stroke) found no difference in the outcome of patients at 14 days and 3 months.[7] There is, therefore, no evidence that heparin is beneficial in the management of acute cardioembolic stroke secondary to atrial fibrillation (see Table 3-1).

Does Warfarin Prevent Stroke in Patients with Atrial Fibrillation?

It is useful to make a distinction between the beneficial effects of warfarin in the primary and the secondary prevention of stroke in nonrheumatic atrial fibrillation. The former has been the subject of four major randomized trials.[7-9] In the Copenhagen Atrial Fibrillation, ASpirin, AntiKoagulation (AFASAK) Study of approximately 1,000 patients, subjects were randomized to receive warfarin, aspirin, or placebo. Warfarin was given openly and the INR maintained between 2.8 and 4.2. Warfarin was associated with a reduced risk of recurrent stroke and death.[8] The Boston Area Anticoagulation Trial for Atrial Fibrillation was also an unblinded randomized trial. A total of 420 patients were randomized to receive either warfarin or control. The INR was maintained between 1.5 and 2.7. The evidence favoring the effect of warfarin in reducing the number of ischemic strokes and deaths was sufficiently strong that the trial was terminated.[9] In the 627 patients eligible for the anticoagulant arm of the Stroke Prevention in Atrial Fibrillation trial, the annual risk of ischemic stroke or systemic embolism was 2.7% in the warfarin group and 7.4% in the placebo group—a relative risk reduction of 67%.[10] There is only one randomized, double-blind, placebo-controlled study of warfarin in patients with atrial fibrillation.[11] In this study, 525 patients were randomized to receive placebo or warfarin, with the INR maintained between 1.4 and 2.8. The annual risk of ischemic stroke was 4.3% in the placebo group and 0.9% in the warfarin group, yielding a relative risk reduction of 79% (Table 3-3). The risk of major hemorrhage was not increased in the warfarin-treated patients.

TABLE 3-3
Warfarin for Primary Prevention of Stroke Due to Atrial Fibrillation

Study	Design	Treatment	Results
Copenhagen Atrial Fibrillation, ASpirin, AntiKoagulation[8]	Randomized, open	Warfarin vs. aspirin vs. placebo	Yearly incidence of thromboembolic complications of 5.5% for placebo and 2.0% for warfarin (RR ↓ of 64%)
Boston Area Anticoagulation Trial for Atrial Fibrillation[9]	Randomized, open	No warfarin vs. warfarin	Yearly incidence of stroke of 2.98% for control and 0.41% warfarin (RR ↓ of 86%)
Stroke Prevention in Atrial Fibrillation[10]	Randomized	Warfarin vs. placebo	Yearly risk of systemic embolism or stroke of 7.4% for placebo and 2.7% for warfarin (RR ↓ of 67%)
Veterans Affairs Stroke Prevention in Nonrheumatic Atrial Fibrillation Study[11]	Randomized, double-blind	Warfarin vs. placebo	Yearly stroke risks of 4.3% for placebo and 0.9% for warfarin (RR ↓ of 79%)

RR = relative risk; ↓ = reduction.

There are two major studies that have examined the use of warfarin in the secondary prevention of stroke in patients with atrial fibrillation. The Veterans Affairs Stroke Prevention in Nonrheumatic Atrial Fibrillation investigators included a small number of patients with recent stroke in their double-blind, placebo-controlled trial.[10] They found warfarin to be effective in reducing the risk of recurrent stroke, but the results did not reach statistical significance because of the small number of patients. The beneficial effect of warfarin in the secondary prevention of stroke, however, was conclusively demonstrated by the European Atrial Fibrillation Trial Study Group.[12] In this study, 669 patients were randomized to receive warfarin (INR of 2.5 to 4.0), aspirin, or placebo, with warfarin being administered in an open fashion. The annual risk of stroke was reduced from 12% in the placebo group to 4% in the warfarin group, and the rate of vascular events (vascular death, nonfatal stroke, myocardial infarction, or systemic embolism) was reduced from 17% to 8%.

The evidence, therefore, supports the use of anticoagulation with warfarin in the primary and secondary prevention of cardioembolic stroke in patients with nonrheumatic atrial fibrillation. With low-intensity anticoagulation (INR of 1.7 to 2.8), this can be accomplished without an excess risk of serious hemorrhage. The risk of serious hemorrhage is increased with more aggressive anticoagulation (INR of 2.5 to 4.0), as was used in the European Atrial Fibrillation Trial.

Does Warfarin Prevent Recurrent Stroke in Patients Whose Initial Stroke Is Not Cardioembolic in Origin?

The question of whether warfarin prevents recurrent stroke in patients whose initial stroke is not cardioembolic in origin has been the subject of a recently completed prospective double-blind, controlled trial, the Warfarin-Aspirin Recurrent Stroke Study (WARSS).[13] Patients between the ages of 30 and 85 years, who had experienced an ischemic stroke within the previous 30 days and were considered "acceptable candidates for warfarin therapy" were eligible for inclusion. Excluded were those in whom the stroke was presumed to be of cardioembolic origin, was due to a high-grade carotid stenosis for which surgery was planned, or was precipitated by a procedure. A total of 2,206 patients were randomized to receive either aspirin or warfarin (adjusted to maintain an INR in the range of 1.4 to 2.8). The mean daily INR for the patients receiving warfarin was 2.1. Patients were followed for 2 years, and the primary endpoint was death from any cause or recurrent ischemic stroke, whichever occurred first. Approximately 55% of strokes were classified as lacunar, with approximately 25% cryptogenic and only 10–13% classified as being due to severe stenosis or occlusion of a large artery. The lower rate of large-artery strokes was likely due to the active exclusion of those with high-grade carotid lesions.

The overall rate of the primary endpoint of death or recurrent ischemic stroke was 16.9%. In the primary intention-to-treat analysis, there were no significant differences between the warfarin and aspirin groups. The rates of major hemorrhage were low and not significantly different between the two groups. Subgroup analysis based on the presumed mechanism of the original stroke (small vessel [lacunar], large-artery stenosis or occlusion, cryptogenic) similarly failed to demonstrate a significant difference in the risk of death or recurrent ischemic stroke, although the study was not powered to detect differences within select subgroups. Moreover, the number of patients with large-artery stroke—who, based on pathophysiology, might be expected to benefit more from anticoagulation—was small. Nevertheless, the overall conclusion from this study is that warfarin does not reduce the risk of recurrent ischemic stroke for noncardioembolic stroke as it does in patients with previous stroke and atrial fibrillation.

Summary

- The International Stroke Trial demonstrated that s.c. unfractionated heparin was associated with a reduction in the incidence of recurrent ischemic stroke, but this benefit was offset by a similar-sized increase in the risk of intracerebral hemorrhage. Overall, the use of heparin was not associated with a reduced risk of dependency at 6 months.

- The use of s.c. low-molecular-weight heparin in the treatment of acute ischemic stroke was examined in the Fraxiparine in Stroke Study and Fraxiparine in Stroke Study–bis (replication study with larger sample size). Although the former suggested that high-dose s.c. low-molecular-weight heparin was associated with a reduced risk of death or dependency at 6 months, it was not borne out by the larger study.
- The use of intravenous low-molecular-weight heparin was the subject of the Trial of ORG 10172 in Acute Stroke Treatment study. In general, there was no significant difference in the functional outcome of the heparin and placebo groups. However, subgroup analysis revealed that the outcome for large-artery atherosclerosis–related strokes was improved by the use of heparin.
- There is no evidence to support the use of heparin in the acute treatment of cardioembolic stroke due to atrial fibrillation.
- Warfarin is beneficial in the primary and secondary prevention of cardioembolic stroke due to atrial fibrillation.
- Compared to aspirin, warfarin does not reduce the risk of death or recurrent ischemic stroke after an initial noncardioembolic ischemic stroke.

References

1. Duke RJ, Bloch RF, Turpie AG, et al. Intravenous heparin for the prevention of stroke progression in acute partial stable stroke: a randomized controlled trial. *Ann Intern Med* 1986;105:825–828.
2. The International Stroke Trial (IST): a randomised trial of aspirin, subcutaneous heparin, both, or neither among 19,435 patients with acute ischaemic stroke. International Stroke Trial Collaborative Group. *Lancet* 1997;349:1569–1581.
3. Kay R, Wong KS, Yu YL, et al. Low-molecular-weight heparin for the treatment of acute ischemic stroke. *N Engl J Med* 1995;333:1588–1593.
4. Hommel M, for the FISS bis Investigation Group. Fraxiparine in Ischaemic Stroke Study (FISS bis). *Cerebrovasc Dis* 1998;(Suppl 4):19.
5. Low molecular weight heparinoid, ORG 10172 (Danaparoid), and outcome after acute ischemic stroke: a randomized controlled trial. The Publications Committee for the Trial of ORG 10172 in Acute Stroke Treatment (TOAST) Investigators. *JAMA* 1998;279:1265–1272.
6. Gubitz G, Counsell C, Sandercock P, Signorini D. Anticoagulants for acute ischemic stroke (Cochrane Review). *Cochrane Database Syst Rev* 2000; CD000024.
7. Berge E, Abdelnoor M, Nakstad PH, Sandset PM. Low molecular-weight heparin versus aspirin in patients with acute ischaemic stroke and atrial fibrillation: a double-blind randomised study. HAEST Study group. Heparin in Acute Embolic Stroke Trial. *Lancet* 2000;355:1205–1210.

8. Petersen P, Boysen G, Godtfredsen J, et al. Placebo-controlled, randomised trial of warfarin and aspirin for prevention of thromboembolic complications in chronic atrial fibrillation. The Copenhagen AFASAK Study. *Lancet* 1989;1:175–179.
9. The effect of low-dose warfarin on the risk of stroke in patients with nonrheumatic atrial fibrillation. The Boston Area Anticoagulation Trial for Atrial Fibrillation Investigators. *N Engl J Med* 1990;323:1505–1511.
10. Stroke Prevention in Atrial Fibrillation Study. Final results. *Circulation* 1991;84:527–539.
11. Ezekowitz MD, Bridgers SL, James KE, et al. Warfarin in the prevention of stroke associated with nonrheumatic atrial fibrillation. Veterans Affairs Stroke Prevention in Non-Rheumatic Atrial Fibrillation Investigators. *N Engl J Med* 1992;327:1406–1412.
12. Secondary prevention in non-rheumatic atrial fibrillation after transient ischemic attack or minor stroke. EAFT (European Atrial Fibrillation Trial) Study Group. *Lancet* 1993;342:1255–1262.
13. Mohr JP, Thompson JL, Lazar RM, et al. A comparison of warfarin and aspirin for the prevention of recurrent ischemic stroke. *N Engl J Med* 2001;345:1444–1451.

CHAPTER 4

Thrombolytic and Antihypertensive Therapy for Acute Stroke

Introduction

Thrombolytic therapy for acute stroke has generated much controversy. Three trials of intravenous streptokinase were terminated prematurely because of the accompanying increased risk of intracerebral hemorrhage. Two further studies have failed to produce evidence of the safety and efficacy of intravenous recombinant tissue-type plasminogen activator (rt-PA). Only the National Institute of Neurological Disorders and Stroke (NINDS) rt-PA Stroke Study of intravenous rt-PA, within 3 hours of the onset of symptoms, yielded clinically significant results. Even these, however, have not been without controversy. Proponents of thrombolysis talk of the 30–50% relative clinical improvement at 3 months in patients who received rt-PA and underplay the increased risk of symptomatic intracerebral hemorrhage with reference to the absence of a significant difference in mortality between the rt-PA and placebo-treated groups. A more cautious description of the results (in terms of absolute rather than relative risk) indicates that the likelihood of an excellent neurologic outcome is increased by 11–13% for those patients who were treated with rt-PA. This potential benefit must be weighed against a 3% chance of death from rt-PA–induced intracerebral hemorrhage.

Some knowledge of how the various thrombolytic trials were performed is necessary to see through the bias of different perspectives. Why did the streptokinase trials fail to demonstrate a beneficial effect on outcome? What is the evidence that rt-PA is safe and effective in the treatment of acute ischemic stroke? What about intra-arterial thrombolysis? These and other questions are the subject of this chapter.

Is Intravenous Streptokinase Safe and Effective in Patients with Acute Stroke?

The safety and effectiveness of intravenous streptokinase in patients with acute stroke has been the subject of study in three prospective randomized trials, two multicenter trials from Europe, and one from Australia. All were terminated prematurely because of the increased mortality in the streptokinase-treated patients.

The Multicentre Acute Stroke Trial–Italy[1] was a multicenter open randomized trial of intravenous streptokinase, aspirin, both, or neither in the management of patients with acute stroke. Patients were eligible for inclusion if they presented within 6 hours of symptom onset and the primary outcome measure was death or disability at 6 months. The study was stopped prematurely after enrollment of 622 patients, 40% of that originally planned, because of an excess of early mortality in the streptokinase-treated patients.

The Multicenter Acute Stroke Trial–Europe[2] was a prospective randomized, placebo-controlled trial of intravenous streptokinase, in which patients with middle cerebral artery (MCA) ischemia were randomized within 6 hours of symptom onset. Primary endpoints were the same as those used in the Multicentre Acute Stroke Trial–Italy. The Multicenter Acute Stroke Trial–Europe was similarly terminated prematurely because of increased mortality due to intracerebral hemorrhage in the streptokinase-treated patients. Moreover, death or disability at 6 months was not significantly different between the placebo and streptokinase groups.

The Australian Streptokinase study was a prospective randomized, double-blind, placebo-controlled trial.[3] Patients between the ages of 18 and 85 with onset of an ischemic stroke within 4 hours were eligible for inclusion. Exclusion criteria, amongst others, included mild deficit and uncontrolled hypertension. Patients were randomized to receive 1.5 million units of intravenous streptokinase or placebo. The primary endpoint was death or disability at 3 months, with a Barthel Index (BI; see Appendix 3 [Barthel Index]) greater than 60 classified as a favorable outcome. It was anticipated that the outcome would be better in patients treated within 3 hours. Therefore, separate analyses were planned for patients who presented within 3 hours and those between 3 and 4 hours. The trial was terminated prematurely because of the significantly worse outcome in patients who received streptokinase more than 3 hours after stroke onset. Only 340 patients had been recruited, including 70 who presented within less than 3 hours of stroke onset. Considering these patients alone, there was a nonsignificant trend towards favorable outcome in the streptokinase-treated patients. A post hoc categorization of patients according to the NINDS BI cutoff score of 95–100 for favorable outcome showed no benefit for streptokinase.

In summary, therefore, there is no good evidence that intravenous streptokinase should be used in the management of patients with acute ischemic stroke. The absence of evidence may, at least in part, reflect the fact that the studies using streptokinase included patients who presented up to 6 hours after the onset of stroke. The only study that showed even a trend towards a better outcome in streptokinase-treated patients was the Australian Streptokinase study in which patients who presented within 3 hours were analyzed separately. It should be borne in mind, however, that this impression is based on a small sample size.

Is Tissue Plasminogen Activator Safe and Effective in Patients with Acute Stroke?

The European Cooperative Acute Stroke Study (ECASS)[4] was the first large placebo-controlled trial of thrombolysis in acute hemispheric stroke. The study aimed to include patients aged 18–80 with a moderate to severe hemispheric stroke syndrome with no or only minor early infarct signs on the initial computerized tomographic (CT) scan, and who could be treated within 6 hours of stroke onset. Patients were randomized to receive either placebo (307 patients) or rt-PA (313 patients) in a dose of 1.1 mg/kg. Primary outcome measures were the BI and the modified Rankin Scale (mRS; see Appendix 28 [Modified Rankin Scale]) at 90 days. Results are reported separately for the intention-to-treat (ITT) analysis (i.e., the results for all patients who were randomized) and for the target population (TP) (i.e., those patients who remained after exclusion of protocol violators). The rationale for separate reporting of the ITT and TP analyses is that the latter provides an indication of whether rt-PA is effective in the specific subgroup of stroke patients for whom it was intended. The ITT analysis, on the other hand, informs on the efficacy of this treatment taking into account the practical difficulties of implementation.

There were no significant differences in the primary outcome measures in the ITT analysis. A difference of one point on the mRS in favor of rt-PA was, however, detected in the TP analysis. The authors developed a combined BI/mRS score to minimize the ceiling effects inherent in each scale, and this was used as a secondary outcome measure. On this combined score, outcome was more favorable for the rt-PA group in both ITT and TP analyses, but this modified scale has not been validated, and so this finding cannot be easily interpreted.

Other secondary outcome measures included repeated assessment, using the Scandinavian Stroke Scale (see Appendix 29 [Scandinavian Stroke Scale]) at 2, 8, and 24 hours and 7 days after treatment, that showed a significantly faster neurologic recovery in patients who received rt-PA. However, the frequency of parenchymal hemorrhage was significantly more frequent, and the 90-day mortality rate was significantly higher in the rt-PA–treated patients. Subgroup analysis also demonstrated that the risk of major intracranial hemorrhage was highest in those patients with extended early CT signs of infarction who received rt-PA.

The ECASS study, therefore, demonstrated the potential for thrombolytic therapy to improve functional outcome in patients with moderate to severe hemispheric stroke without extended infarct signs on initial CT scan. However, the positive effects were outweighed by the increased mortality in the rt-PA–treated patients.

The NINDS study was the first to demonstrate the safety and efficacy of intravenous rt-PA.[5] This was a prospective randomized, placebo-controlled study in which active treatment comprised rt-PA in a dose of 0.9 mg/kg. To be eligible for inclusion in the study, patients had to have had the onset of symptoms of an ischemic stroke within 3 hours and a measurable deficit on the National Institutes of Health Stroke Scale (NIHSS; see Appendix 22 [National Institutes of Health Stroke Scale]). Amongst the exclusion criteria were minor or rapidly improving symptoms, systolic blood pressure greater than 185 mm Hg, the need for aggressive therapy to reduce blood pressure to within the specified limits, and a seizure at the onset of the stroke. There were two parts to the study. Part 1, designed to assess changes in neurologic deficit within 24 hours of stroke onset, used complete recovery or an improvement of four points on the NIHSS as measures of the clinical activity of rt-PA. Part 2 used four outcome measures to determine whether the use of rt-PA resulted in sustained clinical benefit at 3 months. The four outcome measures used were the BI, the mRS, the Glasgow Outcome Scale (see Appendix 10 [Glasgow Outcome Scale]), and the NIHSS. Scores of 95–100 on the BI, less than or equal to 1 on the NIHSS and mRS, and I on the Glasgow Outcome Scale were considered indicative of a favorable outcome.

In part 1, there was no significant difference between the placebo and rt-PA groups in the percentages of patients who recovered completely or improved by at least four points on the NIHSS. In part 2, however, there was a significant increase in the likelihood of favorable outcome in the patients who received rt-PA. Compared to the placebo group and depending on the outcome measure used, there was an 11–13% absolute increase in the number of patients with a favorable outcome at 3 months (Table 4-1).

In a subsequent study, these results were sustained at 6- and 12-month follow-ups. Even though symptomatic hemorrhage occurred more frequently in the rt-PA–treated patients, there was no increase in the proportion of patients with severe disability or death at 3 months.

ECASS II was designed with the results of ECASS and the NINDS studies in mind.[6] The inclusion criteria were similar to ECASS except that more stringent CT criteria were used, and patients with systolic blood pressure greater than 185 mm Hg were excluded. Greater effort was also made to avoid protocol violation with respect to the nature of the findings on CT scan, and a dose of 0.9 mg/kg alteplase was used (to match that used in the NINDS study). As in the first ECASS study, patients who presented within 6 hours of symptom onset were recruited. The primary outcome was the proportion of patients who had a favorable outcome (determined by a score of 0 or 1 on the mRS) at 90 days (one of the endpoints that was used in the NINDS study). All randomized patients were included in an ITT analysis, and both patients and investigators were blinded to the treatment used. A favorable outcome was observed in 40.3% of patients who received alteplase and 36.6% of patients who received placebo, yielding an absolute difference of 3.7% that was not statistically significant. In a post hoc analy-

TABLE 4-1
Recombinant Tissue-Type Plasminogen Activator in Acute Ischemic Stroke: The
National Institute of Neurological Disorders and Stroke Trial

	*Percentage of Patients with a Favorable Outcome**			
	Recombinant Tissue-Type Plasminogen Activator	*Placebo*	*Absolute Risk Reduction (%)*	*Relative Risk Reduction (%)*
Barthel Index	50	38	12	24
Modified Rankin Scale	39	26	13	33
Glasgow Outcome Scale	44	32	12	27
National Institutes of Health Stroke Scale	31	20	11	35

*Defined as Barthel Index = 95–100; modified Rankin Scale ≤1; National Institutes of Health
Stroke Scale ≤1; and Glasgow Outcome Scale = I.

sis based on dichotomization of mRS scores in which outcome was classified in terms of independence (mRS of 0–2), 54.3% and 46.0% of alteplase-
and placebo-treated patients, respectively, had a favorable outcome. Severe
parenchymal hemorrhages were more frequent in the alteplase group, but
this did not lead to an overall increase in morbidity and mortality in the
alteplase group.

The better outcome and lower mortality rate in the placebo group in
ECASS II (compared to both ECASS I and the NINDS trial) (Table 4-2) was
likely due to selection bias, as patients in ECASS II had less severe neurologic deficits at the time of entry into the study. However, the relevance of
care being provided in a stroke unit (which has independently been shown
to impact favorably on outcome) to the improved outcome remains unclear.

Should Hypertension in the Context of Acute Ischemic Stroke Be Treated?

Elevation in blood pressure, sometimes marked, after acute stroke is commonly observed but usually falls to pre-existing levels within a few days
after the stroke.[7] The question arises, however, as to whether there is any
benefit to be gained from antihypertensive therapy in the acute phase after
stroke. Blood pressure parameters were clearly defined in the NINDS trial
of intravenous rt-PA. A systolic blood pressure greater than 185 mm Hg and
the need for aggressive therapy to reduce blood pressure to within the specified limits were amongst the exclusion criteria. For patients with marked

TABLE 4-2
Comparison of the Results of the European Cooperative Acute Stroke Study-II and
the National Institute of Neurological Disorders and Stroke Study

| | Percentage of Patients with a Favorable Outcome* | | Absolute Risk Reduction (%) |
	Placebo	Thrombolytic	
European Cooperative Acute Stroke Study II	36.6	40.0	3.7
National Institute of Neurological Disorders and Stroke Study	26.0	39.0	13.0

*Favorable outcome defined as modified Rankin Scale score of ≤1.

hypertension who present within the 3-hour window for rt-PA, therefore, there is reason to institute measures to reduce systolic blood pressure for the purposes of administering rt-PA.

With the exception of patients in whom antihypertensive therapy is instituted for the purposes of administering intravenous rt-PA, there are essentially no clinical data to answer this question, and so a rational decision must be made on the basis of an understanding of the pathophysiology of cerebral perfusion.[8]

Under normal circumstances, cerebral blood flow (CBF) is determined by the relationship between cerebral perfusion pressure (CPP) and cerebrovascular resistance (CVR), where CBF = CPP ÷ CVR. CPP is determined by the difference between the mean arterial pressure (MAP) forcing blood into the cerebral vasculature and the venous back-pressure. Raised intracranial pressure (ICP) is transmitted to the venous system, raising venous back-pressure. For practical purposes, therefore, CPP = MAP − ICP. Autoregulation describes the process whereby cerebral blood vessels constrict or dilate (to increase or decrease CVR, respectively) in response to changes in CPP to maintain a constant CBF. For example, increased CPP (due to ↑MAP) (↑ = raised; ↓ = lowered) leads to vasoconstriction and ↑CVR. Similarly, a fall in CPP (due to ↓MAP or ↑ICP) leads to vasodilatation and ↓CVR.

Animal studies, together with limited data from human studies, have shown that blood flow through collateral blood vessels, which is responsible for perfusion of the ischemic penumbra after arterial occlusion, is critically dependent on CPP. This is because autoregulation is impaired in ischemic tissue. That is to say, the vasodilator response to a fall in CPP (↓MAP or ↑ICP) is impaired, and so CBF may fall precipitously. A fall in blood pressure, therefore, may lead to an increase in the size or severity of the ischemic zone. This is the theoretical rationale for not lowering blood pressure in the acute phase of ischemic stroke. But it should be recognized that documentation of the actual risks of lowering blood pressure is based largely on case reports. There is a single randomized, double-blind, placebo-controlled trial of antihypertensive therapy after acute ischemic stroke.[9] These authors randomized 16 patients within 72 hours of ischemic stroke to receive either placebo or antihypertensive therapy (with nicardipine, captopril, or clonidine). Single-photon emission CT was performed before the initiation of therapy and after 3 days to evaluate CBF; neurologic deficit on admission and after 3 days was determined using the NIHSS. They observed a greater reduction in blood pressure in the nicardipine-treated patients that was accompanied by a failure of MCA-perfusion to improve with time (as determined by single-photon emission CT scanning). There were no significant changes in NIHSS scores. This study was suboptimal for a range of reasons, including small sample size, use of different antihypertensive agents within the treated group, and failure to specify primary efficacy measures in advance, to name but a few. Nevertheless, it does represent one of the few attempts to correlate acute antihypertensive treatment after ischemic stroke with measures of CBF and clinical outcome.

Proponents of antihypertensive therapy in the context of acute stroke have argued that there are also theoretical benefits to this approach. Reducing blood pressure may decrease the risk of hemorrhagic transformation, prevent further vascular injury, and reduce the formation of edema. However, because the edema is due to ischemia, it seems to make more sense to focus primarily on reducing ischemia. In the absence of another indication for antihypertensive therapy (e.g., eligibility to receive intravenous rt-PA, malignant hypertension, or concurrent myocardial ischemia), there is, therefore, little scientific basis and no clinically proven benefit to lowering blood pressure, no matter how high it is.

Is Thrombolysis Effective Therapy for All Forms of Ischemic Stroke?

The NINDS rt-PA Stroke Study is the only study that provides some information regarding the use of thrombolytic therapy in the various types of ischemic strokes. A priori, it might be expected that thrombolysis would be more effective in large-artery and cardioembolic stroke than in lacunar stroke. Stroke in the NINDS rt-PA Stroke Study was classified as small vessel occlusive, large vessel occlusive, and cardioembolic. The proportion of patients with a favorable outcome (ascertained by each of the four outcome measures used—BI, mRS, Glasgow Outcome Scale, and the NIHSS), were reported separately for those who were treated with rt-PA and those who received placebo. A positive effect of rt-PA on all outcome measures at 3 months was present for all stroke subtypes. Those who caution against the use of rt-PA for lacunar stroke raise a number of objections to these results. The first is that the classification of stroke subtype in the NINDS study was based on the combination of clinical impression and CT scan without the confirmation of magnetic resonance or vascular imaging studies. The second is that the prognosis for favorable outcome in small vessel (lacunar) stroke patients in the NINDS study was worse than is generally recognized for this type of stroke, raising further doubts about the accuracy of the designation of these strokes as being due to small vessel occlusive disease. It is not clear, however, that the latter claim is true. In the NINDS study, 40% of the placebo-treated patients with lacunar stroke achieved a favorable outcome that was defined as an mRS score less than or equal to 1. Other studies of the outcome of lacunar stroke have reported favorable outcome in 73%[10] to 85%[11] of patients, but in these studies, favorable outcome was defined as an mRS less than or equal to 2. The data, therefore, are not directly comparable. Presently, the balance of evidence favors the use of rt-PA even in patients suspected of having lacunar stroke.

Is There a Role for Intra-Arterial Thrombolysis in the Management of Acute Stroke?

The Prolyse in Acute Cerebral Thromboembolism trials (PROACT I and II) are the only randomized, double-blind, controlled trials that have evaluated the efficacy and safety of intra-arterial thrombolysis in acute ischemic stroke.

In both PROACT I[12] and PROACT II,[13] eligibility for inclusion proceeded through two phases. Clinical eligibility required patients aged 18–85, with focal signs attributable to an MCA stroke in whom treatment could be initiated within 6 hours of symptom onset and who had a minimum NIHSS score of 4. These patients then underwent angiography, and only those with complete MCA occlusion (Thrombolysis in Myocardial Infarction [TIMI] 0) or minimal perfusion (TIMI 1) of either the M1 or M2 segments were eligible for randomization to receive recombinant pro-urokinase (rpro-UK). PROACT I included a placebo group who received a saline infusion, but PROACT II did not. All patients also received an infusion of heparin, with a switch being made from high to low dose midway through PROACT 1 because of the high incidence of intracerebral hemorrhage in those who received high-dose heparin. In PROACT I, the primary measure of outcome was recanalization of the M1 or M2 MCA (TIMI 2 or TIMI 3) 2 hours after the start of the infusion. Clinical outcome was assessed using the NIHSS, the mRS, and the BI at 7, 30, and 90 days after treatment. In PROACT II, the primary outcome measure was the percentage of patients achieving an mRS score of 2 or less (signifying slight or no disability) at 90 days. Angiographic recanalization rate was one of the secondary outcome measures.

In PROACT I, 105 patients underwent angiography to identify 40 eligible patients who were treated, 26 with rpro-UK (6 mg) and 14 with placebo.

Partial or complete recanalization occurred in 15 of 26 patients (58%) who received rpro-UK and two of 14 placebo-treated patients. Favorable clinical outcome (NIHSS of 0–1, mRS of 0–1, and BI of 9–10*) occurred approximately 10% more frequently in the rpro-UK–treated patients, but these results did not achieve statistical significance (perhaps because of the small number of patients treated). Intracerebral hemorrhage with clinical deterioration occurred twice as frequently (15% vs. 7%) in the rpro-UK–treated group.

In PROACT II, 474 patients underwent angiography to identify 180 patients who were eligible for randomization to receive rpro-UK (121 patients) at a dose of 9 mg or no treatment. For the primary outcome analysis, 40% of the rpro-UK patients and 25% of controls achieved an mRS score of less than or equal to 2 at 90 days, an absolute risk reduction of 15%. Intracranial hemorrhage with neurologic deterioration within the first 24 hours occurred in 10% and 2% of rpro-UK and control patients, respectively. Recanalization (TIMI 2 or TIMI 3 flow) occurred in 66% of rpro-UK–treated patients and 18% of controls.

PROACT I was a placebo-controlled trial but was not powered to detect a clinical benefit. PROACT II, specifically designed to have sufficient power to detect improved clinical outcome after intra-arterial thrombolysis, was randomized and blinded but not placebo-controlled. With this caveat in mind, the results of PROACT II suggest that patients with acute MCA stroke of less than 6 hours' duration may benefit from intra-arterial thrombolysis.

Summary

- There is no evidence to support the routine use of intravenous streptokinase in the management of acute stroke.
- The NINDS rt-PA Stroke Study supports broad indications for intravenous thrombolysis with rt-PA within 3 hours of the onset of stroke.
- Treatment may be beneficial irrespective of the patient's age, gender, or stroke subtype.
- Patients with a broad spectrum of neurologic deficits may benefit from thrombolysis, with the exception of patients with very mild and resolving deficits.
- The risk of symptomatic intracranial hemorrhage is increased when CT demonstrates early changes of a recent major infarction such as sulcal effacement, mass effect, edema, or hemorrhage. These findings, therefore, contraindicate the use of intravenous thrombolysis.

---

*The authors defined *favorable outcome* as a BI of 9–10, but the BI is a scale from 0 to 100; presumably they mean a BI of 90–100.

- The risk of complications can be reduced by strict adherence to the exclusion criteria used in the NINDS rt-PA Stroke Study:
  ◊ Current use of oral anticoagulants or an INR greater than 1.7
  ◊ Use of heparin within the preceding 48 hours and prolonged partial thromboplastin time
  ◊ Platelet count less than 100,000/mm^3
  ◊ Another stroke or serious head injury within the preceding 3 months
  ◊ Major surgery within the preceding 14 days
  ◊ Pretreatment blood pressure greater than 185/110 mm Hg
  ◊ Prior intracranial hemorrhage
  ◊ Blood glucose less than 50 mg/dL
  ◊ Seizure at stroke onset
  ◊ Recent myocardial infarction or gastrointestinal/genitourinary bleeding within the preceding 21 days
- The American Academy of Neurology has published a practice advisory regarding the use of thrombolytic therapy for acute ischemic stroke,[14] wherein specific guidelines for the use of rt-PA are outlined. Guidelines for the management of arterial hypertension following the administration of rt-PA are also outlined.
- There are some data to suggest that intra-arterial rpro-UK may be safe and effective in patients with moderately severe MCA if administered within 6 hours of the onset of symptoms.
- Antihypertensive therapy in the context of acute ischemic stroke remains controversial except when necessary to permit the use of intravenous rt-PA or when indicated by concurrent medical conditions (acute myocardial infarction or malignant hypertension).

References

1. Randomized controlled trial of streptokinase, aspirin, and combination of both in treatment of acute ischaemic stroke. Multicentre Acute Stroke Trial–Italy (MAST-I) Group. *Lancet* 1995;346:1509–1514.
2. Thrombolytic therapy with streptokinase in acute ischemic stroke. The Multicenter Acute Stroke Trial–Europe Study Group. *N Engl J Med* 1996;335:145–150.
3. Donnan GA, Davis SM, Chambers BR, et al. Streptokinase for acute ischemic stroke with relationship to time of administration. Australian Streptokinase (ASK) Trial Study Group. *JAMA* 1996;276:961–966.
4. Hacke W, Kaste M, Fieschi C, et al. Intravenous thrombolysis with recombinant tissue plasminogen activator for acute hemispheric stroke. The European Cooperative Acute Stroke Study (ECASS). *JAMA* 1995;274:1017–1025.

5. Tissue plasminogen activator for acute ischemic stroke. The National Institute of Neurological Disorders and Stroke rt-PA Stroke Study Group. *N Engl J Med* 1995;333:1581–1587.

6. Hacke W, Maste M, Fieschi C, et al. Randomised double-blind placebo-controlled trial of thrombolytic therapy with intravenous alteplase in acute ischaemic stroke (ECASS II). Second European-Australasian Acute Stroke Study Investigators. *Lancet* 1998;352:1245–1251.

7. Wallace JD, Levy LL. Blood pressure after stroke. *JAMA* 1981;246:2177–2180.

8. Powers WJ. Acute hypertension after stroke: the scientific basis for treatment decisions. *Neurology* 1993;43:461–467.

9. Lisk DR, Grotta JC, Lamki LM, et al. Should hypertension be treated after acute stroke? A randomized controlled trial using single photon emission computed tomography. *Arch Neurol* 1993;50:855–862.

10. Grau AJ, Weimar C, Buggle F, et al. Risk factors, outcome, and treatment in subtypes of ischemic stroke: the German Stroke Data Bank. *Stroke* 2001;32: 2559–2566.

11. Petty GW, Brown RD, Whisnant JP, et al. Ischemic stroke subtypes: a population-based study of functional outcome, survival and recurrence. *Stroke* 2001;31:1062–1068.

12. del Zoppo GJ, Higashida RT, Furlan AJ, et al. PROACT: a phase II randomized trial of recombinant pro-urokinase by direct arterial delivery in acute middle cerebral artery stroke. PROACT Investigators. Prolyse in Acute Cerebral Thromboembolism. *Stroke* 1998;29:4–11.

13. Furlan A, Higashida R, Wechsler L, et al. Intra-arterial prourokinase for acute ischemic stroke. The PROACT II Study: a randomized controlled trial. Prolyse in Acute Cerebral Thromboembolism. *JAMA* 1999;282:2003–2011.

14. Practice advisory: thrombolytic therapy for acute ischemic stroke—summary statement. Report of the Quality Standards Subcommittee of the American Academy of Neurology. *Neurology* 1996;47:835–839.

CHAPTER 5

Carotid Stenosis

Introduction

The European Carotid Surgery Trial (ECST)[1] and the North American Symptomatic Carotid Endarterectomy Trial (NASCET)[2] established a clear indication for carotid endarterectomy (CEA) in patients with symptomatic high-grade stenosis. To appreciate the clinical applicability of this finding, however, it is necessary to understand something about the way in which these studies were performed. What were the inclusion criteria that defined the study populations, and can the results be broadly generalized? Is contrast angiography (CA) necessary to define the degree of stenosis before surgery? What is the risk of recurrent stroke, and does it depend on the degree of stenosis? Are there clinical criteria that can be used to define high- and low-risk patients who might benefit to a greater or lesser extent from endarterectomy? What was the nature of the medical therapies used (against which the effects of CEA were compared)? These and other questions are the subject of this chapter.

What Is the Risk of Stroke in Patients with Carotid Stenosis?

Data from both the NASCET[2] and ECST[1] trials showed that the risk of stroke is related to the degree of stenosis. The data for patients who received best medical therapy are outlined in Table 5-1.

These data represent the risk of ipsilateral stroke when the index event was either a retinal or hemispheric transient ischemic attack (TIA) or stroke. However, there are some data from the NASCET study that suggest that the risk of recurrent stroke is less in patients whose index event was transient retinal ischemia (amaurosis fugax).[3] There is also some indication that the risk of recurrent stroke falls off with time—a phenomenon that may relate to stabilization of the atheromatous plaque with time.

Finally, it is worth noting that approximately 60% of recurrent strokes are related to the same carotid lesion, but a significant minority (40%) are due to either lacunar or cardioembolic stroke. Furthermore, the risk of recurrent cardioembolic stroke might have been even greater if

TABLE 5-1
Risk of Stroke with Symptomatic High-Grade Carotid Stenosis

	Stenosis (%)			
Outcome Measure	70–79	80–89	90–99	Total
North American Symptomatic Carotid Endarterectomy Trial (all ipsilateral stroke at 2 yrs)	19.9	28.5	34.6	26.0
European Carotid Surgery Trial (major ipsilateral stroke at 3 yrs)	8.8	21.4	31.7	26.5

patients with significant cardiac disease had not been excluded from the NASCET study.

What Is the Evidence That Patients with Symptomatic High-Grade Stenosis Should Undergo Carotid Endarterectomy?

There are two major studies that examined the role of CEA in patients with symptomatic carotid stenosis. The preliminary results of the NASCET[2] and the ECST studies[1] published in 1991 provided evidence in favor of CEA in patients with symptomatic high-grade carotid stenosis.

The NASCET study[2] included 659 patients who were randomized to best medical therapy with or without CEA. Medical therapy included aspirin (usually 1,300 mg per day), antihypertensive, antilipid, and antidiabetic therapy, as required. Patients younger than 80 years with a hemispheric TIA, episode of amaurosis fugax, or nondisabling stroke within the previous 120 days were eligible for inclusion. The degree of stenosis was measured on CA. Measurements were made of the luminal diameter at the point of maximal stenosis (M) and at a normal portion of the artery beyond the carotid bulb (D) (Figure 5-1). The degree of stenosis was calculated with the formula ($[1 - M/D] \times 100$). Stenosis of 70–99% was classified as severe or high grade. Uncontrolled hypertension, diabetes mellitus, angina pectoris, or myocardial infarction within the previous 6 months led to exclusion, unless there was resolution of the relevant factor within 120 days of the qualifying TIA or stroke. Patients were also excluded if a more severe intracranial stenosis was identified. No patients were lost to follow-up, and the study was terminated prematurely because of the clearly better outcome in the surgical group.

The combined rate of stroke and death within the perioperative period (time from randomization to 30 days postsurgery) was 5.8%. The rate of stroke and death in a comparable 32-day period was 3.3% in the patients

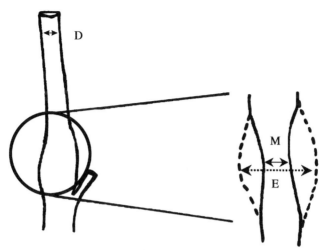

FIGURE 5-1   Measurement of the degree of stenosis in the North American Symptomatic Carotid Endarterectomy Trial (NASCET) and the European Carotid Surgery
Trial (ECST). The dashed line indicates the contour of the normal carotid artery.
The solid line indicates the contour of the stenosed carotid artery. NASCET degree
of stenosis = ([1 – M/D] × 100); ECST degree of stenosis = ([1 – M/E] × 100). (D =
diameter of carotid artery distal to the bulb; E = estimated diameter of normal
carotid artery at the level of the stenosis; M = measured diameter of stenosed internal carotid artery.) (Modified from H Wein, N Bornstein. Stroke prevention. *Neurol
Clin* 2000;18:331.)

treated medically. The 2-year risk of ipsilateral stroke was 9% and 26% in
the CEA and medical groups, respectively. This represents an absolute risk
reduction of 17% with 6 patients being the number needed to treat to prevent one stroke over 24 months* (Table 5-2).

Of additional interest is the observation that the benefit from CEA
was greatest in patients with the highest degrees of stenosis (Table 5-3).
Thus, notwithstanding the increased perioperative morbidity and mortality, the results at 2 years clearly indicated a benefit from CEA.

The European study[1,4] produced similar results. As with NASCET,
patients were eligible for inclusion if they had experienced a retinal infarct,
TIA, or nondisabling stroke within the preceding 6 months. This study
included 455 patients with high-grade stenosis who were randomized to
surgery and 323 patients randomized to avoid surgery. All received appropriate medical therapy, including aspirin, treatment of hypertension, and
advice to stop smoking. As in the NASCET study, all patients underwent
CA. The degree of stenosis was calculated using the diameter at the point of

---

*Number needed to treat is derived from the absolute risk reduction and is calculated as 100 ÷
absolute risk reduction.

TABLE 5-2
North American Symptomatic Carotid Endarterectomy Trial Study Results for
Medical and Surgical Groups

Outcome Measure	Medical Group (%)	Surgical Group (%)
Perioperative stroke[a]	3.3	5.8
Ipsilateral stroke[b]	26.0	9.0
Major or fatal ipsilateral stroke[b]	13.1	2.5
Any stroke[b]	27.6	12.6
Any stroke or death[b]	32.3	15.8

[a]Or equivalent 32-day period in the medical group.
[b]Cumulative risk over 2 yrs.

maximal stenosis (M) and the estimated diameter of the original artery (E)
using the formula ([1 − M/E] × 100) (see Figure 5-1). This method underesti-
mates the degree of stenosis compared to the NASCET study. High-grade
stenosis in the ECST study was defined as greater than 80%, which correlates with greater than 60% in the NASCET study. Using the ECST criteria,
a stenosis of 85% would be equivalent to the lower cutoff of 70% used in
the NASCET study to define high-grade stenosis.

In patients with greater than 80% stenosis, the 30-day risk of the combined endpoint of death or major stroke was 4.5%. At 3 years, the risk of
death or disabling stroke was 14.9% and 26.5% in the surgical and medical
groups, respectively—an absolute risk reduction of 11.6%.

The results of the NASCET and ECST studies were strikingly similar.
Both showed that patients with symptomatic high-grade stenosis benefit
from CEA in terms of a reduced 2- to 3-year risk of death or disabling stroke.
They also both demonstrated that the risk of death or stroke varied with the
degree of stenosis, being greatest in those with the highest degree of stenosis.
These two studies were also similar in that the perioperative risk of death or
stroke was relatively low at 5.8% and 4.5% in the NASCET and ECST studies, respectively. Finally, the magnitudes of the combined risk of death and
stroke at final follow-up were very similar. A direct comparison is difficult
because of the different techniques used for measuring the degree of stenosis
as well as slightly different endpoints. Using roughly comparable degrees of
stenosis, the risks may be summarized as outlined in Table 5-4.

TABLE 5-3
Risk of Stroke Is Increased with Greater Degrees of Stenosis

	Degree of Stenosis (%)		
Outcome measure	70–79	80–89	90–99
Absolute risk reduction of ipsilateral stroke at 2 yrs	12	18	26

TABLE 5-4
Summary of North American Symptomatic Carotid Endarterectomy Trial
(NASCET) and European Carotid Surgery Trial (ECST) Study Results

	NASCET 2-Yr Risk of All Ipsilateral Strokes			ECST 3-Yr Risk of Death or Disabling Ipsilateral Stroke		
Percent Stenosis	Medical (%)	Surgical (%)	Absolute Difference (%)	Medical (%)	Surgical (%)	Absolute Difference (%)
70–79	19.9	7.4	12.5	8.8	5.6	3.2
80–89	28.5	10.6	17.9	21.4	5.2	16.2
90–99	34.6	8.5	26.1	31.7	4.8	26.9
Total	26.0	9.0	17.0	26.5	14.9	11.6

Finally, it should be noted that the morbidity from angiography was not included in these analyses, presumably because this was required of patients in both medical and surgical groups. However, the morbidity from angiography may become relevant if only those patients who are thought to be candidates for endarterectomy are subject to angiography, with the severity of stenosis being evaluated by noninvasive measures in patients who are believed not to be surgical candidates.

The final conclusion from these two important studies is that CEA is safe and effective in reducing the intermediate-term risk of death and stroke in patients with symptomatic high-grade carotid stenosis. This benefit is due in no small part to the low surgical morbidity and mortality in these two studies.

What about Patients with Symptomatic Moderate-Grade Stenosis?

After publication of the preliminary results in patients with high-grade stenosis, NASCET continued to randomize patients with symptomatic moderate grade (less than 70%) stenosis, with these results reported separately.[5] The 30-day perioperative rate of stroke or death was 6.7%, compared to 2.4% in the medical group during a similar period. Long-term outcome data were presented separately for patients with narrowing of 50–69% that was classified as high-moderate stenosis. The 5-year risk of ipsilateral stroke was 22.2% and 15.7% for the medical and surgical groups, respectively. The absolute risk reduction of 6.5% indicates that the number needed to treat with endarterectomy is 15 to prevent one ipsilateral stroke at 5 years. A similar pattern of results was obtained for the other outcome measures of disabling ipsilateral stroke, any stroke, disabling stroke, any stroke or death, and any disabling stroke or death. In general, for symptomatic high-moderate stenosis, the risks were greater for patients treated medically, but the overlapping confidence intervals preclude firm conclusions being drawn about the benefits of surgery.

In an effort to determine whether subgroups of patients with high-moderate stenosis might benefit from CEA, the investigators performed a post hoc univariate analysis of patients' baseline characteristics. This analysis identified seven factors that were associated with a doubled perioperative risk of stroke or death. These included evidence of an infarct on a computerized tomographic scan or magnetic resonance imaging ipsilateral to the carotid stenosis, contralateral carotid occlusion, left-sided carotid disease, diabetes, hypertension, use of less than 650 mg aspirin per day, and absence of a history of myocardial infarction or angina. Regression analysis also identified four characteristics that were associated with greater long-term benefit from surgery: male gender, recent stroke, recent hemispheric symptoms, and use of greater than 650 mg aspirin per day. These results suggest that selected patients with high-moderate stenosis may benefit from endarterectomy, but this benefit is lost if the perioperative risk of disabling stroke or death exceeds the 2% reported in the NASCET study.

How Should Asymptomatic Carotid Stenosis Be Managed?

The issue of how asymptomatic carotid stenosis should be managed has been the subject of a number of studies, including the Carotid Artery Stenosis with Asymptomatic Narrowing: Operation Versus Aspirin (CASANOVA) study, which was inconclusive; the Mayo Clinic Trial, which was terminated prematurely because of increased number of myocardial infarctions in the surgical group; and the Veterans Affairs Cooperative Study, which included TIA with stroke and death in a combined endpoint analysis. The Asymptomatic Carotid Atherosclerosis Study (ACAS)[6] came closest to answering the question of how patients with asymptomatic carotid stenosis should be managed.

The ACAS investigators randomized approximately 800 patients to receive aggressive medical therapy with or without the addition of CEA. To be eligible for inclusion, there had to be a recent Doppler ultrasound demonstrated stenosis of greater than 60%. After randomization to the surgical group, all patients had CA with the degree of stenosis measured by the same technique as that used in the NASCET study. Asymptomatic cerebral infarction demonstrable on computerized tomographic scans was not an exclusion for surgery. All patients received aspirin 325 mg per day as well as aggressive treatment of vascular risk factors like hypertension, diabetes, and hyperlipidemia.

All patients in the surgical group had CA with its attendant stroke complication rate of 1.2%. Including these angiographic complications, the

30-day perioperative risk of stroke or death was 2.7%. The risk of stroke or death was 0.4% in the medical group during a comparable period. Patients were followed for a mean duration of 2.7 years, and outcomes at 5 years were projected from Kaplan-Meier curves. The results of this study are summarized in Table 5-5.

The estimated 5-year combined risk of ipsilateral stroke or perioperative stroke or death was 11.0% for the medical group and 5.1% for the surgical group, yielding an absolute risk reduction of 5.9% (number needed to treat is 17 over 5 years). Given that statistically significant results were obtained only for the category of "ipsilateral stroke" and not "ipsilateral major stroke," it is relevant to know how the ACAS investigators defined "major stroke." They regarded grades II–IV of the Glasgow Outcome Scale (see Appendix 10 [Glasgow Outcome Scale]) as a major stroke (i.e., stroke from which recovery is anything short of a return to normal life).

A superficial glance at the results of ACAS might suggest that patients with asymptomatic high-grade stenosis do benefit from CEA. However, closer inspection reveals a number of issues that should caution against this conclusion. First, surgery did not confer an advantage with regard to the endpoint of disabling stroke. The benefit was seen only in the category of "ipsilateral stroke" that included only those patients with complete recovery. Second, although statistically significant differences were detected for the risks of ipsilateral stroke, perioperative stroke, or death, the absolute difference is small— approximately 1.0% per year. For an individual patient, therefore, the net gain of 1.0% per year may not justify the upfront perioperative risk. Finally, it is worth noting that the perioperative morbidity and mortality were extremely good in the ACAS study and that this most likely biased the results in favor of the surgical group. However, unless similarly good results can be achieved by other centers, it may not be possible to generalize these results.

Given these concerns, the current recommendation is that patients with asymptomatic high-grade carotid stenosis should not undergo endarterectomy. It may be that in the future it will be possible to identify patients with asymptomatic stenosis who are at high risk for ipsilateral stroke and that this subgroup could benefit from CEA.

TABLE 5-5
Results of the Asymptomatic Carotid Atherosclerosis Study

	Medical (%)	Surgical (%)	p Value
30-Day perioperative risk of stroke or death	0.4	2.7	—
5-Yr risk of ipsilateral stroke (including perioperative stroke/death)	11.0	5.1	0.004
5-Yr risk of major ipsilateral stroke (including perioperative stroke/death)	6.0	3.4	0.12

How Should the Presence of Carotid Occlusion Influence the Decision to Proceed with Carotid Endarterectomy?

Follow-up data from the NASCET study indicated that the 5-year risk of ipsilateral stroke in patients with carotid occlusion was 9.4%.[7] The likely explanation for this relatively low rate of stroke relates to the idea that the likelihood of atheroma dislodgement and distal embolization is extremely low in the absence of blood flow through the affected carotid artery. CEA, therefore, should not be performed in those with occlusion of the carotid artery on the side of symptoms.

Some have argued that the presence of contralateral carotid occlusion should influence the decision to proceed with endarterectomy of the patent artery even if it is asymptomatic. Data from the NASCET study, however, indicate that this combination of arterial lesions in symptomatic patients confers a twofold increase in the perioperative risk of stroke or death.

How Should Patients with Crescendo Transient Ischemic Attacks and High-Grade Carotid Stenosis Be Managed?

CEA is ordinarily performed electively once patients are identified as having symptomatic high-grade stenosis. The question arises, however, as to whether management should differ for patients with TIAs of increasing frequency or severity when these are symptomatic of an underlying high-grade carotid stenosis. The two alternatives to elective surgery are emergent endarterectomy and interim anticoagulation before elective surgery. A retrospective review of 29 patients treated with short-term heparinization as a bridge to preoperative evaluation, angiography, and endarterectomy suggested that this approach was safe and effective.[8] However, there are no good-quality data to indicate how these patients are best managed.

Is Contrast Angiography Necessary to Delineate the Degree of Stenosis?

The sensitivity and specificity of magnetic resonance angiography (MRA) and duplex ultrasound (DU), alone and in combination, have been studied using CA as the gold standard for the demonstration of carotid stenosis. Patel et al. performed a blinded comparison of 148 carotid bifurcations that were evaluated using each of three-dimensional time of flight (3D-TOF) MRA, 2D-TOF MRA, DU, and CA.[9] For 70–99% stenosis, they found that 3D-TOF MRA had a sensitivity of 94% and a specificity of 85%. Using the criterion of internal carotid artery peak systolic velocity greater than 2,300 mm per second, DU offered a sensitivity of 94% and a specificity of 83%. When there was agreement between the results of the MRA and DU, the sensitivity and specificity increased to 100% and 91%, respectively. Similar results were obtained by Young et al. in their blinded prospective study of the diagnostic accuracy of MRA and DU compared to CA.[10] They reported a sensitivity and specificity of 86% and 93%, respectively, for MRA and a sensitivity and specificity for DU of 89% and 93%, respectively. Combining MRA and DU yielded slightly improved sensitivity and specificity of 92% and 95%, respectively.

A few other points are worth noting. The first is that 2D-TOF MRA lacked sensitivity and specificity in comparison to 3D-TOF MRA. The combination of 2D- and 3D-TOF MRA, however, proved particularly useful in distinguishing high-grade stenosis from complete carotid occlusion. Second, it should be noted that both DU and MRA provide data about a restricted length of the carotid arteries and may fail to detect significant stenoses that are either proximal or distal to the region imaged by these modalities. Finally, MRA lacks sensitivity for demonstrating tandem intracranial stenosis, which, if more severe than the extracranial stenosis, represented an exclusion-criterion in the NASCET study.

When Should Carotid Endarterectomy Be Performed?

The general recommendation has been to delay endarterectomy for 5–6 weeks after a stroke. The basis for this rationale has been the high morbidity and mortality encountered in those patients who underwent early CEA in the 1960s. More recent case reports and series, however, have highlighted the safety of early endarterectomy in select patient populations. The rationale for early CEA relates to the non-negligible risk of recurrent stroke during the 5- to 6-week interval after the index stroke. In the NASCET study, the 30-day risk of stroke in patients with severe carotid stenosis was 4.9%. Other studies have suggested that the 30-day risk of recurrent large-artery atherothrombotic stroke is around 7.9%. Early surgery might prevent many of these events, and thus offer an even greater benefit over medical therapy, if it could be performed with no greater perioperative risk of stroke or death than when performed after a delay of 5–6 weeks. The question thus becomes focused on the safety of early CEA.

The study by Hoffmann and Robbs[11] is the largest in which the results of early and late surgery are described. They reported their experience with two groups of patients undergoing CEA, with the stratification based on whether endarterectomy was performed within or after 6 weeks after the stroke. Patients were not randomized, but the data were collected prospectively, and there were no significant differences between subjects in the two groups. Patients deemed eligible for early surgery were those with a stable and minor neurologic deficit in the presence of either greater than 60% ipsilateral carotid stenosis or 40–60% stenosis with ulceration. All patients were subject to either computerized tomographic scans or magnetic resonance imaging to document the presence of an infarct. The study included a total of 207 patients, 86 of whom underwent early CEA and 121 of whom were operated on more than 6 weeks after the stroke. There was a trend towards a higher morbidity and mortality in the late surgery group, but these results did not reach significance. This study suggests that early surgery may be even safer than delayed endarterectomy, but in the absence of data from a prospective randomized controlled trial, the most appropriate timing of CEA after a stroke remains controversial.

The etiology of stroke after early CEA is not well established, but hyperperfusion (due to impaired cerebral autoregulation) resulting in cerebral hemorrhage is thought to represent an important factor. The idea had been that autoregulation is likely to be most impaired in the early period after a stroke, and this provided the rationale for delaying surgery. In the more recent studies, however, there was meticulous attention to blood pressure control to avoid excessive hypertension and consequent cerebral hyperperfusion after CEA. This may at least partially explain the lower morbidity and mortality reported in these studies compared to earlier studies.

Thus, although the issue of the timing of endarterectomy after stroke remains an unresolved question, there are limited data to support the safety of early CEA in select patients. Postoperative control of blood pressure to avoid cerebral hyperperfusion is likely an important factor in reducing the risk of stroke.

Summary

- CEA reduces the risk of stroke and death in patients with symptomatic high-grade (greater than 70%) stenosis from 26% to 9% at 2 years.
- There is equivocal evidence that CEA reduces the 5-year risk of ipsilateral stroke in select patients with high-moderate (50–69%) stenosis.
- The data from the ACAS trial suggested a possible benefit from CEA for patients with hemodynamically significant (greater than 60%) asymptomatic stenosis, but caution is required in the interpretation and generalization of this finding.
- The benefits of CEA are critically dependent on a low perioperative morbidity and mortality. Morbidity in excess of that achieved in the NASCET, ECST, and ACAS trials results in loss of any benefit that may have been derived from CEA.
- Contrast angiography remains the gold standard for defining the degree of carotid stenosis, but the combination of DU and MRA suffices when the results of these two studies are congruent.
- CEA offers no benefit to patients with carotid occlusion.
- The appropriate management of patients with crescendo TIAs that are symptomatic of an underlying high-grade stenosis remains

unclear. There is no good evidence either for or against the use of anticoagulation in this context.
- There are limited data to support the safety of early CEA in select patients after a stroke, but resolution of this issue awaits a prospective randomized, controlled study.

References

1. MRC European Carotid Surgery Trial: interim results for symptomatic patients with severe (70-99%) or with mild (0-29%) carotid stenosis. European Carotid Surgery Trialists' Collaborative Group. *Lancet* 1991;337:1235–1243.
2. Beneficial effect of carotid endarterectomy in symptomatic patients with high-grade carotid stenosis. North American Symptomatic Carotid Endarterectomy Trial Collaborators. *N Engl J Med* 1991;325:445–453.
3. Streifler JY, Eliasziw M, Benavente OR, et al. The risk of stroke in patients with first-ever retinal vs hemispheric transient ischemic attacks and high-grade carotid stenosis. North American Symptomatic Carotid Endarterectomy Trial. *Arch Neurol* 1995;52:246–249.
4. Randomized trial of endarterectomy for recently symptomatic carotid stenosis: final results of the MRC European Carotid Surgery Trial (ECST). *Lancet* 1998;351:1379–1387.
5. Barnett HJM, Taylor DW, Eliasziw M, et al. Benefit of carotid endarterectomy in patients with symptomatic moderate or severe stenosis. *N Engl J Med* 1998;339:1415–1425.
6. Endarterectomy for asymptomatic carotid artery stenosis. Executive Committee for the Asymptomatic Carotid Atherosclerosis Study. *JAMA* 1995;273:1421–1428.
7. Inzitari D, Eliasziw M, Gates P, et al. The causes and risk of stroke in patients with asymptomatic internal carotid artery stenosis. North American Symptomatic Carotid Endarterectomy Trial Collaborators. *N Engl J Med* 2000;342:1693–1700.
8. Nehler MR, Moneta GL, McConnell DB, et al. Anticoagulation followed by elective carotid surgery in patients with repetitive transient ischemic attacks and high-grade carotid stenosis. *Arch Surg* 1993;128:1117–1123.
9. Patel MR, Kuntz KM, Klufas RA, et al. Preoperative assessment of the carotid bifurcation. Can magnetic resonance angiography and duplex ultrasonography replace contrast angiography? *Stroke* 1995;26:1753–1758.
10. Young GR, Humphrey PR, Shaw MD, et al. Comparison of magnetic resonance angiography, duplex ultrasound, and digital subtraction angiography in assessment of extracranial internal carotid artery stenosis. *J Neurol Neurosurg Psychiatry* 1994;57:1466–1478.
11. Hoffmann M, Robbs J. Carotid endarterectomy after recent cerebral infarction. *Eur J Endovasc Surg* 1999;18:6–10.

CHAPTER 6

Association between Stroke and Atrial Septal Abnormalities

Introduction

The nature of the association between atrial septal abnormalities, most notably a patent foramen ovale (PFO), and ischemic stroke has been the subject of controversy for some time. The published studies are all limited in some way or another. Most are retrospective, do not include a control group, and comprise only small numbers of patients or used different treatment regimens for secondary prevention of stroke, such that the risk of stroke recurrence or the effects of treatment cannot be reliably disentangled. The recent (2001) publication of the results of a prospective study of young patients with cryptogenic stroke and underlying atrial septal abnormalities has helped to shed light on these long-standing controversies. It is, nevertheless, useful to be aware of these older studies that provide a context within which to evaluate the results of the single prospective study.

This chapter focuses on the association between stroke and the presence of an atrial septal abnormality. What is the nature of this association? What is the risk of recurrent stroke in patients in whom atrial septal abnormalities are detected? What are the available therapeutic options, and do they impact on the risk of stroke recurrence?

What Is the Spectrum of Atrial Septal Abnormalities That May Be Relevant to Stroke?

Atrial septal abnormality is a generic term that includes a number of structural defects including atrial septal aneurysm (ASA), PFO, and atrial septal defect (ASD). The term *ASA* refers to an abnormally redundant and mobile atrial septum that may be defined as greater than 1 cm bulging of the septum beyond the septal plane into either the left or right atrium or greater than 1 cm phasic course of the septum during the cardiorespiratory cycle. There is no uniform consensus on the echocardiographic definitions of PFO and ASD. Certainly, the presence of a visible structural septal defect constitutes evidence of an ASD. The term *atrial septal communication* is sometimes used in the literature and refers to the presence of a visible structural defect (i.e., an ASD). In the absence of such a defect, however, trans-septal blood flow can be measured with both color Doppler and after the injection of agitated saline (microbubbles). The presence of trans-septal flow only with Valsalva, but not at rest, indicates the presence of a PFO. There is some controversy regarding whether the presence of trans-septal flow at rest in the absence of a visible structural defect should be regarded as a PFO or an ASD.

What Is the Nature of the Association between Stroke and the Presence of a Patent Foramen Ovale or Atrial Septal Aneurysm?

The evidence from case-control studies for an association between stroke and PFO or ASA is best summarized in a recent meta-analysis.[1] In this systematic review, Overell and colleagues identified three groups of studies that examined the incidence of PFO or ASA in (1) stroke patients relative to nonstroke subjects, (2) patients with cryptogenic stroke compared to controls with stroke of a known cause, and (3) cryptogenic stroke patients relative to nonstroke control subjects. Their conclusion was that both PFO and ASA are unequivocally associated with ischemic stroke in patients younger than 55 years of age. Although ASA is a less frequent finding, the association with stroke is greater than in patients with only a PFO. The evidence did not clearly support an association between PFO or ASA and stroke in patients older than age 55 years. Of note is that in the older patients, there was no association in studies of all ischemic strokes versus nonstroke patients, but the odds ratio almost reached a significant level when patients with cryptogenic stroke were compared to nonstroke controls. This suggests that there may be an association when other risk factors or more common causes have been excluded, but this observation remains unconfirmed.

However, does the association between stroke and the presence of a PFO or ASA imply causation? The presumptive mechanism for PFO-related stroke is paradoxic embolism from venous thrombi, even though the presence of deep venous thrombosis is infrequently demonstrable. A further possibility is that thrombus may form within the left atrial lumen of the ASA and embolize systemically, even in the absence of a PFO. Some studies have indicated that the risk of first and recurrent stroke is increased in patients with a larger PFO[2] or ASA,[3] suggesting a "dose-response" relationship and thus supporting the causal relationship between the presence of ASA and ischemic stroke. A recent prospective study (summarized in detail later in this chapter)[4] suggests otherwise. These investigators found that the degree of interatrial shunting was not a significant predictor of the risk of recurrent ischemic stroke.

Which Investigative Technique Is Best Suited to Demonstrating a Patent Foramen Ovale or Atrial Septal Aneurysm?

Broadly speaking, there are three techniques available for demonstrating the presence of a PFO, ASA, or their consequence of cerebral embolism. These include transthoracic echocardiography, transesophageal echocardiography (TEE), and transcranial Doppler monitoring for emboli after intravenous injection of agitated saline (microbubbles). The sensitivity of transthoracic echocardiography and TEE has been evaluated prospectively in a series of 79 patients with cryptogenic stroke,[5] with TEE being superior for the detection of both ASA and PFO.

What Is the Risk of Recurrent Stroke in Patients with a Patent Foramen Ovale or Atrial Septal Aneurysm?

Until recently, the question of the risk of recurrent stroke in patients with a PFO or ASA had not been the subject of a prospective study. The retrospective Lausanne study[6] included 140 patients with any ischemic stroke and a PFO. Sixty-six percent of patients received antiplatelet therapy, 21% received long-term anticoagulation, and 8% underwent surgical closure. There were eight further strokes over the 3-year follow-up period, yielding an annual stroke recurrence risk of 1.9%. Multivariate analysis identified four factors associated with stroke recurrence, including the presence of an interatrial communication (i.e., an ASD), coexisting cause of stroke, history of recently active migraine, and a posterior cerebral artery territory stroke as the index event. No data are provided, but the authors note that treatment had no effect on the risk of stroke recurrence.

The French PFO and ASA Study Group[7] was also a retrospective analysis of patients with otherwise unexplained stroke or transient ischemic attack (TIA) and transesophageal echo–demonstrable PFO or ASA. This study included 132 patients, 25% of whom were treated with oral anticoagulants, 45% of whom received antiplatelet agents (aspirin or ticlopidine), 5% of whom were untreated, and the remainder of whom received antiplatelet or anticoagulant therapy for a limited time. There were six recurrent events (two strokes and four TIAs) during the mean follow-up period of 22 months, yielding an annual stroke recurrence risk of 1.2% for the group as a whole but an annual risk of 4.4% in patients with both PFO and ASA.

The French PFO and ASA Study Group recently reported the results of their prospective study.[4] These investigators identified patients between the ages of 18 and 55 who had experienced an ischemic stroke within the preceding 3 months for which no definite cause had been identified. A total of 598 patients were enrolled in the study, but 17 were subsequently excluded for failing to meet inclusion criteria. This population included 304 patients without

TABLE 6-1
Risk of Recurrent Stroke with Patent Foramen Ovale (PFO) and
Atrial Septal Aneurysm (ASA)

Type of Atrial Septal Abnormality	*Cumulative Risk of Recurrent Stroke after the Indicated Period (%)*			
	1 Yr	*2 Yrs*	*3 Yrs*	*4 Yrs*
None	2.0	3.7	4.2	4.2
PFO	1.8	1.8	2.3	2.3
ASA	Few patients and no strokes; unable to calculate			
Combination of PFO and ASA	2.0	4.0	6.3	15.2

and 277 patients with atrial septal abnormalities—216 patients with only PFO, 10 with only ASA, and 51 with both. Ninety-two percent of patients received antiplatelet therapy with aspirin for more than 90% of the follow-up period. Two patients (both without ASA) were lost to follow-up, and the remainder were observed for a mean of 37.8 months. There were 12 recurrent strokes (11 of which were ischemic) amongst the 304 patients with no atrial septal abnormality, six recurrent strokes (all ischemic) amongst the 216 patients with only PFO, and six recurrent strokes (all ischemic) amongst the 51 patients with both PFO and ASA. There were no recurrent strokes amongst those with only ASA. The estimated cumulative risks of recurrent stroke over a 4-year period were estimated from Kaplan-Meier curves and are shown in Table 6-1.

Thus, whereas the combination of PFO and ASA was a significant predictor of an increased risk of recurrent ischemic stroke, the presence of an isolated PFO or isolated ASA was not. The small number of patients with an isolated ASA precluded meaningful analysis of the risk of stroke recurrence amongst these patients.

There was general agreement between this prospective study and the prior retrospective studies with regard to the risk of recurrent stroke, with estimates ranging from 2.0 to 4.4% over the first year. Also notable is that this risk did not substantially increase over subsequent years. It should be noted, however, that the majority of patients in these studies were treated with either antiplatelet agents or oral anticoagulants, and so these studies do not inform on the risk of stroke recurrence if untreated.

What Is the Most Appropriate Treatment for Patients with Patent Foramen Ovale or Atrial Septal Aneurysm and Stroke?

The optimal treatment of patients with cryptogenic stroke and an identified PFO or ASA remains unclear, as there have been no prospective controlled studies. Broadly speaking, there are four possibilities—antiplatelet therapy, oral anticoagulation, transcatheter closure, or surgical closure. There are no randomized prospective studies that have addressed this question. The retrospective Lausanne study[6] suggested that neither antiplatelet therapy nor oral anticoagulants impacted on the risk of recurrent stroke. In the prospective study by Mas et al.,[4] 92% of patients received antiplatelet therapy (with aspirin) for more than 90% of the follow-up period. The risk of recurrent stroke among patients with either isolated PFO or ASA was similar to that among patients with no atrial septal abnormality. Although this study does not demonstrate the efficacy of aspirin therapy, it does indicate that the risk of recurrent stroke, if treated with aspirin, is not increased by the presence of either a PFO or an ASA. In this study, the presence of a combination of a PFO and an ASA was associated with a significantly increased risk of recurrent stroke despite treatment with aspirin. The issue of whether the risk of recurrent stroke might be reduced by a more aggressive form of therapy (e.g., anticoagulation) was not addressed by this study and remains an unanswered question.

The results[7] of surgical closure of PFO have been mixed. Homma et al.[8] reported their results of 28 patients with cryptogenic stroke who underwent closure of PFO by open thoracotomy. There were no significant perioperative complications. Eleven patients received aspirin postoperatively, but the remainder received no medical therapy. There were three TIAs and one stroke during the mean follow-up period of 19 months, yielding a cumulative estimate of the annual risk of recurrent stroke or TIA of 19.5%. Postoperative antiplatelet therapy did not affect the risk of recurrence. The results were more favorable in the prospective study by Devuyst et al.,[9] which included a highly selected group of patients younger than age 60 with recurrent TIA or stroke and both PFO and ASA. There were no operative complications, and antiplatelet or oral anticoagulants were not used after surgery. There were no new clinical or subclinical strokes during the mean follow-up period of 23 months.

More recently, Windecker et al.[10] have reported the safety and efficacy of percutaneous transcatheter closure of PFO. The cohort included 80 patients with either cerebral or extracranial systemic paradoxic embolism who were treated by percutaneous transcatheter closure. Device deployment was unsuccessful in two patients, and there was one perioperative stroke. During the mean follow-up period of 1.6 years, there were eight recurrent thromboembolic events, including six TIAs and two peripheral emboli, yielding annual recurrence risks of 2.5% for TIA and 0.0% for stroke.

The conclusion, therefore, is that patients with an isolated PFO or ASA (but not the combination of the two) can be adequately managed with aspirin. For those with the combination of a PFO and an ASA, the risk of stroke remains increased (rising to approximately 15% at 4 years) despite aspirin therapy, but whether more aggressive therapy should constitute anticoagulation or percutaneous or surgical closure has not been the subject of study. The optimal treatment of these patients remains unknown.

Summary

- Retrospective case-control studies suggested that PFO and ASA are associated with ischemic stroke in patients younger than 55 years of age.
- These case-control studies (summarized in a recent meta-analysis) indicate that the risk of first and recurrent stroke is increased among patients with a larger PFO or ASA, suggesting a "dose-response" relationship and possible causal association. Data from the only prospective study indicate that there is no association between the degree of shunting (i.e., the size of the ASD) and the risk of recurrent stroke.
- The available evidence suggests an annual risk of stroke recurrence of 1–2% for patients with isolated PFO or ASA irrespective of antiplatelet or oral anticoagulant therapy; this risk is no greater than that reported for patients with no atrial septal abnormality.
- Data from the only prospective study indicate that if treated with aspirin, the risk of recurrence after a cryptogenic stroke in young patients with only a PFO is no greater than those among patients with no atrial septal abnormality.
- Both retrospective case-control and prospective studies indicate that the combination of PFO and ASA is associated with an increased risk of recurrent stroke despite antiplatelet therapy.
- TEE is the investigative modality of choice for demonstrating the presence of a PFO or ASA.
- The role of percutaneous transcatheter or surgical closure of PFO remains unclear.
- The optimal treatment of patients with the combination of PFO and ASA remains unclear, but antiplatelet therapy alone is insufficient to reduce the risk to a level that is equivalent to patients without an atrial septal abnormality.

References

1. Overell JR, Bone I, Lees KR. Interatrial septal abnormalities and stroke: a meta-analysis of case-control studies. *Neurology* 2000;55:1172–1179.
2. Stone DA, Godard J, Corretti MC, et al. Patent foramen ovale: association between the degree of shunt by contrast transesophageal echocardiography and the risk of future ischemic neurologic events. *Am Heart J* 1996;131:158–161.
3. Cabanes L, Mas JL, Cohen A, et al. Atrial septal aneurysm and patent foramen ovale as risk factors for cryptogenic stroke in patients less than 55 years of age. A study using transesophageal echocardiography. *Stroke* 1992;24:1865–1873.

4. Mas JL, Arquizan C, Lamy C, et al. Recurrent cerebrovascular events associated with patent foramen ovale, atrial septal aneurysm, or both. *N Engl J Med* 2001;345:1740–1746.
5. Pearson AC, Labovitz AJ, Tatineni S, Gomez C. Superiority of transesophageal echocardiography in detecting cardiac source of embolism in patients with cerebral ischemia of uncertain etiology. *J Am Coll Cardiol* 1991;17:66–72.
6. Bogousslavsky J, Garazi S, Jeanrenaud X, et al. Stroke recurrence in patients with patent foramen ovale: the Lausanne Study. Lausanne Stroke with Paradoxical Embolism Study Group. *Neurology* 1996;46:1301–1305.
7. Mas JL, Zuber M. Recurrent cerebrovascular events in patients with patent foramen ovale, atrial septal aneurysm, or both and cryptogenic stroke or transient ischemic attack. French Study Group on Patent Foramen Ovale and Atrial Septal Aneurysm. *Am Heart J* 1995;130:1083–1088.
8. Homma S, Di Tullio MR, Sacco RL, et al. Surgical closure of patent foramen ovale in cryptogenic stroke patients. *Stroke* 1997;28:2376–2381.
9. Devuyst G, Bogousslavsky J, Ruchat P, et al. Prognosis after stroke followed by surgical closure of patent foramen ovale: a prospective follow-up study with brain MRI and simultaneous transesophageal and transcranial Doppler ultrasound. *Neurology* 1996;47:1162–1166.
10. Windecker S, Wahl A, Chatterjee T, et al. Percutaneous closure of patent foramen ovale in patients with paradoxical embolism: long-term risk of recurrent thrombo-embolic events. *Circulation* 2000;101:893–898.

CHAPTER 7

Intracerebral Hemorrhage

Introduction

Many controversies surround the management of patients with intracerebral hemorrhage (ICH), in large part because of the paucity of prospective randomized, controlled trial data that might more rationally guide therapy. These controversies include, but are not limited to, the optimal acute management of hypertension, the treatment of raised intracranial pressure (ICP), and the appropriate use of surgical techniques to drain intracerebral hematomas. In the absence of quality data, it is appropriate to think in terms of pathophysiology to guide management decisions. It would be useful, therefore, to know something about the time course and prognosis of ICH. This chapter aims to shed light on these and other controversies by reviewing the pertinent literature with due recognition of its limitations.

Which Factors Influence Prognosis of Intracerebral Hemorrhage?

The mortality from ICH is high, and various factors have been identified as predicting a poor outcome, including the volume of parenchymal blood, the volume of intraventricular blood, and the level of consciousness. Broderick et al.[1] developed a simple model to predict 30-day mortality after ICH. They reviewed the clinical data and computerized tomographic (CT) scans of 188 patients with ICH. The volume of ICH was measured by two independent methods. In the first, they employed computerized image analysis to physically measure the volume of hemorrhage. In the second, they estimated the volume of hemorrhage using the formula for an ellipsoid ($4/3 \times \pi \times abc$, where a, b, and c represent the radii in three dimensions). Neurologic function at presentation was documented using the Glasgow Coma Scale (GCS; see Appendix 9 [Glasgow Coma Scale]), and clinical outcome was graded using a modified Oxford Handicap Scale (see Appendix 27 [Oxford Handicap Scale]). Using 30-day mortality as the dependent variable, they analyzed age, race, gender, initial systolic blood pressure, volume of ICH, volume of intraventricular hemorrhage, GCS score, location of hemorrhage, and surgery (yes or no) using univariate regression analysis. Overall, they found a 30-day mortality rate of 44%. In the univariate regression analysis,

TABLE 7-1
Thirty-Day Mortality Rates from Intracerebral Hemorrhage

Volume of Intracerebral Hemorrhage	Lobar Hemorrhage (%)	Deep Hemorrhage (%)
<30 cc	7	23
30–60 cc	60	64
>60 cc	71	93

volume of ICH, volume of intraventricular blood, and initial GCS score were significant predictors of 30-day mortality. For supratentorial hemorrhage, the volume of ICH was the most important predictor of mortality. Thirty-day mortality rates for the different ICH volumes are summarized in Table 7-1. Employing a model that incorporated GCS score on admission and the categorization of ICH volume, they were able to develop a model that could predict 30-day mortality with high sensitivity and specificity.

What Is the Time Course of Primary Intracerebral Hemorrhage?

The pathophysiology of primary ICH is commonly thought to involve an initial brief period of bleeding that quickly tamponades itself via the mass effect created. The neurologic deterioration frequently observed during the first 24 hours after the onset of symptoms has commonly been attributed to the development of edema around the area of hemorrhage. There is some evidence, however, suggesting that this may not be the case. In their prospective observational study, Brott and colleagues[2] tried to determine the proportion of patients with spontaneous ICH who had ongoing bleeding within the first 20 hours after symptom onset. They recruited patients with CT evidence of ICH who presented within 3 hours of symptom onset. Head CT and neurologic examinations were repeated 1 and 20 hours after the baseline evaluation. Hemorrhage growth was operationally defined as an increase in ICH volume by at least 33% and was observed in 39 (38%) of the 103 patients studied. Growth occurred within the first hour in 27 (26%) patients and between 1 and 20 hours in the remaining 12 (12%). Moreover, growth of hemorrhage over the first hour was significantly associated with clinical deterioration as measured by a change in the GCS and National Institutes of Health Stroke Scale scores (see Appendix 22 [National Institutes of Health Stroke Scale]).

The dynamic nature of ICH during the first several hours represents an opportunity to intervene to prevent neurologic deterioration. However, this study failed to reveal any factors clearly predictive of early hemorrhage growth that might be used to select patients for aggressive treatment.

Should Elevated Blood Pressure after Intracerebral Hemorrhage Be Treated?

Marked elevation in systemic blood pressure after ICH is common, and yet there are limited clinical data to help guide decisions about the appropriate management of hypertension in this context. In the absence of data, it seems appropriate to consider treatment options based on an understanding of pathophysiology. One theoretical reason to lower blood pressure after ICH is based on the argument that rebleeding may be more likely if blood pressure remains markedly elevated. It is certainly true that early rebleeding contributes to worsening neurologic condition, but this was not clearly related to elevated blood pressure in the one study that addressed this question.[2] Thus, although rebleeding may be responsible for some of the morbidity and mortality that accompanies ICH, the relationship between acute elevations in blood pressure and the risk of rebleeding remains unclear. Arguments against antihypertensive therapy are based on the recognition that increased local tissue pressure produces a zone of ischemia around the clot and that perfusion of this ischemic zone relies on adequate blood pressure. Furthermore, autoregulation may be impaired with the consequence that decreased cerebral perfusion pressure (CPP) (due to raised ICP because of the mass effect of the hemorrhage) does not trigger the reflex vasodilation necessary to preserve cerebral blood flow when blood pressure is pharmacologically reduced. The data substantiating these various theoretical issues are scant.

Dandapani et al.,[3] in a retrospective study, examined the relationship between blood pressure and outcome in 87 patients after ICH. Blood pressure was recorded regularly during the first 6 hours after presentation, and all patients were treated with a nonstandardized antihypertensive regime that usually consisted of oral nifedipine followed by intravenous sodium nitroprusside. Outcome was assessed using the Glasgow Outcome Scale (see Appendix 10 [Glasgow Outcome Scale]). Case-fatality and combined morbidity and mortality rates were reported based on a stratification using cutoff mean arterial pressure (MAP) of 145 mm Hg within the first 2 hours. Morbidity and mortality were significantly greater amongst those with MAP greater than 145 mm Hg during the first 2 hours after presentation. Between 2 and 6 hours after ICH and after treatment, MAP was measured and stratified as being greater or less than 125 mm Hg. The results of this study are summarized in Table 7-2. In summary, these results suggest that severe morbidity and mortality are higher amongst patients with marked hypertension and that effective antihypertensive therapy has a favorable effect on prognosis.

Recognizing the conflicting theoretical reasons for and against antihypertensive therapy in the context of acute ICH as well as the lack of evidence, the American Heart Association Stroke Council has established a set of guidelines regarding hypertensive therapy in ICH.[4] They have recommended that MAP be maintained below 130 mm Hg in patients with a history of hypertension. For those in whom ICP monitoring is performed, CPP

TABLE 7-2
Effect of Blood Pressure on the Morbidity and Mortality of Intracerebral Hemorrhage

Outcome Measure (30 Days)	MAP within the First 2 Hrs (%)		p Value
	<145 mm Hg	>145 mm Hg	
Mortality	21	47	<0.1
Mortality + severe morbidity	34	65	<0.05

Outcome Measure (30 Days)	MAP between 2 and 6 Hrs (%)		p Value
	<125 mm Hg	>125 mm Hg	
Mortality	21	43	<0.1
Mortality + severe morbidity	34	60	<0.05

MAP = mean arterial pressure.

(MAP – ICP) should be kept greater than 70 mm Hg. They also acknowledge that blood pressure management needs to be individualized based on the presence or absence of chronic hypertension, elevated ICP, age, presumed cause of hemorrhage, and interval since onset.

What Is the Evidence Supporting Nonsurgical Management of the Increase in Intracranial Pressure That Results from Intracerebral Hemorrhage?

ICP is directly related to the volume of the intracranial contents, and the presence of an ICH has the effect of raising ICP. A number of approaches have been used to reduce ICP in patients with ICH, but glycerol and corticosteroids for the reduction of brain edema are the only two agents that have been tested in prospective controlled trials.

The study by Poungvarin et al.[5] is the only randomized double-blind trial of steroids in patients with CT-confirmed diagnosis of ICH. This study included 93 patients who were randomized within 48 hours of stroke onset to receive either placebo or intravenous dexamethasone (10 mg initially, followed by 5 mg every 6 hours for 6 days, 5 mg every 12 hours for 2 days, and 5 mg per day for 1 day). Patients were stratified according to the level of consciousness at the time of randomization. Interim analysis at 21 days revealed similar mortality rates between the two groups and a higher complication rate in those receiving dexamethasone. These findings led to the premature termination of the study with the conclusion that dexamethasone, in the doses used in this study, should not be used for the treatment of acute ICH.

The results of a randomized placebo-controlled trial of intravenous glycerol were similarly disappointing. Yu et al.[6] randomized 216 patients within 24 hours of the onset of CT-confirmed ICH to receive either placebo or intravenous glycerol (500 mL of 10% solution) every 4 hours for 4 days. They found no significant differences in 6-month mortality or outcome using the Barthel Index (see Appendix 3 [Barthel Index]).

The use of other osmotic agents, like mannitol, has not been tested in a prospective randomized fashion, and there are only limited data from uncontrolled trials to support their use. Duff et al.[7] reported their experience with a series of 12 patients with spontaneous supratentorial ICH who were treated with a combination of osmotic agents, controlled ventilation, and continuous monitoring of ICP. They compared their results to a group of historical controls[8] with patients stratified according to the level of consciousness at the time of presentation. For the purpose of ensuring that their patient population was comparable to the historical control group, they excluded patients with small ICH (long axis less than 4 cm), those with mild symptoms, and those who were clearly terminal at the time of presentation. ICP was monitored in all patients and hyperventilation employed for ICP greater than 25 mm Hg to maintain partial pressure of carbon dioxide (Pco_2) at 24–26 mm Hg. The treatment regimen also included the intravenous administration of an osmotic diuretic (either urea or mannitol) when ICP rose above 40 mm Hg or when CPP fell below 50 mm Hg. With these measures, the investigators were able to maintain ICP less than 40 mm Hg and CPP greater than 50 mm Hg. Duration of follow-up varied from 4 months to 6 years. The results are summarized in Table 7-3.

The results are difficult to interpret because the numbers are small and the control group is a historical one. Moreover, the presence and size of the ICH were not confirmed by CT in the study by McKissock et al. However, these are the best available data, and decisions about the use of osmotic agents must be made in the absence of better data.

What Is the Evidence for Benefit from Surgical Evacuation of an Intracerebral Hematoma?

Juvela et al.[9] performed the first prospective randomized study of surgical versus conservative management of patients with spontaneous supratentorial ICH in the post–CT scan era. These authors randomized 52 patients with spontaneous supratentorial ICH who were unconscious or had a severe neurologic deficit and who were evaluated within 24 hours of the onset of symptoms. Operation comprised hematoma evacuation via craniotomy, and the mean time from bleeding to operation was 14.5 hours. Outcome was assessed based on stratification according to admission GCS score. There were no significant differences in mortality rates, survival times, or morbidity between the two treatment groups as a whole, although

TABLE 7-3
Outcome of Intracerebral Hemorrhage Treated Aggressively with Measures to
Reduce Intracranial Pressure

| | Outcome (No. of Patients) | | | |
Initial Level of Arousal	Full Work	Partial Disability	Total Disability	Dead
Duff et al.[7]				
Alert	2 (100%)	—	—	—
Drowsy	1 (20%)	4 (80%)	—	—
Stuporous	1 (33%)	1 (33%)	—	1 (33%)
Comatose	—	1 (50%)	1 (50%)	—
McKissock et al.[8]				
Alert	2 (33%)	2 (33%)	1 (17%)	1 (17%)
Drowsy	6 (11%)	16 (30%)	11 (21%)	20 (38%)
Stuporous	3 (14%)	2 (9%)	2 (9%)	15 (68%)
Comatose	—	—	—	10 (100%)

one-third of the patients in the conservative group, and only one in the surgical group, were independent at the 6-month follow-up evaluation. Prerandomization GCS rather than treatment option was the most powerful predictor of outcome in that all patients with GCS scores of 7–10 were totally disabled at 1 year, whereas those who were independent at 1 year all had prerandomization GCS scores of 11–14.

Batjer et al.[10] conducted a randomized trial of surgical and best medical therapy, with or without ICP monitoring, in patients with hypertensive putaminal hemorrhages at least 3 cm in maximal diameter. They excluded patients with the mildest and most severe deficits. The trial was terminated prematurely after only 21 patients had been randomized when it became clear that the outcome was extremely poor in all treatment groups.

The Surgical Treatment for Intracerebral Hemorrhage (STICH) study by Morgenstern and colleagues[11] included 34 patients with supratentorial hemorrhage who were randomized to receive medical or surgical therapy. They included patients with an ICH volume greater than 9 cc. Medical management was standardized between the two treatment groups, and patients in the surgical group underwent hematoma evacuation via open craniotomy within 12 hours of symptom onset. Survival and functional outcome favored surgery, but the differences between the two treatment groups were not significant. The authors attributed these findings to the limited statistical power of the study to detect significant differences. In a follow-up study, Morgenstern et al.[12] tried to determine whether ultra-early surgical clot evacuation (i.e., within 4 hours of the onset of symptoms) might further improve outcome by preventing early hematoma expansion and the development of surrounding edema. They employed the same methodology used in the STICH study except that the surgical group was treated within 4 hours, rather than 12 hours, of the onset of symptoms. Having previously demonstrated a mortality rate of 29% in medically treated patients and 18% in the 12-hour surgical group, they planned to terminate the trial if mortality in the 4-hour surgery group exceeded 30%. In fact, the trial was stopped at the time of a planned interim analysis (after having enrolled 11 patients) because of a 36% mortality rate amongst the surgical group. This increased mortality rate was thought to be due, at least in part, to the increased risk of rebleeding that resulted from the difficulty encountered in achieving adequate hemostasis at the time of surgery.

The study by Zuccarello et al.[13] was also insufficiently powered to detect significant differences between patients managed medically and surgically. These investigators randomized 20 patients with supratentorial ICH who presented within 24 hours of symptom onset. Eligibility criteria included an ICH volume greater than 10 cc, the presence of focal neurologic deficit, and a GCS greater than 4. Surgery was performed within 3 hours of randomization. The 3-month Glasgow Outcome Scale was the primary endpoint with the Barthel Index and modified Rankin Scale scores (see Appendix 28 [Modified Rankin Scale]) used as secondary measures of outcome. Although a trend towards improved outcome was noted amongst those treated surgically, they found no statistically significant differences in the primary or secondary endpoints.

The study by Auer and colleagues[14] of endoscopic surgery versus medical treatment is the only randomized study to show a benefit in favor of surgery. These investigators randomized 100 patients with neurologic deficit due to ICH with volume greater than 10 cc, who presented within 48 hours of symptom onset, to medical therapy or hematoma evacuation through a burr hole by means of a neuroendoscope. The primary endpoints of the study were the 6-month mortality rate and quality of survival, both of which were improved in the surgical group. Subgroup analysis, however, indicated that the beneficial effect of surgery was only evident in patients younger than 60 years of age, those in whom the ICH was subcortical (rather than thalamic or putaminal) and less than 50 cm^3, and those who were either alert or somnolent (but not stuporous or comatose) preoperatively. These results, therefore, suggest a benefit to endoscopic evacuation of smaller subcortical hematomas. The small size of the subgroups, however, does not permit firm conclusions.

Summary

- There are almost no prospective controlled data that may be useful in guiding the treatment of ICH.

- Prognosis following spontaneous supratentorial ICH is determined predominantly by the volume of the ICH and the level of arousal (measured by the GCS) at the time of initial presentation.
- There are data to support the pathophysiologic concept that there is early growth of ICH and that this contributes to increasing neurologic morbidity.
- There are no data to support the contention that uncontrolled hypertension contributes to the early growth of ICH. This is a largely unstudied question.
- There are data from a single retrospective study suggesting that early treatment of hypertension after ICH is associated with better neurologic outcome. Based on this study, MAP greater than 145 mm Hg should be treated with the aim of lowering MAP to less than 125 mm Hg.
- The American Heart Association Stroke Council has recommended therapy to maintain MAP below 130 mm Hg or CPP greater than 70 mm Hg.
- The use of corticosteroids and glycerol in the management of raised ICP after ICH are not supported based on negative results from prospective randomized placebo-controlled trials.
- The use of osmotic agents like mannitol in combination with intermittent hyperventilation to reduce ICP is supported only by retrospective uncontrolled data.
- Surgical evacuation of ICH has been evaluated in a series of prospective studies, with a beneficial effect demonstrated only in the study of subcortical ICH evacuation using a neuroendoscope within 48 hours of symptom onset.
- Hematoma evacuation via craniotomy does not improve outcome even if performed within 4 hours of the onset of symptoms.

References

1. Broderick JP, Brott TG, Duldner JE, et al. Volume of intracerebral hemorrhage: a powerful and easy-to-use predictor of 30-day mortality. *Stroke* 1993;24:987–993.
2. Brott T, Broderick J, Kothari R, et al. Early hemorrhage growth in patients with intracerebral hemorrhage. *Stroke* 1997;28:1–5.
3. Dandapani BK, Suzuki S, Kelley RE, et al. Relation between blood pressure and outcome in intracerebral hemorrhage. *Stroke* 1995;26:21–24.
4. Broderick JP, Adams HP, Barsan W, et al. Guidelines for the management of spontaneous intracerebral hemorrhage: a statement for healthcare professionals from a special writing group of the stroke council, American Heart Association. *Stroke* 1999;30:905–915.

5. Poungvarin N, Bhoopat W, Viriyavejakul A, et al. Effects of dexamethasone in primary supratentorial intracerebral hemorrhage. *N Engl J Med* 1987;316: 1229–1233.

6. Yu YL, Kumana CR, Lauder IJ, et al. Treatment of acute cerebral hemorrhage with intravenous glycerol: a double-blind, placebo-controlled, randomized trial. *Stroke* 1992;23:967–971.

7. Duff TA, Ayeni S, Levin AB, Javid M. Nonsurgical management of spontaneous intracerebral hematoma. *Neurosurgery* 1981;9:387–393.

8. McKissock W, Richardson A, Taylor J. Primary intracerebral hemorrhage: a controlled trial of surgical and conservative treatment in 180 unselected cases. *Lancet* 1961;2:221–226.

9. Juvela S, Heiskanen O, Poranen A, et al. The treatment of spontaneous intracerebral hemorrhage. A prospective randomized trial of surgical and conservative treatment. *J Neurosurg* 1989;70:755–758.

10. Batjer HH, Reisch JS, Allen BC, et al. Failure of surgery to improve outcome in hypertensive putaminal hemorrhage. A prospective randomized trial. *Arch Neurol* 1990;47:1103–1106.

11. Morgenstern LB, Frankowski RF, Shedden P, et al. Surgical treatment for intracerebral hemorrhage (STICH): a single-center, randomized clinical trial. *Neurology* 1998;51:1359–1363.

12. Morgenstern LB, Demchuk AM, Kim DH, et al. Rebleeding leads to poor outcome in ultra-early craniotomy for intracerebral hemorrhage. *Neurology* 2001;56:1294–1299.

13. Zuccarello M, Brott T, Derex L, et al. Early surgical treatment for supratentorial intracerebral hemorrhage: a randomized feasibility study. *Stroke* 1999;30: 1833–1839.

14. Auer LM, Deinsberger W, Niederkorn K, et al. Endoscopic surgery versus medical treatment for spontaneous intracerebral hematoma: a randomized study. *J Neurosurg* 1989;70:530–535.

CHAPTER 8

Subarachnoid Hemorrhage

Introduction

Aneurysmal subarachnoid hemorrhage (SAH) has a 30-day mortality rate of 45%, and approximately half of the survivors sustain irreversible brain damage. Delayed neurologic deterioration, in part due to the development of vasospasm, is the major cause of disability. Vasospasm typically develops between 3 and 14 days after aneurysmal SAH and is usually recognized by the development of new focal neurologic deficits or a global reduction in the level of consciousness that is not attributable to hydrocephalus or rebleeding. The presence and severity of vasospasm correlate strongly with the amount of blood in the subarachnoid cisterns on initial computerized tomographic (CT) scan.

Many controversies surround the management of patients with saccular aneurysms. For example, there are no prospective randomized trials of surgical or endovascular intervention versus conservative management of unruptured intracranial aneurysms, and so the management of these aneurysms remains controversial. Other controversies relate to the acute management of patients with aneurysmal SAH. What, for example, is the role of the calcium channel antagonist nimodipine in the prevention and management of vasospasm? What is the evidence supporting the use of *h*ypertensive, *h*ypervolemic, and *h*emodilution (triple-H) therapy? These and other questions are the focus of this chapter.

What Is the Appropriate Management of Unruptured Aneurysms?

An unruptured intracranial aneurysm is typically found in one of three general circumstances: the patient may be entirely asymptomatic and the aneurysm is an incidental finding; the patient may be symptomatic for some reason other than rupture; or the patient may have presented with SAH from rupture of one aneurysm, and a second (unruptured) aneurysm is incidentally discovered. Symptoms not due to rupture include mass effect (e.g., cranial nerve compression), cerebrovascular symptoms (e.g., from distal embolization), or headaches. The management of these unruptured intracranial saccular aneurysms remains controversial. The decision whether to treat them and, if so, whether surgically or via an endovascular approach depends on many factors, including the risk of subsequent rupture, the age and comorbidity of the patient, and the available surgical and endovascular expertise. It is also necessary to consider the willingness of the individual patient to accept the immediate risk of the morbidity and mortality that accompany an invasive procedure in exchange for long-term benefit to be gained from removal of the aneurysm.

To make an informed decision, therefore, about the best course of action, it is necessary to know the natural history of unruptured aneurysms (i.e., the risk of subsequent rupture) as well as the morbidity and mortality associated with their repair. There are a number of studies that have addressed the issue of the natural history of these unruptured aneurysms. It is useful to consider these in the light of the important conclusion that emerged from the International Study of Unruptured Intracranial Aneurysms (ISUIA)[1]—that the risk of rupture differs for those with a history of SAH compared to those without such a history.

Wiebers et al.[2] reviewed the records of 65 patients with 81 unruptured intracranial aneurysms (including 19 patients with symptomatic aneurysms and 46 with no symptoms). None of these patients had a history of SAH and none had undergone surgery. All patients were followed until death or until at least 5 years after the aneurysm had been diagnosed. The mean duration of follow-up was 98.5 months, during which time eight aneurysms ruptured. All ruptures involved aneurysms larger than 10 mm. None of the 44 aneurysms smaller than 10 mm ruptured. In a follow-up study of 130 patients with 161 aneurysms (which included the initial cohort), Wiebers et al.[3] extended these initial observations. None of the 102 aneurysms smaller than 10 mm ruptured, whereas 15 of the 51 aneurysms 10 mm or larger did eventually rupture. In this study, the mean size of aneurysms that subsequently ruptured was 21.3 mm. Other studies, while confirming the importance of aneurysmal size, have suggested that a smaller aneurysmal size (approximately 7 mm) may better dichotomize patients into low and high risk of subsequent rupture. In the Cooperative Aneurysm Study,[4] for example, the critical size for aneurysm rupture was 7–10 mm.

ISUIA is the largest study to date to address the issue of how best to treat unruptured aneurysms.[1] It included both retrospective and prospective cohorts. The objective of the retrospective portion of the study was to define the natural history of unruptured saccular aneurysms in two groups of patients, those with and without a history of SAH, and to determine whether there are subgroups of patients who are at increased risk of aneurysmal rupture. Patients were eligible for inclusion in this component of the study if they had at least one unruptured aneurysm, irrespective of whether it was symptomatic. This arm of the study included 1,449 patients with 1,937 unruptured aneurysms. The mean duration of follow-up was 8.3

years, and information for these patients was obtained from the review of medical records and by means of an annual standardized questionnaire. There were 32 confirmed aneurysmal ruptures during the follow-up period. Of the 12 patients in the group with no history of a ruptured aneurysm, only one involved an aneurysm that was less than 10 mm in size. Of the 20 patients in the group with a history of aneurysmal SAH, 17 involved aneurysms that were less than 10 mm in size. Size greater than 10 mm was a risk factor for rupture in the group of patients with no history of SAH but not in the other group. Location of the aneurysm was also predictive of the risk of rupture, with those at the basilar tip and in the posterior circulation posing a greater risk. These and other results are summarized in Table 8-1.

The available data, therefore, support the idea that spontaneous SAH in those without a history of a ruptured aneurysm is most often caused by aneurysms of at least 7–10 mm. There are a number of possible explanations for the discrepant findings between the studies that have suggested 7 mm (vs. 10 mm) as the cutoff for defining aneurysms as being more or less likely to rupture. One possibility is that aneurysm size may decrease at the time of rupture (leading to underestimation of the aneurysm size when determined at the time of SAH) or that the critical size for aneurysmal rupture is smaller at the time of formation or soon thereafter. Presently, there is insufficient evidence to resolve this controversy.

The aim of the prospective component of the ISUIA study was to evaluate the morbidity and mortality associated with the treatment of unrup-

TABLE 8-1

Risk of Rupture of Intracranial Aneurysms: The International Study of Unruptured Intracranial Aneurysm

	No History of SAH (n = 727)	History of SAH (n = 722)
No. ruptured aneurysms during follow-up	12	20
Annual rate of rupture		
Size <10 mm	0.05%	0.5%
Size >10 mm	~1%	~1%
High risk factor for rupture		
Size >10 mm	Yes	No*
Location	Basilar tip, posterior communicating artery, vertebrobasilar, or posterior cerebral artery distribution	Basilar tip

SAH = subarachnoid hemorrhage.
*The risk of rupture is relatively high (and similar) for both small and large aneurysms.

TABLE 8-2
Surgical Morbidity and Mortality of Aneurysmal Repair

Outcome Measure	No History of SAH (n = 798)	History of SAH (n = 198)
30-Day surgical morbidity* and mortality	13.6%	17.5%
1-Yr surgical morbidity* and mortality	13.1%	15.7%

SAH = subarachnoid hemorrhage.
*Morbidity was defined as modified Rankin Scale score ≥3, Mini-Mental State Examination score <24, or a score of <27 on a telephone interview of cognitive status.

tured intracranial aneurysms. Eligibility criteria for the prospective cohort were similar to those used for the retrospective cohort, except that the investigators decided whether individual patients would undergo treatment (surgical or endovascular) of the unruptured aneurysm. A total of 1,172 patients were enrolled in the treatment group, and 996 underwent surgery—198 of whom had a history of SAH and 798 of whom did not. The results are summarized in Table 8-2.

Age was the only predictor of surgical outcome with the surgical morbidity and mortality substantially lower for younger patients. Although the surgical morbidity and mortality rates in this study were higher than those reported previously, the investigators concluded that the surgical morbidity and mortality greatly exceeded the 7.5-year risk of rupture among patients with aneurysms smaller than 10 mm in diameter.

The conclusion is that the morbidity and mortality of surgical repair of an unruptured intracranial aneurysm that is less than 10 mm in size (in a patient without a history of SAH) exceeds the intermediate-term risk of rupture. It makes the most sense, therefore, to follow these aneurysms over time and to intervene only once they exceed approximately 10 mm in diameter. Whether endovascular treatment will offer the prospect of aneurysmal repair with significantly lower morbidity and mortality remains to be proven in a formal study.

What Is the Role of Nimodipine in the Management of Subarachnoid Hemorrhage?

The pathophysiology of vasospasm is poorly understood. One hypothesis is that vasoactive substances in the hemorrhagic cerebrospinal fluid lead to an increase in vascular smooth muscle calcium concentrations and vasoconstriction, hence the rationale for the use of calcium channel antagonists like nimodipine.

Allen et al.[5] were the first to prospectively evaluate the efficacy of nimodipine in preventing or altering the severity of ischemic neurologic deficits due to vasospasm. This was a randomized double-blind, placebo-controlled trial. Only patients regarded as "neurologically normal" who could receive the study medication within 96 hours of the onset of symptoms were eligible for inclusion. Patients were randomized to receive placebo or nimodipine in an initial dose of 0.7 mg/kg and a maintenance dose of 0.35 mg/kg every 4 hours for 21 days. Subjects were evaluated frequently and were investigated with CT scan or angiography within 48 hours of the onset of a new focal deficit. Vasospasm was deemed the cause only if the deficit occurred within the territory of the affected artery and no other cause could be identified. The primary measure of efficacy was neurologic outcome at 21 days, with subjects classified as (1) normal, (2) mild or moderate deficit, and (3) severe deficit. One hundred sixteen patients met eligibility criteria, with 60 randomized to receive placebo and 56 nimodipine.

In analyzing the results of this study, it is worth recollecting the question posed by the investigators: Does nimodipine alter the likelihood of a poor outcome due to vasospasm? The outcome measure used was the probability of a poor outcome due to vasospasm (determined by the absence of any other explanations for the outcome). They found that nimodipine significantly reduced the occurrence of severe neurologic deficits (including death) from vasospasm. Eight of 60 placebo-treated patients either died or had residual severe deficits from spasm at the end of 21 days, in comparison to 1 of 56 patients in the nimodipine-treated group. From these results, the authors conclude that the efficacy of nimodipine was due to its inhibitory effect on cerebral arterial spasm. This conclusion, however, extends beyond the data supplied, as the results do not demonstrate that vasospasm occurs with a lower frequency amongst those treated with nimodipine. Instead, the results are compatible with a slightly different conclusion—that treatment with nimodipine is associated with a more favorable outcome amongst those patients who develop vasospasm. However, this does not equate with a proof of mechanism. The importance of this study lies in its demonstration that the outcome of patients with favorable-grade SAH may be improved by treatment with nimodipine.

The results of this initial study were subsequently extended to patients with poor-grade SAH. Petruk et al.[6] recruited patients with greater than or equal to Hunt and Hess grade III SAH (see Appendix 15 [Hunt and Hess Scale]) who presented within 96 hours of the onset of symptoms and randomized them to receive either placebo or nimodipine (administered orally in a dose of 90 mg every 4 hours). Treatment continued for 21 days. The development of a new neurologic deficit was ascribed only to vasospasm if demonstrated angiographically soon after the deficit appeared and in the absence of an alternative explanation for the clinical deterioration. Three primary endpoints were specified in advance, including (1) the frequency of poor outcome due to a delayed ischemic deficit due to vasospasm alone, (2) the presence of angiographically demonstrable vasospasm, and (3) the incidence and size of hypodensities on the 3-month CT scan. The primary analysis included 154 patients, of whom 82 received placebo and 72 were treated with nimodipine. There were significantly fewer permanent delayed ischemic deficits from vasospasm alone in the nimodipine group compared to those who received placebo (7.9% vs. 29.3%, respectively). With regard to the second primary outcome measure, there was no significant difference in the degree of vasospasm between the nimodipine- and placebo-treated patients. Finally, there was no significant difference between the two groups with regard to the number or size of infarcts. The final conclusion was that oral nimodipine treatment was associated with a decrease in the number of patients who developed delayed ischemic deficits and an overall increase in the likelihood of patients having a good neurologic outcome.

The results of these two smaller studies have since been confirmed in the larger double-blind, placebo-controlled British aneurysm nimodipine trial.[7] In this study, 554 patients with SAH of any clinical grade were randomized to receive placebo or nimodipine (60 mg orally every 4 hours) within 96 hours of the onset of symptoms. Treatment was continued for 21 days. Outcome was assessed according to the five-point Glasgow Outcome Scale (see Appendix 10 [Glasgow Outcome Scale]) at least 3 months after study entry, and the primary endpoint was the number of cerebral infarcts. The results of this study are summarized in Table 8-3. Like the ones that preceded it, this study did not demonstrate a reduction in the frequency or severity of vasospasm, but it does confirm the prior conclusion that nimodipine (administered in a dose of 60 mg every 4 hours for 21 days) reduces

TABLE 8-3
Effects of Nimodipine in Subarachnoid Hemorrhage: The British Aneurysm Nimodipine Trial

	Nimodipine (n = 278)	Placebo (n = 276)	Relative Risk Reduction	Absolute Risk Reduction	p Value
Number of cerebral infarcts	61 (22%)	92 (33%)	34%	11%	0.003
Likelihood of a poor outcome*	55 (20%)	91 (33%)	40%	13%	<0.001

*Defined as dead, persistent vegetative state, or severe disability.

the likelihood of stroke and poor outcome in patients with SAH of any clinical grade.

What Is the Evidence Supporting the Use of Triple-H Therapy in Subarachnoid Hemorrhage?

Hemodynamic augmentation by way of triple-H therapy is one of the many methods that has been investigated and used for the management of vasospasm after SAH. Hyperdynamism (increased cardiac output) is variably included as a component of this form of therapy. The theoretical foundation for triple-H therapy is incomplete but based primarily on the idea that the development of delayed neurologic deficits is due to vasospasm and that these may be overcome by hemodynamic augmentation. Before even considering the evidence describing and supporting the use of triple-H therapy, a few points are worth noting. First, the generation of delayed ischemic deficits in SAH may not be entirely related to the development of vasospasm. Alternative theories include the development of a structural blood-induced arteriopathy (rather than a state of blood vessel spasm) and reperfusion injury. Second, in evaluating the data that support the use of triple-H therapy, a distinction should be made between the use of this therapy for prophylaxis against vasospasm and use of this therapy for the treatment of clinically apparent vasospasm. Finally, data regarding the implementation, application, and monitoring of triple-H therapy as well as the outcome measures that are used remain somewhat arbitrary, variably practiced, and vaguely reported.

For the most part, the use of this hemodynamic therapy has been based on data from retrospective case series with beneficial results reported in 60–80% of patients with clinically apparent vasospasm, but these response rates are difficult to interpret in the absence of control groups. There has only been one prospective controlled trial of triple-H therapy, and in this study, it was used as prophylaxis against the development of vasospasm and its adverse consequences (discussed at the end of this section).[8]

Kassell et al.[9] reported their experience with volume expansion and induced arterial hypertension in a series of 56 patients with progressive neurologic deficits from angiographically proven cerebral vasospasm. The retrospective nature of this study accounts for the heterogeneity of the patients included. The hypervolemic hypertensive therapy was initiated in 40 patients after aneurysm obliteration. Six of the 40 patients also had untreated, incidentally detected aneurysms, and 16 had an untreated ruptured aneurysm. The general approach was to increase intravascular volume with the variable combination of blood, crystalloid, colloid, and fludrocortisone. If this hypervolemic therapy did not result in prompt improvement in neurologic deficit, then hypertension was induced with vasopressors (with dopamine and dobutamine being used most frequently). Specific parameters were not prespecified, and blood pressure was raised to a level required to overcome the neurologic deficit. However, a systolic pressure of 240 mm Hg (or a mean arterial pressure of 150 mm Hg) was not exceeded in those with obliterated aneurysms, and a systolic blood pressure of 160 mm Hg was the limit in those with untreated aneurysms.

Complete or partial resolution of neurologic deficits was observed within 1 hour of commencement of hypervolemic hypertensive therapy in 81% of patients. This improvement was permanent in 74%. Sixteen percent of patients were unchanged, and 10% deteriorated. There were 19 serious complications, the most frequent being pulmonary edema (10 patients) and aneurysmal rebleeding (three patients). The episodes of rebleeding occurred only in patients with unclipped aneurysms, and the pulmonary edema was symptomatic only in two patients. The authors concluded that hypervolemic hypertensive therapy is safe and effective in patients whose aneurysm has been successfully clipped or otherwise removed from the arterial circulation. They did, however, acknowledge the limitation of their study given its retrospective and uncontrolled design.

Awad et al.[10] reported their experience of 42 patients with angiographically confirmed vasospasm after SAH who were treated with a standardized protocol of triple-H therapy. In this series, clinical vasospasm developed and was treated after the aneurysm had been clipped in 27 patients and before surgery in 10 patients. Five patients did not undergo craniotomy (four because of death from vasospasm and one because no aneurysm was identified at angiography). Clinical vasospasm was defined as delayed neurologic deterioration that could not be attributed to other factors. A central venous or Swan-Ganz catheter was placed at the first sign of clinical vasospasm. Hemodynamic objectives comprised raising the central venous pressure to 10–12 mm Hg (or the pulmonary artery wedge pressure to 15–18 mm Hg) and changing the hematocrit to 33–38 g/dL (either via blood transfusion or phlebotomy). Systolic blood pressure was maintained in the 160–200 mm Hg range if the aneurysm had been clipped or in the 120–150 mm Hg range in the presence of an unclipped aneurysm. A dopamine infusion was used when necessary to achieve the desired systolic blood pressure. Response to therapy was measured using the modified Hunt and Hess grading scheme. Sustained improvement by at least one grade was observed in 60% of patients, 24% were unchanged, and 16% deteriorated during triple-H therapy.

Levy and colleagues[11] reported their experience with 23 patients treated for symptomatic vasospasm after SAH that was confirmed by either increased velocities on transcranial Doppler ultrasound or by conventional angiography. The authors note that the majority of patients were managed in the postoperative setting (i.e., postaneurysm clipping), but the proportion of patients in this series with unclipped aneurysms is not clearly stated. All patients had Swan-Ganz catheters placed and were initially treated with hypervolemic therapy. This comprised colloid infusion to attain a pulmonary artery wedge pressure of 12–16 mm Hg. Dobutamine (5–10 µg/kg per minute) was administered to those patients who remained refractory to only hypervolemic therapy (defined as a plateau or decline in neurologic deficit over a period of 6 hours). Eighteen of the 23 (78%) had reversal of ischemic symptoms from vasospasm, with onset of recovery occurring after 4–10 days. The treatment protocol described in this study required frequent clinical evaluation with titration of the dobutamine infusion to clinical response. In general, a cardiac index of 5–6 L per minute per m^2 was required to obtain a clinical response. The rationale for choosing dobutamine, a β-agonist that stimulates B1 receptors (ionotrope) and B2 receptors (vasodilation), is that it produces an increase in cardiac output as well as afterload reduction. These changes lead to an increase in the pulse pressure (pulsatility) that is thought to impact favorably on cerebral perfusion in the context of dysautoregulation. The conclusion, therefore, from this retrospective case series was that an increase in the cardiac index (hyperdynamic therapy) in conjunction with volume loading (hypervolemic therapy) led to improvement or reversal of the neurologic deficit from SAH-induced vasospasm in 78% of patients who did not respond to only hypervolemic therapy. The results of these retrospective studies of triple-H therapy for the treatment of symptomatic vasospasm are summarized in Table 8-4.

TABLE 8-4
Triple-H Therapy for Vasospasm after Subarachnoid Hemorrhage

Study	Treatment Protocol	Sample Size (No. of Patients)	Outcome		
			Improved	No Change	Worse
Kassell[9]	Specific parameters not specified	40	74%	16%	10%
Awad[10]	Central venous pressure 10–12 or PCWP 15–18 cm H_2O; hematocrit 33–38%; systolic blood pressure 160–200[a] or 120–150[b] mm Hg	42	60%	24%	16%
Levy[11]	PCWP 12–16 cm H_2O; dobutamine titrated to clinical and radiographic response (cardiac index ≥5 L/minute/m^2)	23	78%	Not reported	Not reported

PCWP = pulmonary capillary wedge pressure.
[a]Clipped aneurysms.
[b]Unclipped aneurysms.

Finally, Egge et al.[8] performed a prospective randomized, controlled study to evaluate the role of hyperdynamic triple-H therapy in preventing delayed ischemic neurologic deficits after SAH. This trial included 32 patients who were treated surgically within 72 hours after aneurysmal SAH. All patients were in Hunt and Hess grades I–III. Patients were stratified according to the volume of subarachnoid blood and then randomized to receive either normovolemic fluid therapy (aimed to maintain neutral fluid balance) or triple-H fluid management (aimed to keep the central venous pressure between 8 and 12 cm H_2O, hematocrit between 30% and 35%, and mean arterial pressure greater than 20 mm Hg, above baseline preoperative levels). Dopamine (5–15 μg/kg per minute) was used to achieve this blood pressure elevation when necessary. Comparison of physiologic parameters (mean arterial pressure, hematocrit, and central venous pressure) between the two groups confirmed the efficacy of these measures in achieving significant differences between the normovolemic and triple-H fluid therapy groups. There were, however, no significant differences between the two groups on a variety of short- and long-term measures. These included the frequency of clinical or transcranial Doppler ultrasound–evident vasospasm, cerebral blood flow (measured by single-photon emission CT), Glasgow Outcome Scale scores (at 14 days and 1 year), and scores on neuropsychological tests. Caution should be exercised in the interpretation of these results because of the small number of patients included (and consequent lack of power to reliably detect a clinical effect). Furthermore, these findings cannot be readily extrapolated to the treatment of clinically apparent vasospasm.

In conclusion, therefore, there are substantial anecdotal and retrospective data to support the safety and efficacy of triple-H therapy, but a more positive endorsement of this approach to the treatment of clinically apparent vasospasm awaits demonstration of its efficacy in a large prospective controlled trial.

Summary

- The natural history of unruptured intracranial aneurysms is different for patients with no history of SAH compared to those with a history of SAH.
- ISUIA is the largest, most systematic natural history study performed to date, but its retrospective nature does raise concerns about unrecognized bias in patient selection (e.g., bias toward including patients who had been selected for conservative management).
- The available data support the idea that spontaneous SAH is most often caused by aneurysms of at least 7–10 mm.

- Data from the ISUIA study indicate that amongst patients with no history of SAH, the annual risk of rupture of aneurysms less than 10 mm in diameter is exceedingly low at approximately 0.05%.
- Aneurysm size is not a reliable predictor of recurrent SAH in those with a history of SAH; the risk of rupture is relatively high irrespective of size.
- Nimodipine reduces the likelihood of stroke and poor outcome in patients with vasospasm from SAH of any clinical grade.
- There have been no prospective randomized, controlled clinical trials establishing the efficacy of hyperdynamic triple-H therapy in the treatment of patients with vasospasm after SAH.
- Data from uncontrolled retrospective case series suggest that the use of triple-H therapy is associated with a favorable outcome in 60–80% of patients with symptomatic vasospasm after SAH.
- The only prospective randomized, controlled study of hyperdynamic triple-H therapy in the prevention of delayed ischemic neurologic deficits after SAH did not show any benefit on a variety of outcome measures, but this study was limited in size by the small number of patients included.

References

1. Unruptured intracranial aneurysms—risk of rupture and risks of surgical intervention. International Study of Unruptured Intracranial Aneurysms Investigators. *N Engl J Med* 1998;339:1725–1733.
2. Wiebers DO, Whisnant JP, O'Fallon WM. The natural history of unruptured intracranial aneurysms. *N Engl J Med* 1981;304:696–698.
3. Wiebers DO, Whisnant JP, Sundt TM, O'Fallon WM. The significance of unruptured intracranial saccular aneurysms. *J Neurosurg* 1987;66:23–29.
4. Locksley HB. Natural history of subarachnoid hemorrhage, intracranial aneurysms and arteriovenous malformations. *J Neurosurg* 1966;25:321–368.
5. Allen GS, Ahn HS, Preziosi TJ, et al. Cerebral arterial spasm—a controlled trial of nimodipine in patients with subarachnoid hemorrhage. *N Engl J Med* 1983;308:619–624.
6. Petruk KC, West M, Mohr G, et al. Nimodipine treatment in poor-grade aneurysm patients. Results of a multicenter double-blind placebo-controlled trial. *J Neurosurg* 1988;68:505–517.
7. Pickard JD, Murray GD, Illingworth R, et al. Effect of oral nimodipine on cerebral infarction and outcome after subarachnoid haemorrhage: British Aneurysm Nimodipine Trial. *BMJ* 1989;298:636–642.
8. Egge A, Waterloo K, Sjøholm H, et al. Prophylactic hyperdynamic postoperative fluid therapy after aneurysmal subarachnoid hemorrhage: a clinical, prospective, randomized, controlled study. *Neurosurgery* 2001;49:593–605.

9. Kassell NF, Peerless SJ, Durward QJ, et al. Treatment of ischemic deficits from vasospasm with intravascular volume expansion and induced arterial hypertension. *Neurosurgery* 1982;11:337–343.

10. Awad IA, Carter LP, Spetzler RF, et al. Clinical vasospasm after subarachnoid hemorrhage: response to hypervolemic hemodilution and arterial hypertension. *Stroke* 1987;18:365–372.

11. Levy ML, Rabb CH, Zelman V, Giannotta SL. Cardiac performance enhancement from dobutamine in patients refractory to hypervolemic therapy for cerebral vasospasm. *J Neurosurg* 1993;79:494–499.

CHAPTER 9

The Antiphospholipid Syndrome

Introduction

The antiphospholipid syndrome (APS) is characterized by venous and arterial thrombosis, recurrent fetal loss, thrombocytopenia, and the presence of a lupus anticoagulant (LA), anticardiolipin (aCL), or other antiphospholipid (aPL) antibodies. The APS may occur in isolation (primary APS) or in association with an underlying autoimmune disease, most commonly systemic lupus erythematosus (SLE; secondary APS). The criteria for diagnosis of the APS have been revised recently (Table 9-1).

The terminology used in the aPL antibody literature is somewhat confusing. *LA* was the term initially used to describe the factor responsible for an observed prolongation of whole blood clotting time and prothrombin time in the absence of any specific clotting factor deficiency. In contrast to the in vitro prolongation of the activated partial thromboplastin time, this factor was found to be associated with a hypercoagulable state in vivo. Some of these patients were subsequently shown to have antibodies directed against the phospholipid cardiolipin in an enzyme-linked immunosorbent assay. Antibodies directed against other phospholipids (including phosphatidylserine, phosphatidylinositol, phosphatidylethanolamine, and phosphatidylglycerol) have since been described. The term *aPL antibody* is now used as a generic term to describe a variety of antibodies that react with negatively charged phospholipids. The aPLs may be conceptualized as a spectrum of antibodies with overlapping specificities.

Thrombosis in the APS is usually venous, but when it occurs in the arterial system, the brain is the most common site involved. In addition to stroke, it has been suggested that a number of nonthrombotic neurologic disorders may also be associated with aPL antibodies. These include migraine, seizures, chorea, transverse myelitis, Guillain-Barré syndrome, sensorineural hearing loss, transient global amnesia, and dementia.

The primary focus of this chapter is the relevance of aPL antibodies to syndromes of cerebral ischemia. Brief reference, however, is also made to some of the other neurologic syndromes that are reported to be associated with aPL antibodies.

TABLE 9-1
Preliminary Criteria for the Classification of the Antiphospholipid Syndrome

Clinical criteria
   Vascular thrombosis: one or more clinical episodes of arterial, venous, or small
      vessel thrombosis, in any tissue or organ. Thrombosis must be confirmed by
      imaging, Doppler studies, or histopathology with the exception of superficial
      venous thrombosis. For histopathologic confirmation, thrombosis should be
      present without significant evidence of inflammation of the vessel wall.
   Pregnancy morbidity: In studies of populations of patients who have more than
      one type of pregnancy morbidity, investigators are strongly encouraged to
      stratify groups of subjects according to the following criteria:
   One or more unexplained deaths of a morphologically normal fetus at or
      beyond the tenth week of gestation, with normal fetal morphology docu-
      mented by ultrasound or by direct examination of the fetus.
   One or more premature births of a morphologically normal neonate at or before
      the thirty-fourth week of gestation because of severe pre-eclampsia, eclamp-
      sia, or placental insufficiency.
   Three or more unexplained consecutive spontaneous abortions before the tenth
      week of gestation, with maternal anatomic or hormonal abnormalities and
      paternal and maternal chromosomal causes excluded.
Laboratory criteria
   Anticardiolipin antibody of IgG or IgM isotype in blood, present in medium or
      high titer, on two or more occasions, at least 6 weeks apart, measured by a
      standardized enzyme-linked immunosorbent assay for β_2-glycoprotein I–
      dependent anticardiolipin antibodies.
   Lupus anticoagulant present in plasma on two or more occasions at least 6 weeks
      apart, detected according to the guidelines of the International Society of
      Thrombosis and Hemostasis (Scientific Subcommittee on Lupus Anticoagu-
      lants/Phospholipid-Dependent Antibodies) in the following steps:
   Prolonged phospholipid-dependent coagulation demonstrated on a screening
      test (e.g., activated partial thromboplastin time, kaolin clotting time, dilute
      Russell's viper venom time, dilute prothrombin time, and Textarin time).
   Failure to correct the prolonged coagulation time on the screening test by mix-
      ing with normal platelet-poor plasma.
   Shortening or correction of the prolonged coagulation time on the screening
      test by the addition of excess phospholipid.
   Exclusion of other coagulopathies (e.g., factor VIII inhibitor or heparin) as
      appropriate.
Definite antiphospholipid antibody syndrome is considered to be present if at least
      one of the clinical criteria and one of the laboratory criteria are met.

Source: Adapted from WA Wilson, AE Gharavi, T Koike, et al. International Consensus
Statement on preliminary classification criteria for definite antiphospholipid syndrome.
Arthritis Rheum 1999;42:1309–1311.

Which Patients with Transient Ischemic Attack or Stroke Should Be Screened for the Presence of Antiphospholipid Antibodies?

There is evidence that aPL antibodies are more common in young patients with stroke. In the retrospective study of Asherson and colleagues,[1] the mean age of the 35 patients with cerebrovascular disease and aPL antibodies was 39 years. The mean age was 45 years in the 128 patients retrospectively reviewed by the Antiphospholipid Antibodies in Stroke Study (APASS) group,[2] but 39% of the patients in this study were 50–80 years old. Levine and colleagues' prospective study of 81 patients revealed a mean age of 55 years in all patients with aPL antibodies. However, the mean age was only 39 in the subgroup with high titer antibodies. There are a number of possible explanations for these results. It may be that aPL antibodies are an important risk factor for stroke only in young patients. Alternatively, it may be that aPL antibodies are also risk factors in the elderly but that the studies to date have failed to demonstrate this effect because it has been masked by the presence of other (more dominant) risk factors such as age, hypertension, and hypercholesterolemia. Nevertheless, the implication is that the yield of testing for aPL antibodies will be higher in stroke patients of a younger age. This is not to say, however, that aPL antibodies in elderly patients with stroke do not carry the same significance. It seems sensible, therefore, to screen for aPL antibodies in young patients with stroke and in older patients if other risk factors are not present. The presence of other features of the APS, such as thrombocytopenia, livedo reticularis, or recurrent fetal loss, should also prompt a more aggressive search for aPL antibodies.

The available evidence suggests that stroke of any type may occur in association with aPL antibodies. In the 1990 APASS study,[2] 75.5% of patients had either a normal cerebral angiogram or intracranial occlusion (with normal extracranial carotids), suggesting that these strokes were either due to in situ thrombosis or cardioembolism. Fifty-two percent of patients had an abnormal echocardiogram, but in only eight of 72 patients was the abnormality (atrial or ventricular thrombus, akinetic segment, or septal defect) a likely source of embolism. Mitral valve abnormalities (e.g., myxomatous thickening, prolapse) accounted for most of the other abnormalities, but these are less readily identified as the likely source of embolism. In the 1993 APASS study[3] (that included 24 patients with aCL antibodies), 37.5% of strokes were due to small vessel disease, 29.2% secondary to large vessel disease, and 20.8% cardioembolic, but the distribution of stroke types in the aCL antibody–positive patients was not reported. Finally, Levine and colleagues[4] described the recurrent strokes in patients with aPL antibodies as "pial territory infarcts" or as "deep hemispheric or brainstem infarcts that are nonlacunar." The overall impression, therefore, is that all stroke types may occur in patients with the APS and that there is no clear predilection for any particular stroke type.

Which Laboratory Tests Are Appropriate for Use in Screening for the Presence of Antiphospholipid Antibodies?

An enzyme-linked immunosorbent assay is typically used to detect and quantify aPL antibodies. Cardiolipin is used as the antigen for detecting aCL antibodies. A proprietary mix of phospholipids (mostly phosphatidylserine) is used in determining aPL antibody reactivity. These antibody titers are typically expressed in immunoglobulin (Ig) G phospholipid (GPL) and IgM phospholipid units in which an antibody concentration of 1 µg/ml represents one unit. The threshold for distinguishing elevated antibody titers has not been consistent in all studies. The consensus seems to be that titers less than 20 GPL units are regarded as negative, titers greater than 20 units positive, and titers above 100 units highly positive.

A variety of tests are available for demonstrating the LA. These include prolongation of the activated partial thromboplastin time, the Russell's viper venom time, and the tissue thromboplastin inhibition test. These tests have differing sensitivities and specificities. A panel of tests with a platelet neutralization procedure should, therefore, be used to ensure detection of all LA antibodies.

No single aPL antibody assay has sufficient sensitivity and specificity enabling it to be performed in isolation. Typically, a panel of aPL antibody assays should be performed including at least LA, aCL, and aPL antibodies. The role of testing for anti–β_2-glycoprotein I antibodies is less clear. A few preliminary observations are that these antibodies are detected more frequently in the primary APS and that these antibodies may occasionally be detected even in the absence of the LA or other aPL antibodies. Furthermore, there is some evidence with regard to stroke and other neurologic syndromes that anti–β_2-glycoprotein I reactivity has a low positive predictive value and a high negative predictive value. This is to say that a negative result is of greater value in excluding a stroke as being part of the APS than a positive result is in demonstrating that a stroke is a manifestation of the APS.[5]

Are All Antibody Isotypes and Titers of Equal Relevance to Patients with Transient Ischemic Attack or Stroke?

Most studies suggest that only aPL antibodies of the IgG isotype are relevant to discussions of cerebral ischemia. The APASS group,[2] for example, found that most patients with stroke had IgG antibodies, although there were a few patients who only had IgM or IgA aPL antibodies. Levine and colleagues[4] found that only IgG aPL antibodies were predictive of recurrent stroke. They also demonstrated that time to recurrence was shorter in patients with higher-titer aCL antibodies, confirming the results of D'Olhaberriague and colleagues.[6]

Elevated titers of aPL antibodies occur in association with infection, certain drugs, and underlying malignancy. These antibodies are frequently of the IgM isotype and thought not to be associated with an increased risk of arterial or venous thrombosis.

The consensus seems to be that high-titer (e.g., greater than 80–100 GPL units) IgG aPL antibodies are predictive of an increased risk of cerebral ischemia. The recent American College of Rheumatology guidelines[7] indicate that these antibodies should be demonstrated on two occasions 6 weeks apart before attributing significance to them. It is more difficult to know how to respond to persistent low-titer IgG antibodies or even high-titer IgM antibodies. In the absence of other risk factors and the presence of recurrent transient ischemic attack (TIA) or stroke, an argument could be made for regarding these antibodies as indicative of an underlying hypercoagulable state.

Is the Presence of Antiphospholipid Antibodies an Independent Risk Factor for First Stroke?

The APASS group evaluated 255 consecutive first ischemic stroke patients and a similar number of age- and sex-matched controls.[3] Elevated aCL antibody titers were present in 9.7% of stroke patients and 4.3% of controls. The association of aCL antibodies and stroke was independent of other stroke risk factors (age, gender, hypertension, diabetes mellitus, coronary artery disease, and cigarette smoking). IgG aCL antibodies were most commonly detected, but independent analysis for antibody isotype and the risk of stroke was not performed.

What Is the Risk of Stroke Recurrence in Patients with Transient Ischemic Attack or Stroke and aPL Antibodies?

The APASS group performed a retrospective study of 128 patients with ocular or cerebral ischemia and antiphospholipid antibodies. They found that 30% had evidence of prior cerebral infarction and that the risk of recurrent stroke was 9.4% over a mean follow-up period of 16 months.[2] Their conclusion was that patients with aPL antibodies are at risk for recurrent stroke.

However, there was no control group, and so it is not clear from this study whether patients with aPL antibodies are at a greater risk of stroke recurrence than patients without these antibodies. Some years later, the APASS group published their follow-up data on 219 patients with first stroke, of whom only 17 (8%) were positive for IgG aCL antibodies. They did not find an increased risk of recurrent stroke in the aCL antibody–positive group.[8] However, this study was limited by the small sample size, the relatively high frequency of other stroke risk factors in the patients they studied, and the use of a relatively low titer (10 GPL units) as the cutoff for defining the presence of these antibodies.

The study of Levine and colleagues[4] did demonstrate that patients with high-titer IgG aPL antibodies are at an increased risk of stroke recurrence. They studied 81 patients with aPL antibodies and cerebral ischemia and found a stroke recurrence rate of 31% over a 3-year period, with the median time to stroke recurrence being only 7.9 months. The risk of recurrence of any thrombotic event (i.e., not limiting the analysis to stroke recurrence, but including, for instance, deep venous thrombosis) was 56% over 3 years, with a median time to recurrence of 7 months. The risk of stroke recurrence, therefore, depends on the antibody isotype and titer, with the risk being greatest in patients with high-titer IgG aPL antibodies.

How Should Patients with Transient Ischemic Attack or Stroke and Antiphospholipid Antibodies Be Treated?

At least at a theoretical level, it is not clear that patients with aPL antibodies only warrant treatment if the risk of stroke is greater than other populations at risk of stroke. Surely it is sufficient that they simply be at risk and that the risk may be modified by a particular treatment.

The recommendation that patients with stroke and aPL should be anticoagulated with warfarin is based on the study by Khamashta and colleagues.[9] This was a retrospective study of 147 patients with a history of arterial or venous thrombosis and elevated titers of aPL antibodies. Only 56 of these patients presented with cerebral ischemia (TIA or stroke). Separate analyses were not performed for patients with thrombotic events involving different arterial or venous circulations. Compared to patients who received neither aspirin nor warfarin, the relative risk among patients with high-intensity anticoagulation (international normalized ratio greater than 3) of a recurrent thrombotic event was 0.05 (significant risk reduction relative to no treatment; $p < 0.001$). Low-intensity warfarin therapy (international normalized ratio less than 3) with or without aspirin resulted in a relative risk of around 0.79 (not statistically significant from the no-treatment group). The relative risk of recurrent thrombosis was highest in the first 6 months after warfarin was discontinued.

The conclusion, therefore, is that high-intensity warfarin therapy represents effective prophylaxis against recurrent arterial and venous thrombosis in patients with the APS. Even if this study did not demonstrate that the risk of stroke or TIA per se was reduced by high-intensity anticoagulation, it does provide reasonable evidence that such therapy reduces the risk of an unspecified recurrent thrombotic event. Finally, lifelong therapy may be required, given that warfarin therapy reduces the likelihood of recurrent thrombosis and that the risk of recurrence was highest shortly after warfarin was discontinued.

Is There an Association between Multiple Sclerosis and the Antiphospholipid Syndrome?

A definitive answer to the question of whether there is an association between multiple sclerosis (MS) and APS is not yet available. However, a number of recent studies have suggested that the APS may closely mimic multiple sclerosis and should be considered in the differential diagnosis.[10–12] Karussis and colleagues provided a detailed account of 20 patients with probable or definite MS (according to Poser's criteria) who were also found to have persistently elevated IgG aCL antibodies. As a group, these patients were atypical by virtue of their presentation with progressive myelopathy or spinocerebellar syndrome, the high frequency of headaches, and the absence of cerebral spinal fluid oligoclonal bands.[10] This was not an isolated report. Ijdo and colleagues,[11] for example, reported 23 patients with aPL who presented with MS or MS-like syndromes. In this series, IgM aCL antibodies were detected in the majority of patients.

Are Other Neurologic Conditions Also Associated with Antiphospholipid Antibodies?

Lavalle and colleagues[13] described transverse myelitis in 12 patients with SLE in association with aPL antibodies. The presentation with transverse myelitis was the initial manifestation of SLE in five of these patients. IgG aCL antibodies were present in nine patients (medium to high titer in seven); IgM aCL antibodies were similarly detected in nine patients (medium to high titer in five). Eight patients had both IgG and IgM aCL antibodies, and these were of medium to high titer in four. Transverse myelitis is an uncommon manifestation of SLE (occurring in approximately 1% of cases), but this report establishes that transverse myelitis in SLE may be associated with elevated titers of aCL antibodies. However, the relative frequency of aCL antibodies in patients with transverse myelitis and SLE remains unclear. It is also not clear whether transverse myelitis may occur as a manifestation of the primary APS.

Chorea is an infrequent but well-recognized manifestation of SLE (occurring in 1–4% of cases). Cervera and colleagues[14] presented six of their own cases and reviewed 44 additional cases from the literature of APS-associated chorea. The LA was present in 92% of cases. IgG aCL antibodies were detected in 39 of 43 cases tested and IgM aCL antibodies in 15 of 22 cases. IgM antibodies alone or in higher titer than the IgG aCL antibodies were detected in six cases. Chorea occurred as part of the primary APS in 15 patients (30%) and as a manifestation of the secondary APS in 35 (70%). For the most part, the mechanism of chorea could not be established. Acute infarction in the basal ganglia was demonstrated in only three patients. Treatment varied, including steroids, haloperidol, or antiplatelet/anticoagulants, and response was generally good. In summary, therefore, chorea (unilateral or bilateral) may occur in association with the APS (either primary or secondary). The association is stronger, but not exclusively, for IgG (rather than IgM) aCL. There are insufficient data to make definitive treatment recommendations.

There has been repeated suggestion of an association between aPL antibody positivity and migraine. The expectation is that this association would be difficult to demonstrate given the high frequency of migraine and the low frequency of aPL antibody reactivity in the general population. Nevertheless, this issue was well addressed in the large prospective study of Tietjen and colleagues.[15] They found that the frequency of aCL antibody positivity is not increased in young people with migraine with or without aura. Although large enough to exclude a strong association, the study was of insufficient size to completely exclude any association at all. There is, however, some evidence to suggest that aPL antibodies are more common in young patients with migrainous stroke.[16] In this study, aPL antibodies (LA or IgG aCL) were detected in six out of 16 patients with migrainous stroke.

Summary

- The presence of aPL antibodies represents an independent risk factor for TIA and stroke.
- The association between aPL antibodies and increased risk of stroke has been established for IgG antibodies and is strongest for high antibody titers.
- The available evidence suggests that β_2-glycoprotein I–dependent aPL antibodies are likely to be more predictive of this increased risk.
- IgM aPL antibodies do not constitute a risk factor for ischemic stroke.
- High-intensity anticoagulation with warfarin (to maintain the international normalized ratio above 3) is indicated if the antibody titers are persistently elevated.

- The duration of therapy is unclear but should probably continue indefinitely.
- aPL antibodies may also be present in patients with other neurologic conditions, notably chorea (in both primary and secondary APS) and transverse myelitis (in APS secondary to SLE). Although these aPL antibodies are usually of the IgG isotype, the data are insufficiently conclusive to dismiss IgM antibodies as irrelevant.
- The APS (with IgM aPL antibodies) should be considered in the differential diagnosis of MS and MS-like illnesses, particularly when the presentation and course of the disease is atypical.
- aPL antibodies may be found in patients with migrainous stroke but, otherwise, are not more prevalent amongst patients with migraine (with or without aura).

References

1. Asherson R, Khamashta M, Gil A, et al. Cerebrovascular disease and antiphospholipid antibodies in systemic lupus erythematosus, lupus-like disease, and the primary antiphospholipid syndrome. *Am J Med* 1989;86:391–399.
2. Clinical and laboratory findings in patients with antiphospholipid antibodies and cerebral ischemia. The Antiphospholipid Antibodies in Stroke Study Group. *Stroke* 1990;21:1268–1273.
3. Anticardiolipin antibodies are an independent risk factor for first ischemic stroke. The Antiphospholipid Antibodies in Stroke Study (APASS) Group. *Neurology* 1993;43:2069–2073.
4. Levine SR, Brey RL, Sawaya KL, et al. Recurrent stroke and thrombo-occlusive events in the antiphospholipid syndrome. *Ann Neurol* 1995;38:119–124.
5. Day HM, Thiagarajan P, Ahn C, et al. Autoantibodies to beta2-glycoprotein I in systemic lupus erythematosus and primary antiphospholipid antibody syndrome: clinical correlations in comparison with other antiphospholipid antibody tests. *J Rheumatol* 1998;25:667–674.
6. D'Olhaberriague L, Levine SR, Salowich-Palm L, et al. Specificity, isotype, and titer distribution of anticardiolipin antibodies in CNS diseases. *Neurology* 1998;51:1376–1380.
7. Wilson WA, Gharavi AE, Koike T, et al. International Consensus Statement on preliminary classification criteria for definite antiphospholipid syndrome: report of an international workshop. *Arthritis Rheum* 1999;42:1309–1311.
8. Anticardiolipin antibodies and the risk of recurrent thrombo-occlusive events and death. The Antiphospholipid Antibodies in Stroke Study Group (APASS). *Neurology* 1997;48:91–94.
9. Khamashta MA, Cuadrado MJ, Mujic F, et al. The management of thrombosis in the antiphospholipid-antibody syndrome. *N Engl J Med* 1995;332:993–997.
10. Karussis D, Leker RR, Ashkenazi A, Abramsky O. A subgroup of multiple sclerosis patients with anticardiolipin antibodies and unusual clinical mani-

festations: do they represent a new nosological entity? *Neurology* 1998;44: 629–634.

11. Ijdo JW, Conti-Kelly AM, Greco P, et al. Anti-phospholipid antibodies in patients with multiple sclerosis and MS-like illnesses: MS or APS. *Lupus* 1999;8:109–115.

12. Cuadrado MJ, Khamashta MA, Ballesteros A, et al. Can neurologic manifestations of Hughes (antiphospholipid) syndrome be distinguished from multiple sclerosis? Analysis of 27 patients and review of the literature. *Medicine* 2000;79:57–68.

13. Lavalle C, Pizarro S, Drenkard C, et al. Transverse myelitis: a manifestation of systemic lupus erythematosus strongly associated with antiphospholipid antibodies. *J Rheumatol* 1990;17:34–37.

14. Cervera R, Asherson RA, Font J, et al. Chorea in the antiphospholipid syndrome. Clinical, radiologic and immunologic characteristics of 50 patients from our clinics and the recent literature. *Medicine (Baltimore)* 1997;76:203–212.

15. Tietjen GE, Day M, Norris L, et al. Role of anticardiolipin antibodies in young persons with migraine and transient focal neurological events: a prospective study. *Neurology* 1998;50:1433–1440.

16. Silvestrini M, Matteis M, Troisi E, et al. Migrainous stroke and the antiphospholipid antibodies. *Eur Neurol* 1994;34:316–319.

CHAPTER 10

Optic Neuritis

Introduction

The majority of cases of idiopathic optic neuritis are due to demyelination, and in a significant proportion of patients, it may represent the first manifestation of multiple sclerosis (MS). Is it possible to predict which patients with optic neuritis will subsequently develop MS? What is the relative value of magnetic resonance imaging (MRI) of the optic nerves and the brain? Does treatment affect visual outcome? Is there any form of treatment that reduces the risk of subsequent MS or the development of disability in MS? These are the important questions that the physician must address when faced with a patient who presents with an attack of optic neuritis.

Do Steroids Affect Visual Outcome in Patients with Optic Neuritis?

The Optic Neuritis Treatment Trial (ONTT)[1] was a prospective randomized, placebo-controlled trial that was designed specifically to answer this question. Patients between the ages of 18 and 46 years with the diagnosis of acute unilateral optic neuritis and visual symptoms of less than 8 days' duration were included in the study. They were randomized to receive intravenous methylprednisolone (IVMP) (250 mg every 6 hours for 3 days, followed by prednisone, 1 mg/kg per day for 11 days), oral prednisone (prednisone, 1 mg/kg per day for 14 days), or placebo (oral placebo for 14 days). Patients in the first two groups also received a brief prednisone taper.

Although a slight visual benefit was observed in the IVMP group at 6 months,[2] visual acuity and other clinical measures of visual function were no different between the three treatment groups at 1 year. Visual acuity, in fact, was 20/40 or better in 95% of the placebo group, 94% of the intravenous group, and 91% of the oral prednisone group. The conclusion, therefore, was that IVMP hastened visual recovery but had no effect on ultimate visual function.

Is There a Reason to Obtain Magnetic Resonance Imaging of the Optic Nerves?

Some authors have suggested that long lesions of the optic nerve, especially if there is involvement of the intracanalicular portion of the nerve, portend a poor prognosis for visual recovery after an attack of optic neuritis. It was reasoned that swelling of the intracanalicular portion of the optic nerve might lead to irreversible ischemic damage. This issue has been the subject of a recent prospective study, in which an effort was made to determine whether patients with involvement of the intracanalicular portion of the optic nerve might benefit particularly from treatment with intravenous steroids.[3] This study included 66 patients—46 with isolated optic neuritis and the remainder with optic neuritis as a manifestation of MS. In this study, lesion length and involvement of the intracanalicular portion of the optic nerve at the time of initial MRI (i.e., at the time of presentation with optic neuritis) predicted neither visual recovery nor response to therapy.

What Is the Risk of Subsequent Multiple Sclerosis after an Attack of Optic Neuritis?

The risk of developing MS after an episode of optic neuritis has been the subject of numerous studies with variable results. In Kurtzke's review,[4] for example, the risk was estimated as ranging from 7% to 41% at 5 years, 10% to 64% at 10 years, and 13% to 78% at 15 years. Although not specifically designed to address this question, the ONTT provided extremely useful data that shed light on this question. The original cohort from the ONTT included 457 patients, but those in whom the diagnosis of MS was already established had to be excluded for the purpose of determining the risk of developing MS after an attack of isolated optic neuritis. The remaining 389 patients formed the cohort for the study of the risk of subsequent MS.[5] In the placebo group, definite MS developed in 17% within 2 years and in 31% within 5 years.

What Is the Value of Brain Magnetic Resonance Imaging in Patients with Optic Neuritis?

Having established the general risk of MS after an episode of optic neuritis, the question arises as to whether there is any way to recognize those at high risk of developing MS. Do abnormalities on MRI identify such patients? MRI was obtained in 352 of the 389 patients in the study of the risk of MS after an episode of acute unilateral optic neuritis. In

TABLE 10-1
Five-Year Risk of Multiple Sclerosis

Patient Group	5-Yr Risk of Multiple Sclerosis (%)
All-comers (untreated)	31
Normal MRI or ≤1 lesion*	16
History of nonspecific neurologic symptoms	44
≥3 Lesions on MRI*	51
≥3 Lesions on MRI* as well as a history of nonspecific neurologic symptoms	66

MRI = magnetic resonance imaging.
*Relevant lesions are those that are ≥3 mm in diameter.

the initial 2-year follow-up study,[5] lesions were characterized on the basis of the size (either less than 3 mm or greater than 3 mm), their location in the periventricular white matter, and their ovoid shape. The 2-year risk of subsequent MS increased depending on the nature and number of abnormalities on MRI. In the placebo group, the 2-year risk of MS was 3% in those with either a normal MRI or with lesions meeting none of the criteria outlined above (i.e., less than 3 mm and neither periventricular in location nor ovoid in shape). The risk of MS increased to 17% amongst those with a single periventricular or ovoid lesion of at least 3 mm and to 36% in those with more than one such lesion.

Careful evaluation of the brain MRI, therefore, is particularly helpful in quantifying the subsequent risk of developing MS. In the 5-year follow-up study,[6] MRI abnormalities were classified purely on the basis of their size, being counted as "lesions" if at least 3 mm. The presence and number of MRI lesions remained the most important prognostic indicators of the risk of MS at 5 years, with the cumulative probability increasing from 16% in those with no lesions on the initial MRI to 51% in those with three or more lesions (Table 10-1).

The presence and number of lesions on the initial MRI were also predictive of the severity of disability at 5 years.[6] Only 7% of those with no brain MRI lesions developed moderate or severe disability (Expanded Disability Status Scale [EDSS] score greater than or equal to 3; see Appendix 17 [Kurtzke Expanded Disability Score]) compared to 24% of those who had at least three lesions on the initial MRI. MRI, therefore, is of value in patients with optic neuritis in that it helps to predict the risk of subsequent MS as well as the long-term disability in those patients who go on to develop MS.

Are There Any Other Factors That Predict the Development of Multiple Sclerosis after an Initial Episode of Optic Neuritis?

Independent of MRI findings, a history of nonspecific neurologic symptoms (predominantly paresthesiae) is also associated with an increased risk of developing MS.[6] Among the patients with optic neuritis and no lesions on brain MRI, the risk of subsequent MS over 5 years was 44% and 15%, respectively, in those with and without prior nonspecific neurologic symptoms. The combination of prior neurologic symptoms and an abnormal MRI increases the risk even further to as high as 66% (in those with at least three lesions) (see Table 10-1).

Amongst those patients with optic neuritis and neither a history of nonspecific neurologic symptoms nor an abnormal brain MRI, certain clinical features of the attack of optic neuritis are also predictive of a low subsequent risk of developing MS. These include the lack of pain, the presence of optic disk swelling, and the presence of relatively mild loss of visual acuity.[6]

What Is the Effect of Steroid Treatment of Optic Neuritis on the Subsequent Risk of Multiple Sclerosis?

The ONTT was a randomized, controlled trial of corticosteroid treatment of optic neuritis, the details of which have already been summarized. Briefly, patients were randomized to receive IVMP, oral prednisone, or placebo. Because patients in the IVMP group were hospitalized for 3 days, they were not blinded to the treatment they received. Although blinding was not strictly enforced and no blinding analysis performed, the authors state that patients in the other groups and the study physicians were generally unaware of treatment assignments. Although the ONTT was designed to evaluate the effects of corticosteroid treatment on visual outcome in optic neuritis, it also provided valuable information about the subsequent risk of MS. For the purposes of this study, the development of MS was determined solely on the basis of clinical criteria with definite MS diagnosed when there was a second episode with new neurologic abnormality confirmed on examination. Recurrent episodes of optic neuritis in either eye were not considered diagnostic of MS.

Considering all patients with unilateral optic neuritis in the ONTT,[5] irrespective of MRI findings, definite MS developed within 2 years in 17.0% of the placebo group, 15.0% of the oral prednisone group, and 7.5% of the IVMP group. The beneficial effect of IVMP on the subsequent risk of MS after an attack of optic neuritis was mostly seen in patients with at least two lesions greater than or equal to 3 mm in size and either periventricular

TABLE 10-2
Effect of Steroid Treatment on the Two-Year Risk of Multiple Sclerosis after
Optic Neuritis (ON)

Category of Patient	Placebo	Prednisone	Methylprednisolone
ON with any magnetic resonance imaging	17%	15%*	7.5%*
ON with at least two lesions ≥3 mm and either periventricular or ovoid	36%	32% (p = 0.62)	16.0% (p = 0.04)

*Statistical comparison to placebo not reported.

in location or ovoid in shape.[5] Amongst patients with these abnormalities on MRI, the 2-year risk of MS was 36% in the placebo group, 32% in the oral prednisone group, and 16% in the IVMP group (Table 10-2).

The beneficial effect of IVMP was no longer apparent after 5-year follow-up, with the cumulative probability of MS being 31% in the placebo group, 32% in the oral prednisone group, and 27% in the IVMP group.[6]

Opponents and proponents of the use of IVMP for the treatment of optic neuritis have emphasized different aspects of these results. Those against treatment point to the lack of an effect of IVMP on the development of MS at 5 years and argue for the lack of a treatment effect. Those in favor of the use of IVMP emphasize how a single 3-day course of IVMP delayed the development of MS over a 2-year period. That is to say, a single course of steroids prevented the occurrence of a further clinical event that would be diagnostic of MS. The fact that this effect was lost by 5 years of follow-up, they argue, is not surprising. They even suggest that this provides a rationale for the intermittent use of a 3-day course of IVMP to prevent flares in patients with already established MS.

In summary, therefore, a 3-day course of IVMP followed by an 11-day course of oral prednisone does delay the occurrence of a second clinical event (that would be diagnostic of MS) for up to 2 years.

Does Treatment with Intravenous Methylprednisolone for Initial Episode of Optic Neuritis Influence the Development of Disability from Multiple Sclerosis?

In the ONTT,[6] moderate or severe disability (EDSS greater than or equal to 3) developed in 14% of the placebo group, 18% of the oral prednisone group, and 16% of the IVMP group. Treatment, therefore, has no effect on the development of MS or of disability from MS at 5 years. The question of whether disability might be reduced by intermittent courses of IVMP over an extended period has not been the subject of prospective study and remains an unanswered question, at least for now.

Does It Matter Whether Oral or Intravenous Steroids Are Used in the Treatment of Optic Neuritis?

In the ONTT, oral prednisone had no effect on the subsequent risk of developing MS, irrespective of MRI findings.[5] However, within 2 years, recurrent optic neuritis occurred in 16% of the placebo group, 13% of the IVMP group, and 30% of the oral prednisone group. Intravenous steroids, therefore, were not protective against subsequent episodes of optic neuritis in either eye, but the use of oral prednisone appeared to double the risk over the subsequent 2 years.

The debate about the implications of the route of steroid administration is clouded by the different dosages used. In the ONTT, patients in the (oral) prednisone group received significantly less corticosteroid (prednisone, 1 mg/kg per day for 14 days) compared to those in the IVMP group (IVMP, 1 g per day for 3 days, followed by prednisone, 1 mg/kg per day for 11 days).*

High-dose oral methylprednisolone has been shown in a randomized, placebo-controlled trial to be effective in improving short-term visual recovery without an adverse effect on subsequent attack frequency over an 8-week period.[7] Although the duration of follow-up in this study was limited to 8 weeks, these results suggest that the differential effect observed in the ONTT may have been due more to the difference in dosages used rather than the route of administration.

Summary

- Treatment of optic neuritis with IVMP improves the rate of visual recovery but has no effect on visual outcome at 1 year.
- Treatment with intermediate-dose oral prednisone alone does not affect visual recovery and is associated with an increased risk of recurrent attacks of optic neuritis.
- The number of MRI lesions greater than or equal to 3 mm in size that are also periventricular in location or ovoid in shape at the time of the first episode of optic neuritis is the single most important predictor of both the development of MS and of disability from MS at 5 years.

---

*Four mg of methylprednisolone has equivalent potency to 5.0 mg of prednisone; the methylprednisolone group, therefore, received the equivalent of approximately 3.5 g more prednisone than the oral prednisone group.

- The presence and nature of abnormalities on optic nerve MRI are not predictive of visual prognosis or the response to treatment.
- Prior nonspecific neurologic symptoms (notably paresthesiae) also increase the risk of subsequent MS. The combination of prior nonspecific neurologic symptoms and an abnormal MRI increases the risk even further.
- IVMP reduces the risk of developing MS at 2 years, but this beneficial effect is lost by 5 years.
- Treatment with steroids has no effect on the development of disability from MS at 5 years.

References

1. Beck RW, Cleary PA. Optic Neuritis Treatment Trial: one year follow-up results. *Arch Ophthalmol* 1993;111:773–775.
2. Beck RW, Cleary PA, Anderson MM, et al. A randomized, controlled trial of corticosteroids in the treatment of acute optic neuritis. The Optic Neuritis Study Group. *N Engl J Med* 1992;326:581–588.
3. Kapoor R, Miller DH, Jones SJ, et al. Effects of intravenous methylprednisolone on outcome in MRI-based prognostic subgroups in acute optic neuritis. *Neurology* 1998;50:230–237.
4. Kurtzke JF. Optic neuritis or multiple sclerosis. *Arch Neurol* 1985;42:704–710.
5. Beck RW, Cleary PA, Trobe JD, et al. The effect of corticosteroids for acute optic neuritis on the subsequent development of multiple sclerosis. The Optic Neuritis Study Group. *N Engl J Med* 1993;329:1764–1769.
6. The 5-year risk of MS after optic neuritis. Experience of the optic neuritis treatment trial. The Optic Neuritis Study Group. *Neurology* 1997;49:1404–1413.
7. Sellebjerg F, Nielsen HS, Frederiksen JL, Olesen J. A randomized, controlled trial of oral high-dose methylprednisolone in acute optic neuritis. *Neurology* 1999;52:1479–1484.

CHAPTER 11

Acute Disseminated Encephalomyelitis

Introduction

There are no generally accepted diagnostic criteria for acute disseminated encephalomyelitis (ADEM). It may, therefore, be extremely difficult to distinguish ADEM from the first episode of multiple sclerosis (MS). If there is one outstanding feature, however, that distinguishes ADEM from MS, it is the monophasic course of ADEM. The problem, of course, is that this feature can only be recognized in retrospect and, therefore, is not helpful at the time of initial presentation.

The major shortcoming of most reports of patients with ADEM is that it is not possible to be sure that patients do in fact have ADEM. The only reliable way to gather information about the clinical features of ADEM is to collect data from patients who present with an episode of central nervous system demyelination and then to re-evaluate these patients after a prolonged interval. Only those who have remained free of relapse can reliably be said to have ADEM. The clinical features of their initial presentation should then be analyzed and described in detail. There are only two sizable series that have adopted this approach,[1,2] and these form the basis for the descriptions that follow.

What Are the Clinical Features That Distinguish Acute Disseminated Encephalomyelitis from a First Attack of Multiple Sclerosis?

Dale et al.[1] studied a group of children who presented with an episode of disseminated demyelination. The children whose illness remained monophasic at follow-up (after a mean of 5.6 years) were classified as having ADEM. The clinical features of the initial illness were compared to those children who subsequently developed clinically definite MS (according to the criteria of Poser). The results of this study are summarized in Tables 11-1 and 11-2.

These data indicate that there is no single feature or combination of features that facilitates an absolute distinction between ADEM and MS.

TABLE 11-1
Comparison of the Clinical Features in Acute Disseminated
Encephalomyelitis and Multiple Sclerosis

Clinical Feature	Acute Disseminated Encephalomyelitis	Multiple Sclerosis	p Value
Preceding illness within 1 mo of neurologic illness	74%	38%	<0.05
Latency from predemyelinating to neurologic illness (days)	13 (2–31)	9 (1–21)	—
Latency from onset neurologic illness to maximum deficit (days)	7 (1–31)	9 (1–60)	—
Signs or symptoms of systemic disease			
Headache	58%	23%	—
Fever	43%	15%	—
Meningism	31%	8%	—
Seizures	17%	0%	Not significant
Polysymptomatic neurologic illness	91%	38%	<0.002
Encephalopathy	69%	15%	<0.002
Pyramidal signs	71%	23%	<0.01
Cerebellar signs	49%	23%	—

— = statistical comparison not reported.

However, a polysymptomatic neurologic illness with encephalopathy and evidence of systemic disease such as headache, fever, and meningism is most likely to represent an instance of ADEM. Although findings on cerebrospinal fluid (CSF) analyses are not helpful in making the distinction, the presence of large (greater than 1 cm) lesions on magnetic resonance imaging (MRI), with sparing of the periventricular white matter and involvement of the cortex or thalamus, lend additional support to the diagnosis of ADEM. Convalescent CSF and MRI findings may also be helpful. The disappearance of CSF oligoclonal bands supports the diagnosis of ADEM, and the appearance of new MRI lesions during the period of convalescence is only seen in MS.

Schwarz et al.[2] performed a similar study in adults. They included 40 adults who were thought to have ADEM and re-evaluated them after a mean duration of follow-up of 38 months. Fourteen patients had experienced a second clinical episode and were thus reclassified as having MS. The remaining 26 patients were classified as having ADEM. The clinical features of the initial episode of demyelination in these two groups were

TABLE 11-2
Comparison of the Results of Investigations in Acute Disseminated
Encephalomyelitis and Multiple Sclerosis

Investigation	Acute Disseminated Encephalomyelitis (%)	Multiple Sclerosis (%)	p Value
Cerebrospinal fluid analysis			
Lymphocytosis	64	42	NS
Elevated protein	60	33	NS
Oligoclonal bands	29	64	NS
Magnetic resonance imaging			
Absolute sparing of periventricular white matter	56	8	—
Cortical gray matter lesions	12	0	—
Basal ganglia lesions	28	8	—
Thalamic lesions	41	25	—
Scans with at least one lesion >1 cm	82	58	—

— = statistical comparison not requested; NS = not significant.

compared. Patients with ADEM were more likely to have had a preceding infection, and the onset of neurologic symptoms was more abrupt. The incidence of systemic symptoms (headache, fever, meningism) and encephalopathy was low but was unique to the patients with ADEM. The claim is made, but the evidence is not clearly provided, that the patients with ADEM were more likely to have a polysymptomatic illness. Brainstem symptoms were present in 62% of patients with ADEM compared to 21% of MS patients ($p = 0.02$). The results of CSF analysis were not helpful in making the distinction between ADEM and MS. Patients with MS were more likely to have periventricular lesions on MRI, and there were no differences in the frequency or pattern of lesion enhancement with gadolinium between the two groups of patients. The results of this study of adult patients are in general agreement with the aforementioned study of children with ADEM.

Is There Such an Entity as Recurrent Acute Disseminated Encephalomyelitis?

The question of whether there is such an entity as recurrent ADEM is extremely difficult to answer in the absence of clear diagnostic criteria for ADEM. At the extremes of central nervous system (CNS) demyelination are the prototypic illnesses of ADEM and MS. ADEM is conceptualized as an acute monophasic illness, often with a good prognosis especially when treated. At the other end of the spectrum is MS that is typically character-ized by recurring episodes of multifocal demyelination over a prolonged period. Clearly, there are patients whose clinical course falls somewhere in between these two extremes. There are numerous reports of patients with what has been labeled *multiphasic* or *recurrent ADEM*.[3,4] Typically, these are descriptions of patients with recurrent episodes of CNS demyelination, with each episode reminiscent more of ADEM than MS. Usually, this means that there is a history of a recent flu-like illness, an explosive onset of a polysymptomatic neurologic illness with systemic features like head-ache and fever, a CSF pleocytosis that is felt to be atypical for MS, and the presence of large confluent tumor-like areas of demyelination visible on MRI. The difficulty is that none of these clinical features reliably distin-guishes ADEM from MS, as evidenced by the data from the recently pub-lished longitudinal studies of patients with CNS demyelination.[1,2]

The study by Dale et al.[1] identified patients with relapses immedi-ately after ADEM. They used the designation *multiphasic disseminated encephalomyelitis* to describe those patients whose relapses were thought to represent part of the same acute monophasic immune process. In this study, relapses that were designated *multiphasic disseminated encephalo-myelitis* occurred within 8 weeks of the initial neurologic illness. But what of patients who present with a second illness, very much like the first, after a prolonged interval? Are these patients appropriately classified as having recurrent ADEM, or do they have MS? Also controversial are patients who develop asymptomatic new lesions on MRI during follow-up after an initial episode of CNS demyelination. In the study by Schwarz et al.,[2] these patients were also classified as having ADEM.

In all likelihood, this will remain a controversial subject until a clearer definition of what constitutes ADEM emerges. For now, the best cri-terion is the monophasic nature of the illness, as determined by the absence of recurrence over prolonged duration of follow-up.

What Are the Treatment Options for Patients with Acute Disseminated Encephalomyelitis?

There are no controlled treatment trials in patients with ADEM. All of the available data are derived from case reports and series. An attempt is not made to refer to every published case report. Instead, a selection has been made based on the sample size and the inclusion of sufficient data to evalu-ate the response to treatment. None of the available reports has included predefined criteria by which outcome or response to treatment is judged. It is necessary to recognize these limitations in evaluating the available data.

Steroids have been used most commonly. Ziegler[5] reported four patients who were treated successfully with corticotropin, Pasternak et al.[6]

described five patients treated with dexamethasone (Decadron), and there are numerous references to the successful use of methylprednisolone.[1,2,7] There are reports of patients who relapsed clinically after early discontinuation of steroids but who responded to reinitiation of steroids and a more gradual taper. The approach adopted by many is to begin with a 3- to 5-day course of intravenous methylprednisolone and then to switch to oral prednisone, which can be tapered gradually over 4–6 weeks. For the most part (when this information is included in the case reports), some clinical improvement is usually noted within 1–2 days of starting high-dose steroids. Moreover, there are many reports of patients who showed no sign of clinical improvement within the first 3–5 days of steroid treatment but subsequently responded well to treatment with either plasma exchange (PE)[8–11] or intravenous immunoglobulin (IVIg).[12,13] The implication would appear to be that an alternative or additional form of immunotherapy should be employed if there is progression of symptoms or if no clinical improvement is noted within the first 3–5 days of intravenous steroid therapy. In these reports, the latency to the onset of clinical improvement was typically 1–4 days after initiation of treatment with PE or IVIg. There is no evidence to support the use of PE rather than IVIg, or vice versa, but in the absence of a clinical response to one method within 4–5 days, the other should be tried.

The ability to make recommendations is severely limited by the poor quality of the available data. However, there is the most (anecdotal) evidence to support the use of steroids as first-line therapy; methylprednisolone has been used most commonly, but decadron and corticotropin may be equally efficacious. Methylprednisolone has been used in high doses (approximately 15 mg/kg per day) for a period of 5–7 days and then gradually tapered. If the clinical response is inadequate within this period, then either PE or IVIg could be tried. Although there are no good data to support this claim, it is probably prudent to continue the steroids (on a gradual taper) while the PE or IVIg is being administered. IVIg is typically used at a dose of 0.4g/kg per day for 5 days, and the course of PE used in the literature has varied from daily exchanges over 5 days to alternate daily exchanges over a more prolonged period. The response to IVIg or PE is typically seen within 1–4 days. If there is no response to either treatment within the 5 days of therapy, then it is reasonable to proceed directly to the alternate modality. There are no data to indicate how patients should be treated if they do not respond to the combination of steroids, PE, and IVIg. The available data do not support a different therapeutic approach based on the age of the patient.

Summary

- There are no clinical, CSF, or MRI features that permit an absolute distinction between MS and ADEM to be made at the time of initial presentation.

- The defining feature of ADEM is its monophasic course, a determination that can only be made after prolonged follow-up.
- A polysymptomatic neurologic illness with encephalopathy and evidence of systemic disease such as headache, fever, and meningism is more likely to represent an instance of ADEM; brainstem symptoms and signs are also more common in ADEM than in MS.
- The presence of large (greater than 1 cm) lesions on MRI with absolute sparing of the periventricular white matter and involvement of the cortex or thalamus are more suggestive of ADEM than MS.
- There are no data from controlled treatment trials to guide the treatment of ADEM.
- There are the most data (from case reports) to support the use of steroids as first-line therapy, with methylprednisolone the agent that has been used most frequently.
- Anecdotal evidence suggests that plasmapheresis and IVIg are equally efficacious.

References

1. Dale RC, de Sousa C, Chong WK, et al. Acute disseminated encephalomyelitis, multiphasic disseminated encephalomyelitis and multiple sclerosis in children. *Brain* 2000;123:2407–2422.
2. Schwarz S, Mohr A, Knauth M, et al. Acute disseminated encephalomyelitis: a follow-up study of 40 adult patients. *Neurology* 2001;56:1313–1318.
3. Cohen O, Steiner-Birmanns B, Biran I, et al. Recurrence of acute disseminated encephalomyelitis at the previously affected brain site. *Arch Neurol* 2001;58:797–801.
4. Modi G, Mochan A, Modi M, Saffer D. Demyelinating disorder of the central nervous system occurring in black South Africans. *J Neurol Neurosurg Psychiatry* 2001;70:500–505.
5. Ziegler DK. Acute disseminated encephalitis. Some therapeutic and diagnostic considerations. *Arch Neurol* 1966;14:476–488.
6. Pasternak J, De Vivo DC, Prensky AL. Steroid-responsive encephalomyelitis in childhood. *Neurology* 1980;30:481–486.
7. Hynson JL, Kornberg AJ, Coleman LT, et al. Clinical and neuroradiologic features of acute disseminated encephalomyelitis in children. *Neurology* 2001;56:1308–1312.
8. Kanter DS, Horensky D, Sperling RA, et al. Plasmapheresis in fulminant acute disseminated encephalomyelitis. *Neurology* 1995;45:824–827.
9. Shah AK, Tselis A, Mason B. Acute disseminated encephalomyelitis in a pregnant woman successfully treated with plasmapheresis. *J Neurol Sci* 2000; 174:147–151.

10. Cotter FE, Bainbridge D, Newland AC. Neurological deficit associated with Mycoplasma pneumoniae reversed by plasma exchange. *BMJ* 1983;286:22.
11. Dodick DW, Silber MH, Noseworthy JH, et al. Acute disseminated encephalomyelitis after accidental injection of a hog vaccine: successful treatment with plasmapheresis. *Mayo Clin Proc* 1998;73:1193–1195.
12. Pradhan S, Gupta RP, Shashank S, Pandey N. Intravenous immunoglobulin therapy in acute disseminated encephalomyelitis. *J Neurol Sci* 1999;165:56–61.
13. Sahlas DJ, Miller SP, Guerin M, et al. Treatment of acute disseminated encephalomyelitis with intravenous immunoglobulin. *Neurology* 2000;54:1370–1372.

CHAPTER 12

Multiple Sclerosis

Introduction

Multiple sclerosis (MS) is an inflammatory demyelinating disorder of the central nervous system. Recent research into disease modifying therapy has been dominated by clinical trials of interferon-β, but other immunomodulatory therapies have also been subjects of study. Difficulty arises in deciding how the efficacy of these therapies should be evaluated. Is it enough that they delay the time to relapse or reduce the frequency of relapses? Is it not more important that any therapy, especially if it carries the risk of toxic side effects and significant cost, be shown to reduce the accumulation of disability? Is it possible to predict who will develop MS after a single episode of central nervous system demyelination? And is there any benefit to early immunomodulatory therapy in these at-risk patients? These and other questions are the focus of this chapter.

What Are the Diagnostic Criteria for Multiple Sclerosis?

The International Panel on the Diagnosis of MS recently published revised guidelines for the diagnosis of MS.[1] The cornerstone of these criteria remains the demonstration of dissemination of clinical events and lesions in space and time. The panel emphasized the need for objective clinical evidence of attacks or progression (i.e., symptoms alone are insufficient). An *attack* is defined as an episode of neurologic disturbance of the kind seen in MS that lasts for at least 24 hours. For the purposes of documenting separation in time of such events, there should be an interval of 30 days between the onset of the first event and the onset of the second event.

Of the available laboratory investigations, magnetic resonance imaging (MRI) is regarded as having the greatest sensitivity and specificity. MRI findings can be used to provide evidence of dissemination of lesions in both time and space; the relevant criteria are summarized in Table 12-1.

Thus, in the context of two or more clinical attacks (i.e., dissemination in time) but only objective clinical evidence of a single lesion, the MRI may provide the necessary evidence for dissemination in space. Similarly, if there has been only a single clinical attack but objective evidence of at least two lesions (i.e., dissemination in space), then the MRI may provide the

TABLE 12-1
Magnetic Resonance Imaging (MRI) Criteria for Dissemination in Space and Time

---

MRI criteria for dissemination in space (at least three of the following are required)*
    One gadolinium-enhancing lesion or nine T2 hyperintense lesions
    At least one infratentorial lesion
    At least one juxtacortical (i.e., involving subcortical U-fibers) lesion
    At least three periventricular lesions
MRI criteria for dissemination in time (either of the following two are required)
    Gadolinium-enhancing lesion on a scan performed 3 mos after the onset of the
        clinical attack
    The presence of a new T2 hyperintense lesion on an MRI performed at least 3 mos
        after the first MRI scan

---

*Based on the criteria of F Barkhof, M Filippi, DH Miller, et al. Comparison of MRI criteria at first presentation to predict conversion to clinically definite multiple sclerosis. *Brain* 1997;120:2059–2069.

necessary evidence for dissemination in time. Finally, there is the common clinical situation of the patient who presents with a clinically isolated syndrome suggestive of MS (the so-called monosymptomatic presentation). The diagnosis of MS would then require ancillary evidence of dissemination in both time and space. In the absence of MRI findings that fulfill the criteria for dissemination in space, the presence of two or more MRI-detected lesions consistent with MS as well as abnormalities in the cerebrospinal fluid (either oligoclonal bands or an elevated immunoglobulin [Ig] G index) may suffice. But it is still necessary to garner evidence of dissemination in time, either by awaiting a second clinical attack or by the presence of new T2 or gadolinium-enhancing lesions on an MRI performed 3 months later.

According to these new criteria, the patient should be classified as having MS or as not having MS. The designation *possible MS* should be reserved for the individual whose evaluation meets some but not all of the necessary criteria. The old terminology of *clinically definite MS* and *laboratory-supported MS* should no longer be used.

Which Features on Brain Magnetic Resonance Imaging Are Predictive of the Development of Multiple Sclerosis after an Episode of Monosymptomatic Demyelination?

MRI is the most sensitive paraclinical test that may assist in making the diagnosis of MS. The criteria that may be used to demonstrate dissemination in time or place are outlined in the preceding section. MRI, however, may also be useful in predicting the progression to MS after presentation with a clinically isolated neurologic syndrome that is suggestive of MS—this has been the subject of a number of studies, one of which is reviewed.[2] Patients with clinically isolated syndromes suggestive of MS (brainstem, cerebellar, or spinal cord syndromes or optic neuritis) were identified prospectively. MRI was performed at the time of initial presentation, and the patients were then followed until the development of new symptoms or signs that permitted the clinical diagnosis of MS. Regression analysis was then performed to identify which imaging parameters were predictive of the progression to MS.

Imaging data were collected in 74 patients, 33 of whom developed MS after a median of 9 months' follow-up. Those who did not develop MS were followed for a median of 39 months. Brain MRI was normal in 13 patients; only one patient developed MS. The presence of gadolinium enhancement and the juxtacortical location of lesions were identified as most important, but periventricular lesions, infratentorial lesions, hypo-intense T1 lesions, large enhancing lesions, and the total number of T2 lesions were also significant. The presence of any T2 lesions provides high sensitivity for conversion to MS, but the specificity is low. Increasing the number of lesions to classify a scan as abnormal leads to increasing specificity but declining sensitivity. Accuracy was found to be optimal at a minimum of nine T2 lesions. In the investigator's final model, four MRI parameters (gadolinium enhancement, infratentorial, juxtacortical, and periventricular location) were used to build a model with an accuracy of 80%.* On the basis of this model, the likelihood of conversion to MS can be calculated based on the number of MRI parameters identified on initial MRI (Table 12-2).

What Is the Effect of Corticosteroids on Acute Multiple Sclerosis Flares?

Corticosteroids and adrenocorticotropic hormone (ACTH) have long been the mainstay of treatment of MS relapses, but it was only relatively recently that intravenous methylprednisolone was compared to placebo in a prospective randomized trial.[3] This study included 50 patients, only 22 of whom were entered into the study at the time of an acute relapse (the remainder had chronic progressive disease). Patients were randomized to receive 500 mg intravenous methylprednisolone daily for 5 days or placebo. Expanded Disability Status Scale (EDSS) scores (see Appendix 17 [Kurtzke Expanded Disability Score]) at 1 and 4 weeks were significantly reduced in

---

*Accuracy = (TP + TN)/(TP + TN + FP + FN), where TP = true positive, TN = true negative, FP = false positive, and FN = false negative.

TABLE 12-2

Risk of Multiple Sclerosis Depends on the Number of Abnormalities on Magnetic Resonance Imaging

Number of Abnormal Magnetic Resonance Imaging Criteria*	Risk of Developing Multiple Sclerosis (%)
0	14
1	28
2	55
3	64
4	84

*Criteria indicate gadolinium enhancement, infratentorial lesion, juxtacortical lesion, or periventricular lesion.

the intravenous methylprednisolone group. Intravenous methylprednisolone, therefore, enhances the rate of recovery from a relapse.

An important issue that has emerged is whether the beneficial effects of steroids are the result of the high dose used, the intravenous route of administration, or a combination of the two. There are two studies that have addressed these issues. In a small randomized, double-blind, placebo-controlled trial, Alam et al.[4] randomized 38 patients with MS who presented in relapse to receive either 500 mg intravenous methylprednisolone (with five placebo tablets) or five 100-mg tablets of methylprednisolone (with a 100-ml placebo solution administered intravenously). Three patients were withdrawn. At 4 weeks, the EDSS scores were improved in 16 out of 20 (80%) in the intravenous group and 10 out of 15 (67%) in the oral group. The degree of EDSS improvement is not stated. Mean EDSS scores for the two groups were similar, but the utility of this measure is controversial. There were no statistically significant differences between the two treatment groups, and the authors concluded that acute flares of MS could be equally well treated with oral or intravenous steroids. In a larger study, Barnes et al.[5] recruited 80 patients with an acute exacerbation of MS "of sufficient severity to justify steroid treatment" and randomized them to receive a more commonly used lower-dose oral regimen or traditional high-dose intravenous methylprednisolone. The oral regimen comprised 48 mg methylprednisolone per day (equivalent to 60 mg prednisolone) for 7 days, followed by 24 mg per day for 7 days, and finally 12 mg per day for 7 days. The intravenous regimen consisted of 1 g per day for 3 days. Patient blinding was maintained by the concurrent administration of either placebo tablets or a placebo infusion, depending on the active treatment assignment. Effective blinding was confirmed with a post hoc unblinding analysis. The primary outcome measure was the number of patients improving by greater than or equal to one EDSS point 4 weeks after trial entry. Secondary outcome measures included a difference of at least one grade on an ambulation index at 4 weeks or of EDSS scores 12 weeks after randomization. They found no significant differences on any of these measures between the two treatment groups.

The conclusion from these studies is that steroids are effective in the treatment of acute relapses of MS. The available evidence seems to suggest that oral steroids (even in the dosages commonly used) are as effective as high-dose intravenous methylprednisolone. These data notwithstanding, high-dose intravenous steroid therapy remains the most commonly used regimen.

What Is the Difference between the Various Formulations of Interferon-β?

There are three forms of interferon-β presently available. Interferon-β1b (Betaseron) is a recombinant product produced in *Escherichia coli* that differs from natural interferon-β by two amino acids and its lack of a glycosylated side chain. It is administered via the subcutaneous route. Interferon-β1a (Avonex) is produced in mammalian cells and has the same amino acid sequence and carbohydrate side chains as natural interferon-β. Rebif is a different form of interferon-β1a that is also produced in Chinese hamster ovary cells. It has the same amino acid sequence and glycosylation pattern as human interferon-β. Avonex is administered via the intramuscular route and Rebif subcutaneously.

What Is the Role of Interferon Treatment in Relapsing-Remitting Multiple Sclerosis?

The beneficial effect of interferon-β treatment on relapse frequency has been demonstrated in a number of recent trials. Each of the formulations of interferon-β (described above) has been studied in a prospective randomized trial.

The IFNB Multiple Sclerosis Study Group was the first to report the results of a prospective randomized, placebo-controlled trial of interferon-β in MS.[6] They recruited 372 patients with MS who were ambulatory with Kurtzke EDSS scores of less than or equal to 5.5 and who had experienced at least two flares within the preceding 2 years. The patients were randomized to receive either placebo or one of two doses of Betaseron administered by subcutaneous injection every other day. Both patients and physicians were blind to the treatment received. The primary endpoints were annual exacerbation rate and the proportion of exacerbation-free patients. Secondary endpoints included the time to first exacerbation, exacerbation severity, change in EDSS from baseline, and quantitative disease burden as measured by annual MRI. The results are summarized in Table 12-3.

TABLE 12-3
Effect of Interferon-β1b (IFN-β1b; Betaseron) on the Course
of Multiple Sclerosis

3-Yr Endpoint	Placebo	1.6 mIU IFN-β1b	8 mIU IFN-β1b	p Value
Annual exacerbation rate	1.21	1.05	0.84	0.0004
Exacerbation-free patients (%)	17.0 (14)	23.0 (18)	27.0 (22)	0.097
Time to first exacerbation (days)	147	199	264	0.028
Mean change in lesion area on magnetic resonance imaging	+17.1%	+1.1%	–6.2%	—

mIU = million international units.

Significant effects of interferon-β1b on both primary and secondary endpoints were demonstrated at both 2- and 3-year follow-up intervals. However, notwithstanding the effects of reducing annual relapse rate by approximately 30% and of diminished mean lesion area on MRI, there was no effect on EDSS scores. Worsening of at least one EDSS point was confirmed in 28% of the placebo and 1.6-mIU (million international units) groups but only 20% of the 8.0-mIU group. There was, therefore, a trend towards reduced disability in the high-dose interferon-β group, but these results did not reach statistical significance ($p = 0.161$). The absence of an effect on disability was confirmed in the open-label extension phase of this study.[7] For the most part, the alternate-day subcutaneous injections were well tolerated without major side effects, although neutralizing antibodies did develop in approximately 45% of patients in the high-dose interferon-β1b group.

The discovery of a therapy that reduced the frequency of relapses represented a major advance in the therapeutic armamentarium of the physician treating patients with MS. However, it is the accumulation of disability rather than the frequency of relapses that is more significant to the long-term well-being of patients with MS. With this in mind, the Multiple Sclerosis Collaborative Research Group designed a study to investigate whether systemically administered interferon-β1a could slow the progression of irreversible neurologic disability associated with relapsing-remitting MS.[8] This was a double-blind, placebo-controlled, randomized trial of Avonex administered intramuscularly at a dosage of 6 mIU (30 μg) weekly. The study recruited 331 patients with relapsing-remitting MS, baseline EDSS of 1.0–3.5, and at least two relapses in the preceding 3 years. The primary outcome measure was the time to onset of sustained worsening in disability that was defined as deterioration from baseline of at least one point on the EDSS that persisted for at least 6 months. Treatment and follow-up duration were variable, with the majority of patients followed for

TABLE 12-4
Effect of Interferon-β1a (Avonex) on the Course of Multiple Sclerosis

Outcome Measure at 2 Yrs	Placebo	Interferon-β1a	p Value
Percentage with sustained progression of disability*	33.9%	21.2%	<0.005
Percentage of patients worsening by ≥2.5 points on Expanded Disability Status Scale	17.9%	3.6%	<0.05
Annual exacerbation rate	0.9	0.61	≤0.05

*Primary outcome measure.

at least 2 years. The time interval to sustained progression of disability was significantly prolonged in interferon-β1a–treated patients compared to those who received placebo (Table 12-4).

This was the first study to demonstrate a reduction in the probability of sustained progression among interferon-β–treated patients. It also confirmed the approximately 30% reduction in the annual exacerbation rate that was observed in the IFNB Multiple Sclerosis Study Group Trial of interferon-β1b.

Finally, the Prevention of Relapses and Disability by Interferon-β1a Subcutaneously in Multiple Sclerosis (PRISMS) study examined the effects of Rebif administered subcutaneously three times per week.[9] This study included 560 patients with relapsing-remitting MS who had had at least two relapses in the preceding 2 years and had Kurtzke EDSS scores of 0–5. Patients were randomized to receive interferon-β1a 22 μg (6 mIU), 44 μg (12 mIU), or placebo given three times per week via subcutaneous injection. The primary outcome measure was the number of relapses over the course of the study. Other outcome measures included the time to first relapse, the proportion of patients who remained relapse-free, and progression to disability (measured by an increase of EDSS score of at least one point that was sustained over at least 3 months). As summarized in Table 12-5, treatment with interferon-β1a was associated with a reduction in the relapse rate, a prolongation in the time to sustained progression, and a reduction in the change in EDSS over the 2-year study period.

These three studies have in common their effect in reducing the rate of relapse by approximately 30%. Both the Avonex and Rebif studies demonstrated that interferon-β treatment is associated with an increase in the time interval to the development of sustained disability and a reduction in the change in EDSS scores over time. In the Betaseron trial, however, the accumulation or progression of disability was a secondary rather than a primary endpoint, and a statistically significant effect on disability was not observed.

TABLE 12-5
Effect of Interferon-β1a (IFN-β1a; Rebif) on the Course of Multiple Sclerosis

Outcome Measure at 2 Yrs	Placebo	6 mIU IFN-β1a	12 mIU IFN-β1a
Mean number of relapses	2.56	1.82[a]	1.73[a]
First quartile time to progression (mos)	11.9	18.5[b]	21.3[b]
Mean change in Expanded Disability Status Scale scores	0.48	0.23[b]	0.24[b]

mIU = million international units.
[a]$p < 0.005$ compared with placebo.
[b]$p \leq 0.05$ compared with placebo.

Is Interferon-β Effective in Patients with Secondary Progressive Multiple Sclerosis?

The European Study Group performed a double-blind, placebo-controlled trial of interferon-β1b in patients with secondary progressive MS (SP-MS).[10] The study included 718 patients with SP-MS and baseline EDSS scores of 3.0–6.5 who were randomized to receive either placebo or 8-mIU interferon-β1b administered subcutaneously on alternate days. The primary outcome measure was the time from baseline to the first visit at which an increase of at least one point on the EDSS (or 0.5 points if baseline EDSS score was 6.0 or 6.5) was recorded (provided that this increase was confirmed 3 months later). Over the 36-month period of follow-up, 49.7% of patients in the placebo group and 38.9% of the interferon-treated patients met the criteria outlined above for progression of disability. The time to progression (for the 40% quartile) was 549 days in the placebo group and 893 days in the interferon-treated group, which amounts to a delay in progression of disability by approximately 12 months. Mean annual relapse rate was also reduced by about 30% in the interferon-treated group, although this beneficial effect dropped annually. Of note is that these benefits were observed in patients with both mild and severe disability. These results confirm prior observations of the beneficial effect of interferon-β in slowing the accumulation of disability in MS and support its use in patients with SP-MS.

The SPECTRIMS (Secondary Progressive Efficacy Clinical Trial of Recombinant Interferon-beta-1a in MS) study did not confirm these results.[11] This was a double-blind, placebo-controlled trial that involved 618 patients with SP-MS who were randomized to receive one of two doses of interferon-β-1a (22 µg or 44 µg) three times per week or placebo. The primary outcome measure was the time to progression of disability (defined as a sustained increase from baseline of at least one EDSS point). On this measure, there were no significant differences between the interferon- and placebo-treated patients. Possible explanations include the shorter observation period in the European study, the shorter duration of the prerandomization secondary progressive phase in the European study, and the higher proportion of patients in the European study with relapses in the 2 years before study entry. The SPECTRIMS study, however, did find a benefit of interferon-β on secondary outcome measures including various measures of relapse rate and severity. Interferon-β therapy, therefore, is effective in reducing relapse frequency in patients with SP-MS, but its utility in preventing the progression of disability remains controversial.

Is There a Role for Interferon Treatment in Patients at High Risk for Developing Multiple Sclerosis?

Two recent studies have addressed the question of what the role is for interferon treatment in high-risk patients. CHAMPS[12] (Controlled High-Risk Subjects Avonex Multiple Sclerosis Prevention Study) recruited patients at the time of their first demyelinating event (optic neuritis, incomplete transverse myelitis, brainstem or cerebellar syndrome) in whom the MRI demonstrated evidence of prior demyelination (i.e., two or more clinically silent lesions on MRI that were at least 3 mm in size, one of which had to be either periventricular in location or ovoid in shape). All patients were treated with intravenous methylprednisolone followed by an oral prednisone taper, but the 383 study patients were randomized to receive either placebo or weekly intramuscular injections of 30 μg of Avonex. The primary endpoint was the development of clinically definite MS. The cumulative probability of developing MS during the 3-year follow-up period was 35% in the interferon-treated group and 50% in the placebo-treated group. The effect of treatment was similar among subgroups classified according to the type of initial event and the number of lesions on the initial T2-weighted MRI scan. Lesion load on MRI was a prespecified secondary endpoint, and this was similarly significantly reduced in the interferon-treated compared to the placebo-treated group.

The Early Treatment of Multiple Sclerosis Study[13] (ETOMS) was designed with a similar goal in mind, but the population recruited was slightly different. Patients were eligible at the time of their first neurologic episode, whether it was unifocal (as in the CHAMPS study) or multifocal, provided that the MRI was also abnormal. For an MRI to be classified as *abnormal*, there had to be either at least four white-matter lesions on T2-weighted scans or at least three such lesions if one was either infratentorial or enhanced with gadolinium. Patients were randomized to receive either 22 μg Rebif weekly or placebo, and the primary endpoint was conversion to clinically definite MS. Secondary endpoints included various MRI measures. The protocol permitted steroid treatment if the initial attack was of a moderate or severe degree. This led to steroid treatment in 68% of the interferon-treated group and 73% of the placebo-treated group. During the 2-year study, 34% of the interferon-treated patients and 45% of the placebo group developed MS. The rate of conversion to clinically definite MS was higher in patients with multifocal onset and in those with more than eight lesions on initial MRI. Significantly fewer new T2 lesions developed in the interferon-treated group compared to the placebo-treated group.

The implications of CHAMPS and ETOMS are similar even though the treatment effect was slightly greater in CHAMPS. This difference may relate to a variety of factors, including the recruitment of patients with multifocal disease at onset, the use of a lower dose of interferon-β1a, and the use of more stringent (i.e., greater lesion load) MRI criteria for study entry in ETOMS.

In view of the already established effect of interferon-β in reducing relapse rate, the results of CHAMPS and ETOMS were perhaps not surprising. Implicit in the effect of suppressing the relapse rate is a prolongation of the time to development of clinically definite MS. It is also unclear whether the early initiation of treatment with interferon-β at the time of the first episode of demyelination has any effect on the ultimate development or accumulation of disability. Although enthusiasts cite the data from CHAMPS and ETOMS to support the early initiation of interferon-β therapy, this conclusion is probably premature.

Does Glatiramer Acetate Impact on the Natural History of Multiple Sclerosis and the Development of Disability?

Glatiramer acetate (Copaxone) was studied by the Copolymer 1 Multiple Sclerosis Study Group in a prospective randomized, placebo-controlled trial.[14] Patients with MS who were ambulatory with EDSS scores of 0–5 and a history of at least two relapses within the preceding 2 years were eligible for inclusion. Two hundred fifty-one patients were randomized to receive either placebo or 20 mg of copolymer 1 (glatiramer acetate) administered daily by subcutaneous injection. The primary outcome measure was the mean number of relapses over the 2-year study period. Secondary outcome measures included the proportion of patients with sustained disease progression (defined as an increase of one point on the EDSS that was sustained for 90 days) and the mean change in EDSS scores from baseline to conclusion of the study. The annualized relapse rates were 0.59 for the copolymer 1–treated group and 0.84 for the placebo-treated group. This therapeutic effect was most pronounced in the patients with lower EDSS scores at entry. There was no significant difference between the two treatment groups in the proportion of patients with sustained progression. In terms of the mean change in EDSS scores from baseline to conclusion, more patients in the copolymer 1 group were improved and fewer were worse, but the use of mean EDSS scores as outcome measures is of questionable validity. The reason is that the EDSS is not a linear scale (i.e., a one-point change from 2 to 3 is not equivalent to a one-point change from 5 to 6). The use, therefore, of linear statistics (i.e., calculation of the mean) for a nonlinear scale is dubious.

This study demonstrated that the effects of copolymer 1 were similar to those of interferon-β with respect to the reduction in relapse rate by approximately 30%. The effects of copolymer 1 on the development of disability, however, are less clear.

Is There a Role for Intravenous Immunoglobulin in the Treatment of Multiple Sclerosis?

The potential benefit of intravenous immunoglobulin (IVIg) in patients with relapsing-remitting MS has been the subject of a number of open trials as well as two prospective randomized, placebo-controlled trials. In the Austrian Immunoglobulin in Multiple Sclerosis Study Group Trial,[15] 150 patients were randomized to receive either monthly IVIg (0.15–0.20 g/kg) or placebo for 2 years. The primary outcome measures were the change in mean EDSS score and the proportion of patients with improved, stable, or worse disability (as defined by an increase or decrease of one point on the EDSS score by the end of the study period). Annual relapse rate was one of the secondary outcome measures. Benefit from IVIg was observed in terms of changes in mean EDSS scores, but these results are difficult to interpret because of the questionable validity of mean EDSS score as an outcome measure, as explained previously (see preceding section). Annual relapse rate, one of the secondary outcome measures, was 0.52 in the IVIg-treated group, compared to 1.26 in the placebo-treated group. This study, therefore, suggested a benefit from IVIg in terms of annual relapse rate, even if the data on disability are difficult to interpret.

Achiron et al.[16] confirmed the benefit of IVIg on relapse rate in their prospective double-blind, placebo-controlled trial. They randomized 40 patients with relapsing-remitting MS to treatment with IVIg or placebo. Patients with yearly exacerbation rates of 0.5–3.0 and EDSS scores of 0–6 were eligible for inclusion. The IVIg-treated group received a loading dose of 0.4 g/kg per day for 5 consecutive days, followed by booster doses of 0.4 g/kg per day every 2 months for 2 years. Patients and physicians were blinded to treatment allocation, and the efficacy of patient blinding was confirmed with a blinding analysis. The primary outcome measures were the yearly exacerbation rates, the proportion of exacerbation-free patients, and the time until the first exacerbation. The 2-year results are summarized in Table 12-6.

TABLE 12-6
Effects of Intravenous Immunoglobulin on the Course of Multiple Sclerosis

	Intravenous Immunoglobulin	*Placebo*	p *Value*
Annual exacerbation rate	0.59	1.61	0.0006
Percentage of exacerbation-free patients	6.0	0.0	0.001
Time to first exacerbation	233 days	82 days	0.003

The beneficial effects of IVIg on relapse rate are comparable to those found in the trials of interferon-β and copolymer 1 and, therefore, support the use of monthly IVIg in patients with relapsing-remitting MS.

Is There a Role for Cyclophosphamide in the Treatment of Multiple Sclerosis?

The question of whether there is a role for cyclophosphamide in the treatment of MS has been the subject of four major studies, and there is no agreement between the various investigators.

In the first study by Hauser et al.,[17] 58 patients with severe progressive MS were randomized to 2–3 weeks of treatment with one of three regimens. Twenty patients received intravenous ACTH, 20 were treated with high-dose intravenous cyclophosphamide plus ACTH, and 18 received a combination of low-dose oral cyclophosphamide, plasma exchange, and ACTH. A variety of quantitative scoring systems including the Kurtzke EDSS were used to evaluate whether patients were improved, unchanged, or worse after treatment. Over the 1-year period of follow-up, progression of disease was stabilized (unchanged or worse) in 80% (n = 16) of patients treated with high-dose cyclophosphamide plus ACTH, as compared to 50% (n = 9) in the plasma exchange group and 20% (n = 4) in the intravenous ACTH alone group. The beneficial effect in the first year was not sustained during more prolonged follow-up.

On the basis of these positive preliminary results, the Northeast Cooperative Multiple Sclerosis Treatment Group was formed to evaluate further the therapeutic potential of cyclophosphamide.[18] These investigators randomized 261 patients with progressive MS to one of four treatment groups. All patients received induction therapy with cyclophosphamide/ACTH with one of two regimens. Groups 1 and 2 received 125 mg cyclophosphamide intravenously four times a day over 8–18 days until the white blood cell count fell to below 4,000/mm³ plus intravenous ACTH (this was the regimen used in the study by Hauser et al.[17]). Groups 3 and 4 received cyclophosphamide at a dose of 600 mg/m² intravenously on days 1, 2, 4, 6, and 8 as well as intramuscular ACTH for 14 days. After this induction therapy, patients in groups 2 and 4 received 700 mg/m² intravenously every 2 months over a 2-year period, whereas patients in groups 2 and 3 received no further therapy. In this way, the two different induction regimens both with and without intermittent pulse therapy could be compared. The EDSS and the ambulation index were used to monitor the progression of disability. Follow-up was performed at 12 and 24 months, with patients categorized as *stabilized* (no change in EDSS score), *improved* (one-point decrease on the EDSS), or as *not responding to treatment*.

There were no differences in the response to treatment with the two induction regimens. However, the administration of intermittent pulse therapy was associated with a small but significant slowing of disease progression at 24 months (that was not apparent before 18 months). For those receiving pulse therapy, 16% had improved and 22% were stable compared to 9% improved and 15% stable in those who received no further therapy after cyclophosphamide/ACTH induction.

These findings need to be balanced against the evidence provided by two other studies that found no benefit from cyclophosphamide. The Canadian Cooperative Multiple Sclerosis Study Group[19] recruited 168 patients who were randomized to receive one of two active treatments or placebo. The intravenous cyclophosphamide group received 1 g daily on alternate days, until white blood cell count fell below 4,500/mm³, plus oral prednisone; the plasmapheresis group received weekly exchanges for 20 weeks as well as oral cyclophosphamide for 22 weeks and alternate-day prednisone for 22 weeks. The primary outcome analysis was based on treatment failure, defined as a worsening of one point on the EDSS that was sustained for at least 6 months. All patients were followed for at least 1 year (and others for up to 30 months). There were no statistically significant differences in the cumulative proportion of treatment failures between the different treatment groups—35% in the cyclophosphamide-treated group, 32% in the plasma exchange group, and 29% in the placebo-treated group.

One possible explanation for the discrepant results between the Canadian and Northeast Cooperative studies is the relatively poor outcome in the control group in the latter study. Hauser and colleagues found that only four (20%) of ACTH-treated patients (controls) were stable or improved at 1 year compared to 36 patients (75%) in the placebo-treated group in the Canadian study. The 75% stabilization rate is more consistent with that reported in other treatment trials and studies of the natural history of MS.[20]

The data, therefore, supporting the use of cyclophosphamide in patients with progressive disease remain controversial. Any decision to use cyclophosphamide should be made with this in mind with a clear understanding of the toxicity and potential long-term complications.

Does Monthly Mitoxantrone Therapy Have an Effect on Relapse Rate or Progression of Disability?

Edan et al. evaluated the efficacy of mitoxantrone in a group of patients with very active disease.[21] Patients were identified by a two-step selection process. The clinical inclusion criteria required the presence of at least two exacerbations or progression of two EDSS points within the previous year. Eligible patients had three MRI scans performed monthly, and only those with at least one active MRI lesion during this period were finally admitted to the study. In this way, 21 patients were randomized to receive monthly intravenous mitoxantrone (20 mg) and intravenous methylprednisolone (1 g), and 21 patients were randomized to receive only intravenous methylprednisolone (1 g). The primary outcome measure was the proportion of patients developing new enhancing lesions on monthly gadolinium-enhanced scans performed during the 6-month follow-up period. The results are summarized in Table 12-7.

Adverse events occurred more frequently in the mitoxantrone group, with eight out of 15 women developing amenorrhea that was permanent in one patient. No cardiotoxicity was observed. These results suggest some efficacy of mitoxantrone on both clinical and MRI measures, but they should be interpreted with caution given that neither patients nor investigators were blinded during the study.

In a second controlled trial of mitoxantrone, Millefiorini et al.[22] randomized 51 patients to receive either monthly intravenous mitoxantrone (8

TABLE 12-7
Effects of Mitoxantrone and Steroids on the Course of Multiple Sclerosis

Outcome Measure	Mitoxantrone + IVMP	IVMP	p Value
Percentage of patients without new enhancing lesion (mo 6)	90.5	31.3	<0.001
Range of mean number of new enhancing lesions per month (mos 0–6)	0.1–2.6	2.9–12.3	<0.001 to <0.05
Change in EDSS score (mo 6)	−1.1	−0.1	0.05
Percentage of patients with one EDSS point improvement (mo 6)	57.0	14.3	<0.01
Number of exacerbations (during 6-mo period)	5	19	—
Exacerbation-free patients (during 6-mo period)	14	7	—

EDSS = Expanded Disability Status Scale; IVMP = intravenous methylprednisolone.

TABLE 12-8
Effects of Mitoxantrone on the Course of Multiple Sclerosis

Outcome Measure	Mitoxantrone	Placebo	p Value
Percentage of patients with ≥1 Expanded Disability Status Scale point progression (over 2 yrs)	2/27 (7%)	9/24 (37%)	0.02
Mean number of annual exacerbations*	0.89	2.62	0.0002
Exacerbation-free patients*	17/27 (63%)	5/24 (21%)	0.006
Mean number of new T2 lesions (over 2 yrs)	3.5	7.3	0.05

*Evaluating physicians were not blinded for these outcome measures.

mg/m^2) or placebo for 1 year. They recruited patients with relapsing-remitting MS with at least two exacerbations within the previous 2 years and EDSS scores of 2–5. The primary outcome measure was the proportion of patients with confirmed progression of at least one EDSS point. Evaluating physicians were blinded to treatment, and an effort was also made to blind patients to the treatment allocation. There was, however, no post hoc blinding analysis to determine the efficacy of the measures taken to ensure blinding. The results of this study are summarized in Table 12-8.

These two studies were somewhat different in their design and the patient populations studied. Patients in the Edan study had more severe disease than those in the Millefiorini study. The latter was also a placebo-controlled trial with blinding for the primary outcome measure. There was no placebo arm in the former study, and mitoxantrone was used in combination with methylprednisolone. The duration of follow-up was also brief in the study by Edan and colleagues, making it difficult to be sure whether the beneficial effects observed over a short period of follow-up would be sustained over a longer period. In this sense, these two studies are complementary and suggest that monthly mitoxantrone may be of benefit in reducing the relapse rate and the progression of disability in patients with relapsing-remitting MS and SP-MS.

Summary

- The MRI characteristics of lesions that are most likely to reflect their being a manifestation of MS are gadolinium enhancement and infratentorial, juxtacortical, or periventricular location.
- Intravenous methylprednisolone enhances the rate of recovery from MS flares.
- Oral steroid regimens may be as effective as high-dose intravenous methylprednisolone in the treatment of acute relapses of MS.

- Systemic interferon-β reduces the annual risk of relapse by about 30%.
- Systemic interferon-β reduces the accumulation of disability in patients with both relapsing-remitting MS and SP-MS.
- Early initiation of interferon-β therapy at the time of first presentation in patients at high risk of developing MS slows the rate of progression to MS, but whether this will translate into a beneficial effect on disability remains unclear.
- Copolymer 1 (glatiramer acetate) reduces the rate of relapse by approximately 30%, but its effect on the accumulation of disability remains unclear.
- Monthly administration of IVIg reduces the rate of relapse to an extent similar to that of interferon-β and glatiramer acetate.
- The evidence for a beneficial effect of cyclophosphamide in reducing the accumulation of disability remains controversial.
- There are two randomized controlled trials (one with a placebo arm) that suggest a benefit of monthly mitoxantrone on both clinical and MRI outcome measures.

References

1. McDonald WI, Compston A, Edan G, et al. Recommended diagnostic criteria for multiple sclerosis: guidelines from the international panel on the diagnosis of multiple sclerosis. *Ann Neurol* 2001;50:121–127.
2. Barkhof F, Filippi M, Miller DH, et al. Comparison of MRI criteria at first presentation to predict conversion to clinically definite multiple sclerosis. *Brain* 1997;120:2059–2069.
3. Milligan, NM, Newcombe R, Compston DA. A double-blind controlled trial of high dose methyl-prednisolone in patients with multiple sclerosis: 1. Clinical effects. *J Neurol Neurosurg Psychiatry* 1987;50:511–516.
4. Alam SM, Kyriakides T, Lawden M, Newman PK. Methylprednisolone in multiple sclerosis: a comparison of oral with intravenous therapy at equivalent high dose. *J Neurol Neurosurg Psychiatry* 1993;56:1219–1220.
5. Barnes D, Hughes RA, Morris RW, et al. Randomised trial of oral and intravenous methyprednisolone in acute relapses of multiple sclerosis. *Lancet* 1997;349:902–906.
6. Interferon beta-1b is effective in relapsing-remitting multiple sclerosis. I. Clinical results of a multicenter, randomized, double-blind, placebo-controlled trial. The IFNB Multiple Sclerosis Study Group. *Neurology* 1993;43:655–661.
7. Interferon beta-1b in the treatment of multiple sclerosis: final outcome of the randomized controlled trial. The IFNB Multiple Sclerosis Study Group and the University of British Columbia MS/MRI Analysis Group. *Neurology* 1995;45:1277–1285.

8. Jacobs LD, Cookfair DL, Rudick RA, et al. Intramuscular interferon beta-1a for disease progression in relapsing multiple sclerosis. The Multiple Sclerosis Collaborative Research Group. *Ann Neurol* 1996;39:285–294.

9. Randomised double-blind placebo-controlled study of interferon beta-1a in relapsing/remitting multiple sclerosis. PRISMS (Prevention of Relapses and Disability by Interferon beta-1a Subcutaneously in Multiple Sclerosis) Study Group. *Lancet* 1998;352:1498–1504.

10. Placebo-controlled multicentre randomised trial of interferon-β1b in treatment of secondary progressive multiple sclerosis. European Study Group on Interferon-beta-1b in Secondary Progressive MS. *Lancet* 1998;352:1491–1497.

11. Randomized controlled trial of interferon-beta-1a in secondary progressive MS: clinical results. Secondary Progressive Efficacy Clinical Trial of Recombinant Interferon-beta-1a in MS (SPECTRIMS) Study Group. *Neurology* 2001;56:1496–1504.

12. Jacobs LD, Beck RW, Simon JH, et al. Intramuscular interferon beta-1a therapy initiated during a first demyelinating event in multiple sclerosis. CHAMPS Study Group. *N Engl J Med* 2000;343:898–904.

13. Comi G, Filippi M, Barkhof F, et al. Effect of early interferon treatment on conversion to definite multiple sclerosis: a randomized study. *Lancet* 2001;357:1576–1582.

14. Johnson KP, Brooks BR, Cohen JA, et al. Copolymer 1 reduces relapse rate and improves disability in relapsing-remitting multiple sclerosis: results of a phase III multicenter, double-blind, placebo-controlled trial. The Copolymer 1 Multiple Sclerosis Study Group. *Neurology* 1995;45:1268–1276.

15. Fazekas F, Deisenhammer F, Strasser-Fuchs S, et al. Randomized placebo-controlled trial of monthly intravenous immunoglobulin therapy in relapsing-remitting multiple sclerosis. Austrian Immunoglobulin in Multiple Sclerosis Study Group. *Lancet* 1997;349:589–593.

16. Achiron A, Gabbay U, Gilad R, et al. Intravenous immunoglobulin treatment in multiple sclerosis: effect on relapses. *Neurology* 1998;50:398–402.

17. Hauser SL, Dawson DM, Lehrich JR, et al. Intensive immunosuppression in progressive multiple sclerosis. A randomized, three-arm study of high-dose intravenous cyclophosphamide, plasma exchange and ACTH. *N Engl J Med* 1983;308:173–180.

18. Weiner HL, Mackin GA, Orav EJ, et al. Intermittent cyclophosphamide pulse therapy in progressive multiple sclerosis: final report of the Northeast Cooperative Multiple Sclerosis Treatment Group. *Neurology* 1993;43:910–918.

19. The Canadian cooperative trial of cyclophosphamide and plasma exchange in progressive multiple sclerosis. The Canadian Cooperative Multiple Sclerosis Study Group. *Lancet* 1991;337:441–446.

20. Weinshenker BG, Bass B, Rice GP, et al. The natural history of multiple sclerosis: a geographically based study. I. Clinical course and disability. *Brain* 1989;112:133–146.

21. Edan G, Miller D, Clanet M, et al. Therapeutic effect of motoxantrome com-
    bined with methylprednisolone in multiple sclerosis: a randomized multicen-
    tre study of active disease using MRI and clinical criteria. *J Neurol Neurosurg
    Psychiatry* 1997;62:112–118.
22. Millefiorini E, Gasperini C, Pozzilli C, et al. Randomized placebo-controlled
    trial of mitoxantrone in relapsing-remitting multiple sclerosis: 24-month clin-
    ical and MRI outcome. *J Neurol* 1997;244:153–159.

CHAPTER 13

Guillain-Barré Syndrome

Introduction

The Guillain-Barré syndrome (GBS) is classically an acute demyelinating polyradiculoneuropathy, characterized clinically by the acute onset of symmetric weakness and areflexia with relatively minor sensory impairment. Cerebrospinal fluid analysis characteristically yields an elevated protein concentration but little or no pleocytosis, and the electrophysiology reveals evidence of demyelination. Over the years, however, unusual variants of this syndrome have been recognized, including an axonal form.

GBS is the most common cause of acute neuromuscular paralysis in developed countries, affecting one to two people per 100,000 annually. The mortality is approximately 10%, and approximately 20% of patients are left with significant motor disability. Plasmapheresis and intravenous immunoglobulin (IVIg) have become the mainstay of therapy, and steroids are thought not to be beneficial. What is the evidence that plasmapheresis and IVIg are beneficial to patients with GBS, and what is the nature of this benefit? Do these forms of treatment affect the ultimate degree of disability, or do they simply hasten recovery? Are there any clinical parameters that may be used to predict prognosis? These and other questions are the subjects of this chapter.

Is There a Role for Steroids?

A role for intravenous methylprednisolone in the treatment of patients with GBS was investigated in the Guillain-Barré Syndrome Steroid Trial Group study.[1] This was a double-blind, placebo-controlled trial in which the active treatment comprised intravenous methylprednisolone, 500 mg per day for 5 days. Patients were eligible for inclusion if disease was of sufficient severity to preclude running and if neurologic symptoms had begun within the preceding 15 days. The study randomized a total of 240 patients, and disease severity was scored on a six-point scale (see Appendix 11 [Guillain-Barré Syndrome Six-Point Scale]). The predetermined primary outcome measure was a 0.5-grade difference in disability grade between the

TABLE 13-1
Effects of Steroids on Outcome in the Guillain-Barré Syndrome

Outcome Measure	Steroids	Placebo
Mean change in disability grade at 4 wks	0.8	0.73
Median time to discontinue ventilation (days)	18	27
Median time to reach grade 2/walk unaided (days)	38	50

steroid- and placebo-treated groups at 4 weeks (as used by the Plasma Exchange/Sandoglobulin Guillain-Barré Syndrome Trial Group). The results of this study are summarized in Table 13-1.

None of these results reached statistical significance. It is relevant to note, however, that 53% of patients in the steroid-treated group and 65% of patients in the placebo-treated group also received plasmapheresis. It is at least theoretically possible that the greater use of plasmapheresis in the placebo-treated group may have biased the study against a therapeutic benefit of steroids. The investigators dismiss this possibility based on their multiple regression analysis that did not reveal a significant beneficial effect of plasmapheresis.

What Is the Role of Plasmapheresis?

The two major prospective randomized studies that compared plasmapheresis with best supportive care in patients with the GBS were performed by the American Guillain-Barré Syndrome Study Group[2] and the French Cooperative Study Group.[3]

The American Guillain-Barré Syndrome Study randomized 245 patients to plasmapheresis versus best conventional therapy. Patients with mild disease or those younger than 12 years were excluded. Clinical evaluation comprised assessment on a six-point scale (with grade 2 representing the ability to walk without assistance). Primary outcome measures were specified in advance as (1) number of patients who improved one grade at 4 weeks after randomization, (2) the time taken to improve by one grade, and (3) the time taken to reach grade 2. The intention to evaluate clinical outcome at 6 months was planned in advance, but the nature of the measures used at this time was not specified. Neither patients nor physicians were blinded to the treatment used. Both groups were equivalent in terms of demographic profile. The results are summarized in Table 13-2.

This study clearly demonstrated that plasmapheresis increases the rate of clinical recovery, and this effect was particularly marked in patients who were treated within 7 days of the onset of symptoms and in those who

TABLE 13-2
Effects of Plasmapheresis on Guillain-Barré Syndrome (the American Guillain-Barré Syndrome Study Group)

Outcome Measure	Best Conventional Therapy	Plasmapheresis	p Value
No. of patients improving one grade at 4 wks	39%	59%	<0.01
Time to improve one grade (days)	40	19	<0.001
Time to reach grade 2 (days)	85	53	<0.001
Duration of ventilation (days)*	23	9	<0.05
Failure to improve one clinical grade at 6 mos	13%	3%	<0.01
Improved by one clinical grade at 6 mos	75%	74%	Not significant
Unable to walk without assistance at 6 mos (i.e., failure to reach grade 2)	29%	18%	<0.05

*In patients who required ventilation only after randomization.

required a ventilator after randomization. The outcome measures at 6 months, however, are more difficult to interpret, with results reported in terms of the number of patients who did not improve one clinical grade, with a smaller proportion (3% vs. 13%) in those who received plasmapheresis. However, closer inspection reveals that a similar proportion (75% vs. 74%) in each group did improve by one clinical grade. The difference between those who did improve by one grade in the conventional treatment group and those who did not, comprises those patients who are listed as "treatment failures" in the plasmapheresis-treated group. These "treatment failures" represent those patients who did not complete the course of plasmapheresis. The second outcome measure reported at 6 months was the number of patients who did not reach grade 2 (i.e., able to ambulate without assistance). Here the percentages were 18% and 29% for plasmapheresis and conventional therapy, respectively—a difference that is statistically significant (p <0.05). It is perhaps surprising that the results were not expressed as the number of patients who reached grade 2, but these numbers cannot be calculated from the data provided. The overall impression is that the data for better final outcome in those treated with plasmapheresis are not very convincing.

The French Cooperative Study randomized 220 patients to treatment with or without plasmapheresis. Patients with disease of any severity were included (although, by happenstance, there was a tendency to recruit patients with more severe disease), provided that age was older than 16

TABLE 13-3
Effects of Plasmapheresis on Guillain-Barré Syndrome (French Cooperative Study)

Outcome Measure	Control	Plasmapheresis	p Value
Time to recover walking with assistance (days)*	44	30	<0.011
Time to onset of motor recovery (days)	13	6	<0.005
Time to begin ventilatory wean (days)	31	18	<0.01
Time to recover walking without assistance (days)	111	70	<0.001

*Primary outcome measure.

years and motor symptoms had begun within the preceding 17 days. Neither patients nor physicians were blinded. Clinical assessment was made using binary measures on 28 tests of motor function (see Appendix 7 [French Cooperative Guillain-Barré Syndrome Study: Functional Testing Scale]). The primary outcome measure was the time to recover the ability to walk with assistance. Secondary outcome measures included (1) change in score, (2) number of patients requiring ventilation after randomization, (3) time to onset of motor recovery (defined as a gain of two items on the functional score), (4) time to begin ventilatory wean, and (5) time to walk without assistance. There were no differences in patient demographics between the treatment and control groups, with mean time from symptom onset to randomization of 6.5 days, mean functional score of 48, and 37% already ventilated at the time of randomization. The results are summarized in Table 13-3. The results of 1-year follow-up of the patients from the French Cooperative Study were subsequently published[4] and are summarized in Table 13-4.

This study also provided clear evidence of an increased rate of recovery in patients treated with plasmapheresis. The evidence for improved

TABLE 13-4
Effects of Plasmapheresis on Guillain-Barré Syndrome (French Cooperative Study)

Outcome Measure at 1 Yr	Control (%)	Plasmapheresis (%)	p Value
Complete recovery	37	60	0.001
Return to work	67	76	NS
Full muscular strength recovery	52	71	0.007
Severe disability	11	11	NS

NS = not significant.

final outcome, however, is again less convincing in part because there was no clear explanation for the difference between the percentage of patients who made a complete recovery and the percentage who were able to return to work. It is possible that inability to make a complete recovery might simply have entailed an absent reflex or mild sensory disturbance, which might not represent a clinically important difference. This, however, is purely speculative, as adequate data are not provided.

What Is the Role of Intravenous Immunoglobulin?

The evidence for the benefit of IVIg is derived from two prospective randomized studies that compared plasmapheresis and IVIg. The first of these was published by the Dutch Guillain-Barré Syndrome Study Group.[5] This trial randomized 150 patients to receive either plasmapheresis or IVIg. Only patients who were unable to walk without assistance and whose symptoms had begun within the preceding 2 weeks were eligible for randomization. Children younger than 4 years were excluded. Clinical assessment was made using the same six-point scale used by the American Guillain-Barré Syndrome Study Group, supplemented by a 60-point Medical Research Council grading system (six muscles on each side, with strength graded from 0 to 5). The last follow-up was performed 6 months after randomization. Physicians were partially blinded (i.e., one of two physicians were blinded at the time of evaluation, and the blinded and nonblinded scores were compared). The primary outcome measure was improvement of at least one grade on the six-point functional scale 4 weeks after randomization. Secondary outcome measures included the time required to improve at least one functional grade and the time required to recover independent ambulation (these outcome measures were all also used by the American Guillain-Barré Syndrome Study Group). The results are summarized in Table 13-5.

TABLE 13-5
Effect of Intravenous Immunoglobulin on Guillain-Barré Syndrome (the Dutch Guillain-Barré Syndrome Study Group)

Outcome Measure	Plasma Exchange	Intravenous Immunoglobulin	p Value
Number improved by one grade at 4 wks	34%	53%	0.024
Time to improve one grade (days)	41	27	0.05
Time to recover independent ambulation (days)	69	55	0.07
Number requiring assisted ventilation	42%	27%	<0.05

TABLE 13-6
Plasma Exchange (PE)/Sandoglobulin Guillain-Barré Syndrome Trial Group

Outcome Measure	PE	IVIg	PE + IVIg
Mean change in disability grade at 4 wks	0.9	0.8	1.1
Time to discontinuation of ventilation (days)	29	26	18
Time to walk unaided (days)	49	51	40

IVIg = intravenous immunoglobulin.

This study clearly demonstrated the efficacy of IVIg in the treatment of patients with severe GBS. Furthermore, the data suggest that IVIg might be even more efficacious than plasma exchange (PE). The nature of the benefit, however, is explicit in terms of rate of recovery but not in terms of whether treatment alters the ultimate outcome or degree of recovery.

It is interesting to note that only 34% of patients treated with PE had improved by one grade at 4 weeks after randomization. In comparison, in the American Guillain-Barré Syndrome Study Group, 59% of patients treated with PE improved by one grade at 4 weeks. The authors of this study suggest that this discrepancy might have been due to their enrolling patients sooner after the onset of their illness. The implication is that patients in the early stages of the disease may still deteriorate further and, therefore, take longer to recover to an equivalent functional grade.

The Plasma Exchange/Sandoglobulin Guillain-Barré Syndrome Trial Group[6] randomized 383 patients to receive PE, IVIg, or a combination of the two (PE followed by IVIg).*

Only patients older than 16 years and with severe disease (unable to walk without assistance) were eligible for inclusion in the study. The six-point disability scale used by the American and Dutch Guillain-Barré Syndrome Study groups was used to evaluate patients clinically. Patient demographics at randomization were similar in all treatment groups, with average duration of illness before randomization being 1 week. The aim of the study was to determine whether IVIg was equivalent or superior to PE and whether PE followed by IVIg was superior to either treatment alone. A difference of half a grade at 4 weeks between two treatment groups was specified in advance as being indicative of a difference in treatment-related outcome. Secondary outcome measures included time to walking unaided, time to discontinuation of ventilatory support, and the average rate of recovery. The results are summarized in Table 13-6.

There were no significant differences in any of the outcome measures between the plasmapheresis-treated and the IVIg-treated groups. As in the

*The results of the combination therapy are discussed in the next section.

Dutch study, patients with a longer duration of disease before randomization had a better outcome at 4 weeks. The explanation offered is that these patients were further along the natural history of the disease and, hence, more likely to show spontaneous recovery. In addition, patients with more severe disease would be expected to present early (and, therefore, be randomized sooner in the course of the disease).

Is There a Role for Combining Plasmapheresis and Intravenous Immunoglobulin?

The Plasma Exchange/Sandoglobulin Guillain-Barré Syndrome Trial Group Study[6] included three treatment arms with some patients receiving only plasmapheresis, others receiving IVIg alone, and yet others receiving plasmapheresis followed by IVIg. As shown in Table 13-6, there were no significant differences in any of the outcome measures between any of the different treatment groups. Taking into account various prognostic factors, repeat statistical analysis suggested that there were marginal benefits to the combination of PE and IVIg with regard to the primary outcome measure (disability at 4 weeks).

Which Factors Affect Prognosis?

The issue of prognosis in GBS has been addressed by a number of studies. Presented here are the results of the two studies that examined prognosis in the prospective randomized treatment trials.

McKhann et al.[7] performed a multivariate analysis on the data obtained from the American Guillain-Barré Syndrome Study Group's prospective randomized investigation of plasmapheresis in GBS.[1] This study identified severely reduced (less than 20% of normal) distal compound muscle action potential amplitude as the most important prognostic factor, with (1) the requirement for mechanical ventilation at the time of randomization, (2) shorter (fewer than 7 days) duration of illness before randomization, and (3) older age, also independently predictive of a worse outcome. Apart from age, which was analyzed as a continuous variable, the other three prognostic factors were analyzed in a dichotomous fashion. Over and above each of these prognostic variables, the outcome was better in patients who received plasmapheresis. Of note is that the outcome was better in patients treated with continuous rather than intermittent cycle exchange.

Visser et al.[8] examined the data of the Dutch Guillain-Barré Syndrome Trial[3] to identify prognostic factors. Potential factors identified in a univariate analysis were then tested in a multivariate analysis in rank order according to the sequence in which they became available in the clinical setting. Using this novel approach, they identified a preceding gastrointestinal illness, older age (older than 50 years), presence of more severe disease, and a recent cytomegalovirus infection as predictive of a poor early (8-week) outcome. The same clinical features were identified at the 6-month endpoint, with the additional factor of a rapid (fewer than 4 days) onset of weakness.

The results of these two studies are largely in agreement with each other, identifying older age, the rapidity of progression of symptoms, and the presence of more severe disease (measured by the requirement for mechanical ventilation in the American study) as poor prognostic indicators. These studies differed, however, in that distal compound muscle action potential amplitude was identified as an important prognostic indicator in the American study but not the Dutch study. Similarly, the nature of the antecedent infectious illness appeared to be significant only in the Dutch study.

Summary

- The available evidence suggests that intravenous methylprednisolone is ineffective in the treatment of patients with GBS.
- There is good evidence that PE and IVIg are each effective forms of therapy in patients with GBS, as measured by the rate of clinical recovery.
- PE is most effective when performed early in the course of the illness.
- There is no good evidence that the combination of PE and IVIg is superior to either treatment alone.
- In some of the studies, the complication rate associated with IVIg was lower than that associated with PE, suggesting that this should be the first line of treatment.
- Outcome measures and methods of clinical evaluation have differed between the studies; their results are summarized in Table 13-7.
- The evidence that final outcome is improved by any form of treatment is less clear. The follow-up data from the French Cooperative

TABLE 13-7
Summary of the Effects of Plasmapheresis in Guillain-Barré Syndrome

Outcome Measure	American[2]	French[3,4]	Dutch[5]
Number of patients improved one grade at 4 wk	59%	Not applicable	34%
Time to independent ambulation (days)	53	70	69

Study suggest that this is the case, but the outcome measures used are a little dubious.

- There is no clear advantage to the use of one type of replacement fluid (albumin or fresh frozen plasma) during PE, but continuous cycle exchange is superior to intermittent cycle.

References

1. Double-blind trial of intravenous methylprednisolone in Guillain-Barré syndrome. Guillain-Barré Syndrome Steroid Trial Group. *Lancet* 1993;341:586–590.
2. Plasmapheresis and acute Guillain-Barré syndrome. The Guillain-Barré Syndrome Study Group. *Neurology* 1985;35:1096–1104.
3. Efficiency of plasma exchange in Guillain-Barré syndrome: role of replacement fluids. French Cooperative Study on Plasma Exchange in Guillain-Barré Syndrome. *Ann Neurol* 1987;22:753–761.
4. Plasma exchange in Guillain-Barré syndrome: one-year follow-up. French Cooperative Group on Plasma Exchange in Guillain-Barré Syndrome. *Ann Neurol* 1992;32:94–97.
5. van der Meche FG, Schmitz PI. A randomized trial comparing intravenous immune globulin and plasma exchange in Guillain-Barré syndrome. Dutch Guillain-Barré Syndrome Study group. *N Engl J Med* 1992;326:1123–1129.
6. Randomized trial of plasma exchange, intravenous immunoglobulin, and combined treatments in Guillain-Barré syndrome. Plasma Exchange/Sandoglobulin Guillain-Barré Syndrome Trial Group. *Lancet* 1997;349:225–230.
7. McKhann GM, Griffin JW, Cornblath DR, et al. Plasmapheresis and Guillain-Barré Syndrome: analysis of prognostic factors and the effect of plasmapheresis. *Ann Neurol* 1988;23:347–353.
8. Visser LH, Schmitz PI, Meulstee J, et al. Prognostic factors of Guillain-Barré syndrome after intravenous immunoglobulin or plasma exchange. Dutch Guillain-Barré Study Group. *Neurology* 1999;53:598–604.

CHAPTER 14

Chronic Inflammatory Demyelinating Polyradiculoneuropathy

Introduction

Chronic inflammatory demyelinating polyradiculoneuropathy (CIDP) is an acquired immune-mediated sensorimotor demyelinating polyneuropathy. It is characterized clinically by fairly symmetric motor and sensory deficits in the proximal and distal limbs. The onset is usually insidious over months to years. The course either may be relapsing and remitting or chronically progressive. CIDP may occur in isolation or in the context of a number of systemic disorders, including human immunodeficiency virus, hepatitis C infection, inflammatory bowel disease, lymphoproliferative disease, and osteosclerotic myeloma. The importance of distinguishing CIDP from other causes of peripheral neuropathy lies in the observation that a significant proportion of patients with CIDP may respond to immune-modifying therapy. Which forms of immunotherapy should be used in the treatment of patients with CIDP, and what is their relative efficacy? Are there any clinical features that may help to predict which patients are likely to respond to immunotherapy? These and other questions are the subject of this chapter.

What Is the Evidence That Steroids Are of Benefit to Patients with Chronic Inflammatory Demyelinating Polyradiculoneuropathy?

The utility of prednisone in the treatment of CIDP was demonstrated by Dyck et al.[1] in a prospective randomized, but uncontrolled, trial. Patients with CIDP who had not previously received immunosuppressive therapy were eligible for inclusion in this study. Patients who fulfilled entry criteria were matched for age and duration of symptoms and then randomized to receive either prednisone or no treatment. Prednisone was initiated at 120 mg every other day, with 5 mg per day on the alternate days, and was tapered over a period of 13 weeks. There were 28 patients who completed

TABLE 14-1
Effects of Steroids on the Outcome in Chronic Inflammatory
Demyelinating Polyradiculoneuropathy

Change in Neurological Disability Score	No-Treatment Group*	Prednisone Group*
Worse	8	2
Unchanged	1	0
Improved	5	12

*Values refer to numbers of patients.

the trial with 14 in each group. The Neurological Disability Score (NDS; a summed score of muscle strength, reflexes, and sensory loss; see Appendix 24 [Neurological Disability Score]) was used as a measure of outcome, with patients evaluated at 6 weeks and then at 3 months. The results are summarized in Table 14-1. In the no-treatment group, the mean NDS change was –1.5 compared with +10 points in the prednisone-treated group. The conclusion was that prednisone leads to a small but significant improvement in disability in previously untreated patients with CIDP.

Is Plasmapheresis Effective in the Treatment of Patients with Chronic Inflammatory Demyelinating Polyradiculoneuropathy?

The role of plasmapheresis has been examined in two prospective placebo-controlled trials.[2,3] In the first, Dyck et al.[2] randomized 34 patients with CIDP to receive plasma exchange (PE) or sham exchange. Randomization was restricted according to age (younger than 50 years or 50 years and older), gender, and NDS (less than 100 or at least 100). The controlled trial lasted 3 weeks, whereafter those who received sham exchange were offered PE (open trial). Neurologic evaluation was performed at weekly intervals for the duration of the controlled and open trials. Evaluation included measurement of NDS, dynamometer measurement of maximal handgrip strength, maximal finger pinch, and maximal inspiratory and expiratory pressures as well as sensory thresholds. Nerve conduction studies were performed both before and after PE. Twenty-nine patients completed the controlled study—15 assigned to PE and 14 to sham exchange. No subjective differences were reported between patients randomized to the two treatment groups. At 3 weeks, five patients receiving PE had an improvement in NDS compared to baseline (change in NDS) that exceeded the largest improvement attained by any patient who received sham exchange. The authors describe these results as "striking differences . . . between the two treatment groups," but it should be noted that there was significant overlap in the change in NDS between the two treatment groups and results for mean change in NDS for the two treatment groups not reported. Improvement in nerve conduction indexes favored PE, but this observation is tempered by the observation of almost significant differences in these indexes between the treatment groups at baseline.

Building on these results, Hahn et al.[3] designed a double-blind, placebo-controlled trial of PE in patients with CIDP. They recruited only patients who had not previously and were not concurrently receiving other forms of immunosuppressive therapy. Eighteen patients were randomized to receive either PE or sham exchange (10 exchanges over a 4-week period), followed by a washout phase; patients were then crossed over for 1 month of the alternate therapy, followed by a second washout phase. The outcome measures employed were similar to those used in the Mayo study[2] to facilitate comparison of the results of the two studies. Three of the 18 patients did not complete the trial, but the results are reported in an intention-to-treat analysis. With PE, significant improvement was observed on all outcome measures. A substantial improvement in neurologic function was found in 12 of 15 (80%) patients with a mean NDS change of 38 points for the group as a whole. This improvement was typically evident within days of starting treatment. Significant improvements in electrophysiologic measures (motor nerve conduction velocity, distal latency, and compound muscle action potential amplitude) were also found. Eight of the 12 patients (66%) who improved with PE subsequently relapsed after stopping PE, with the deterioration occurring within 7–14 days of the last exchange. The authors conclude that a beneficial effect from PE could be expected early in the course of CIDP provided that the clinical, electrophysiologic, and histologic features were those of primary demyelination without secondary axonal loss. The results of this study were more impressive than the initial study of PE by Dyck et al.[2] (80% vs. 33% rate of improvement). This difference may relate, at least in part, to the more aggressive schedule of PE employed in this study.

Is Intravenous Immunoglobulin Effective in the Treatment of Patients with Chronic Inflammatory Demyelinating Polyradiculoneuropathy?

The efficacy of intravenous immunoglobulin (IVIg) in the treatment of patients with CIDP has been the subject of two double-blind, placebo-controlled studies.[4,5] The earlier study (1996),[4] which employed a crossover design, included 30 patients (16 with chronic progressive and 14 with relapsing disease) who were randomized to receive either 0.4 g/kg of IVIg or placebo for 5 consecutive days. Patients remained in a particular treatment arm for 28 days and were then crossed over to receive the alternate treatment. Prior immunosuppressive therapy did not constitute an exclusion criterion, but concurrent immunosuppressive therapy (except for low-dose prednisone) was not permitted. The same outcome measures employed in the PE studies (NDS, grip strength, clinical grade, and electrophysiologic parameters) were used in this study. There was a significant improvement in all outcome measures amongst those treated with IVIg. A response to IVIg treatment was observed in 19 of 30 patients (63%), and the mean NDS improvement was 24.4 points for all patients who received IVIg.

Open follow-up was available for all but one patient after completion of the controlled trial. It became apparent that patients with relapsing CIDP obtained only temporary benefit from any single course of IVIg. A response to repeat courses of IVIg, however, was consistently observed. Although the duration of treatment benefit varied considerably, it could be fairly reliably predicted for each patient. In this way, nine patients were maintained on long-term IVIg pulse therapy, with infusions administered either at the earliest sign of relapse or just before the anticipated relapse. The dose of IVIg could usually be tapered down to less than or equal to 1 mg/kg body weight and administered as a single-day infusion. A few patients required the addition of a small dose of prednisone to their regular IVIg infusions.

More recently (2001), Mendell and colleagues[5] performed a randomized, placebo-controlled trial of IVIg in patients with CIDP who had not previously received any form of immunosuppressive therapy. Patients were randomized to receive either placebo or IVIg (1 g/kg per day) for 2 days. Muscle strength was assessed using a Modified Medical Research Council scale. Other outcome measures included the Hughes Functional Disability Scale (a seven-point scale ranging from healthy to death; see Appendix 14 [Hughes Functional Disability Scale]) as well as various electrophysiologic parameters. Improvement in strength was observed in 76% of IVIg-treated patients, and this improvement was generally notable early (within 10 days). Functional evaluation using the Hughes Functional Disability Scale also favored the IVIg-treated group, with 38% of patients improving at least one functional grade compared to 10% in the placebo-treated group. Trends towards improvement in electrophysiologic measures (distal latency and conduction velocity) were also observed in the IVIg-treated patients. These results support the findings of the study by Hahn,[4] with benefit observed in a similar proportion of patients (63% vs. 76%). The key difference was the inclusion in this latter study of only patients with CIDP who had not previously received any form of immunosuppressive therapy. The study by Mendell et al.[5] also differed in the dose and duration of IVIg as well as the outcome measures used.

How Does Intravenous Immunoglobulin Compare to Plasma Exchange in the Treatment of Patients with Chronic Inflammatory Demyelinating Polyradiculoneuropathy?

IVIg and PE were compared head-to-head in a single (observer) blinded study.[6] This trial included patients with static or worsening disability who had not received PE or IVIg in the preceding 6 weeks and in whom there had been no change in their maintenance immunotherapy within the same time period. PE was performed twice weekly for the first 3 weeks and once weekly for the second 3 weeks. IVIg was administered at a dose of 0.4 mg/kg once per week for the first 3 weeks and 0.2 mg/kg once per week for the second 3 weeks. The 6-week course of PE or IVIg was followed by a washout period of variable duration. Those who did not respond to the initial therapy or who relapsed (to their original level of disability) were then crossed over to receive the alternative therapy. In total, 17 patients were treated with PE and 15 received IVIg. Primary endpoints included NDS, the weakness subset of the NDS, and the summated compound muscle action potential of ulnar, median, and peroneal nerves. Secondary endpoints were the summated sensory nerve action potential of median and sural nerves and vibratory detection threshold of the great toe. Endpoints were examined at the end of each 6-week study period. Patients who received either PE or IVIg (as either the first or second treatment) showed significant and comparable improvement from baseline in all three primary endpoints. Of the 17 patients who received PE in either phase, the mean NDS improvement was 38.3 points. Of the 15 patients who received IVIg in either phase, the mean NDS improvement was 36.1 points. The similar degree of improvement observed with each treatment modality suggests that they are of equal efficacy.

Summary

- The efficacy of the oral prednisone in the management of previously untreated patients with CIDP has been demonstrated in a single randomized, but uncontrolled, trial.
- The efficacy of plasmapheresis in the management of previously untreated patients with CIDP has been demonstrated most convincingly in a prospective placebo-controlled crossover study. Patients received a course of 10 exchanges over 4 weeks, and improvement, discernible within days of starting treatment, was observed in 80%.
- The efficacy of IVIg has been demonstrated in two prospective double-blind, placebo-controlled trials. These two studies differed

in design, dose, and duration of treatment with IVIg as well as outcome measures employed, but the results were similar, with improvement reported in 63–76% of patients. The benefits were generally observed within 10–14 days of the initiation of treatment.
- PE and IVIg were compared head-to-head in a single prospective, randomized study. The treatment regimens used in this study differed from those in the placebo-controlled trials of each of these therapies. Comparable rates of improvement were observed for PE and IVIg based on both clinical and electrophysiologic measures of outcome.

References

1. Dyck PJ, O'Brien PC, Oviatt KF, et al. Prednisone improves chronic inflammatory demyelinating polyradiculoneuropathy more than no treatment. *Ann Neurol* 1982;11:136–141.
2. Dyck PJ, Daube J, O'Brien P, et al. Plasma exchange in chronic inflammatory demyelinating polyradiculoneuropathy. *N Engl J Med* 1986;314:461–465.
3. Hahn AF, Bolton CF, Pillay N, et al. Plasma-exchange therapy in chronic inflammatory demyelinating polyneuropathy. A double-blind, sham-controlled, cross-over study. *Brain* 1996;119:1055–1066.
4. Hahn AF, Bolton CF, Zochodne D, Feasby TE. Intravenous immunoglobulin treatment in chronic inflammatory demyelinating polyneuropathy. A double-blind, placebo-controlled, cross-over study. *Brain* 1996;119:1067–1077.
5. Mendell JR, Barohn RJ, Freimer ML, et al. Randomized controlled trial of IVIg in untreated chronic inflammatory demyelinating polyradiculoneuropathy. *Neurology* 2001;56:445–449.
6. Dyck PJ, Litchy WJ, Kratz KM, et al. A plasma exchange versus immune globulin infusion trial in chronic inflammatory demyelinating polyradiculoneuropathy. *Ann Neurol* 1994;36:838–845.

CHAPTER 15

Myasthenia Gravis

Introduction

Myasthenia gravis (MG) is an autoimmune disorder in which antibodies are either directed against the muscle nicotinic acetylcholine receptor itself or against other postsynaptic targets that indirectly reduce nicotinic acetylcholine receptor numbers. It is the prototypic neurologic autoimmune disorder in which both antigen and antibody have been identified, removal of antibody has been shown to lead to clinical improvement, and the disease can be recreated in mice after passive transfer of the autoantibody. Understandably, therefore, immunosuppressive therapy forms the mainstay of disease-modifying treatment, with acetylcholinesterase inhibitors being reserved for symptomatic management. Notwithstanding the obvious theoretical grounds for using immunosuppressive therapy, it is useful to consider the evidence that supports their use. Which immunosuppressive therapies have been shown to be beneficial in MG? Are the beneficial effects of the different treatment strategies comparable? Is there a role for immunosuppressive therapy in patients who have only ocular disease? These and other questions are the subjects of this chapter.

What Is the Evidence That Steroids Are of Benefit in Patients with Myasthenia Gravis?

The use of corticosteroids in the treatment of MG is an excellent example of a treatment that has become established without ever having been subjected to the rigorous evaluation of a large prospective, placebo-controlled trial. Nevertheless, it is useful to reflect on some of the literature that describes the utility of corticosteroids.

The study by Howard et al.,[1] published in 1976, was the closest approximation to a placebo-controlled trial. Thirteen patients with mild to moderate generalized MG were randomized to receive either prednisone 100 mg on alternate days or placebo. At a 2-year follow-up, three of the six patients in the prednisone-treated group and three of the seven patients who were placebo-treated were improved. The four patients in the placebo group who were unchanged were then treated with prednisone, and an improvement was noted in three of the four. Overall, therefore, 70% of patients who were treated responded to prednisone, but this response rate was not significantly different from that in the placebo group. The failure of this study to demonstrate a beneficial effect of alternate-day prednisone may have been the consequence of its small sample size. Notwithstanding the results of this study, prednisone continued to be used in the treatment of MG.

Sghirlanzoni and colleagues[2] described their experience with 60 patients whom they treated with steroids. They did not use a uniform steroid dosing schedule. Some were treated with a slowly increasing dosage; others received high-dose therapy on alternate days or every day. Once sustained improvement was achieved and maintained for 3–4 months, the dose was gradually reduced by 10% every 5–7 weeks until the lowest maintenance dose was reached. The response to therapy was described as *complete remission* (recovery with no requirement for medication), *pharmacologic remission* (clinical recovery but still requiring pharmacotherapy of some sort), *improvement*, or *nonresponsive*. Overall, improvement was noted in 72% of patients. Those who received higher dosages achieved a clinical response more rapidly, but by 6 months, the response rates were similar in the two treatment groups provided that a dose of 100 mg prednisone on alternate days had been reached. The only baseline characteristic predictive of a better response to corticosteroid therapy was age of onset after the age of 40 years.

Pascuzzi et al.[3] studied 116 patients with MG who were treated with the same steroid regimen and were followed for between 8 months and 17 years. They designated the response to treatment as *satisfactory* (remission or marked improvement) or *unsatisfactory* (unimproved or only moderate improvement). Treatment was initiated with prednisone, 60–80 mg for 3 consecutive days, after which the dosage was changed to an equivalent alternate-day schedule. Dose reductions occurred at a rate of approximately 10 mg every 2 months provided that the patient maintained clinical response. The response was satisfactory in 80% of patients, with marked improvement in 53% and remission in 27%. In those with a satisfactory response, the onset of sustained improvement occurred after a mean of 13 days, and the median time to maximal improvement was 5–6 months. Older age was the strongest predictor of a better response to steroid therapy, but the presence of milder disease and symptoms of shorter duration were also important.

More recently (1992), Evoli and colleagues[4] reported their experience with 104 patients with MG who were treated with steroids. The initial prednisone dose varied from 0.8 to 1.5 mg/kg per day, with the higher doses used for patients with more severe disease. This dose was maintained until improvement was obvious (usually approximately 3 weeks) and was then gradually changed to an alternate-day regimen. Patients were followed for at least 2 years. The response to treatment was classified as *improved* (complete remission, pharmacologic remission, or marked improvement) or *unresponsive* (moderate improvement, no improvement of deterioration).

TABLE 15-1
Summary of Data Relating to the Use of High-Dose Oral Steroids

Response to treatment with high-dose oral steroids	
Frequency of improvement (%)	80[a]–94[b]
Latency to onset of sustained improvement (days)	13[a]–16[b]
Median time to maximal improvement (mos)	5–6[a]
Early deterioration with high-dose oral steroids	
Frequency (%)	21[b]–48[a]
Severe (%)	7.0[b]–8.6[a]
Mean latency to onset of deterioration (days)	4–5[a,b]

[a]Data from RM Pascuzzi, HB Coslett, TR Johns. Long-term corticosteroid treatment of myasthenia gravis: report of 116 patients. *Ann Neurol* 1984;15:291–298.
[b]Data from A Evoli, AP Batocchi, MT Palmisani, et al. Long-term results of corticosteroid therapy in patients with myasthenia gravis. *Eur Neurol* 1992;32:37–43.

Improvement was noted in 98 patients (94%), and the mean time to onset of objective improvement was 16 days. The effects of high-dose steroids in MG are summarized in Table 15-1.

How Problematic Is the Early Clinical Deterioration That May Accompany the Initiation of Steroid Therapy?

The phenomenon of transient worsening of myasthenic symptoms shortly after the initiation of corticosteroid therapy is well recognized. Pascuzzi et al.,[3] for example, reported an early deterioration in 48.0% of patients, in 10 (8.6%) of whom it was severe. The exacerbation occurred between 1 and 17 days after the initiation of therapy (mean onset on day 5). In the retrospective series of Evoli et al.,[4] transient early deterioration with initiation of steroid therapy was observed in 22 patients (21%), in approximately one-third of whom it was severe. Typically, the deterioration occurred at a mean of 4 days after the start of therapy. In the study by Sghirlanzoni and colleagues,[2] a transient deterioration was observed in 38% of patients treated initially with a high dose compared to 19% in those who received a slowly increasing dose. This observation—that the incidence of transient deterioration could be reduced by a gradual initiation of steroid therapy—was not a new one. Seybold and Drachman[5] had previously reported their experience with 12 patients in initiating treatment with low-dose steroids. Transient worsening of myasthenic symptoms was not observed in any of their patients.

In these four series, therefore, the incidence of early deterioration varied from 0% to 48%, with some indication that early deterioration occurred more frequently in those who were treated with early, high-dose steroids.

What Is the Optimal Dosing Schedule When Steroid Therapy Is Initiated?

Broadly speaking, there are two options for the initiation of steroid therapy, high dose and low dose. The philosophy behind initiating therapy with high-dose steroids (e.g., prednisone 1 mg/kg per day) is that the clinical response is more rapid, and lack of response to therapy is not due to "under dosing." The competing argument for initiation with low-dose steroid (e.g., approximately 25 mg prednisone every other day) followed by gradual dosage increments is that the incidence of early deterioration (which may require mechanical ventilation if severe) appears to be less frequent than when therapy is started with high-dose steroids. Other factors that may enter the equation are the severity of the disease (although there is no good evidence indicating whether patients with less severe disease are less likely to experience a marked deterioration) and whether therapy is being initiated in an inpatient or outpatient setting. Although it is difficult to make an evidence-based recommendation, it seems reasonable to begin steroid therapy with a high-dose regimen when patients can be closely monitored and promptly treated if myasthenic symptoms worsen. Low-dose therapy seems more prudent when steroid therapy is initiated in a less-controlled or less-supervised environment.

Is High-Dose Intravenous Methylprednisolone of Any Benefit?

Arsura and colleagues[6] reported rapid improvement in 12 of 15 patients with rapidly progressive severe MG who were treated with high-dose intravenous methylprednisolone (IVMP). Patients received an infusion of 2 g over 12 hours, and this was repeated every 5 days if improvement was limited. Those who improved clinically also received 30 mg prednisone followed by a gradual taper. Satisfactory improvement (defined as being asymptomatic or having only minor symptoms that do not interfere with daily activities) occurred in 10 of 15 patients after the second infusion and in 2 more after the third infusion. Improvement began a mean of 3 days after the first infusion and 2 days after the second infusion and was maximal at approximately 9 days after the last infusion. The latency to clinical improvement, therefore, was substantially shorter than in the studies by Pascuzzi and Evoli, in which the latencies were 13 and 16 days, respectively. At follow-up 15 months later, 10 patients had maintained their level of satisfactory functioning while continuing a prednisone taper.

The efficacy of IVMP in MG was recently evaluated in a small double-blind, placebo controlled trial.[7] Twenty patients with moderate to severe generalized MG with clinical deterioration despite optimal antiacetylcholinesterase therapy were randomized to receive either IVMP (2 g per day for 2 days) or placebo. Apart from two patients in the IVMP group who were taking azathioprine at the time, none of the other patients was receiving any other form of immunosuppressive therapy. A beneficial response to treatment was found in one of nine patients who received placebo and in eight of 10 patients treated with IVMP. The duration of clinical response varied from 4 to 14 weeks. In this study, the degree of initial deterioration after IVMP was not systemically evaluated, but one patient did report moderate worsening of myasthenic symptoms.

These studies show that although the degree and duration of response is variable, high-dose IVMP may be of benefit in a significant proportion of patients with worsening MG. The available data do not adequately inform on the frequency or severity of early deterioration, and a decision to use IVMP in patients with severe MG should also be tempered by the potential for the development of a severe myopathy.

How Effective Is Azathioprine as a Steroid-Sparing or Adjunctive Agent?

In general, the frequency of response to steroids has varied between approximately 70% and 90%. In many of these studies, however, relapses have occurred during attempts to wean the steroid dose. The long-term toxicity associated with prolonged use of relatively high-dose steroids has led to a search for other treatment strategies.

The use of azathioprine in MG has been the subject of many retrospective uncontrolled studies as well as two prospective controlled studies. The Myasthenia Gravis Clinical Study Group[8] randomized patients with severe MG to receive prednisone or azathioprine. Because of the anticipated delayed response to azathioprine, these patients also received prednisone for the first 4 months. Accordingly, the authors felt that the primary outcome of the study should be a measure of long-term outcome that would not be influenced by the early short-term use of prednisone in the azathioprine group. The main endpoint was the time that elapsed before the first episode of meaningful clinical deterioration over the 5-year duration of the study. There were 20 patients in the prednisone group and 21 in the azathioprine group. In total, there were 21 events that met the endpoint criterion of a meaningful clinical deterioration; 12 of these occurred in the prednisone group and nine in the azathioprine group. Although there was no significant difference between the two treatment groups with respect to the time to the first deterioration, the deterioration rate was estimated at 52% and 37% in the prednisone and azathioprine groups, respectively. There are, however, many reasons to be cautious in attributing too much significance to the apparent benefit of azathioprine over prednisone, and the conservative conclusion from this study is that long-term therapy with azathioprine alone is at least as effective as prednisone alone.

In a smaller study of only 10 patients, Bromberg et al.[9] randomized patients with MG previously untreated with immunosuppression to receive either prednisone or azathioprine. Two patients randomized to receive azathioprine were crossed over to receive prednisone because of an idiosyncratic drug response to azathioprine. Only one of the remaining two patients responded to azathioprine. Four patients in the prednisone group responded well to treatment. The two patients who were crossed over early also responded to prednisone, as did the two patients who did not respond to azathioprine within the first year of treatment. The authors concluded that prednisone was of greater benefit than azathioprine as a single agent in the treatment of MG.

A related issue is whether the combination of prednisone and azathioprine offers even greater benefit than either treatment alone. The Myasthenia Gravis Study Group performed a randomized double-blind, controlled trial comparing prednisolone (100 mg on alternate days) plus placebo to the combination of prednisolone and azathioprine (2.5 mg/kg per day).[10] Patients with MG in whom disabilities interfered with normal activities were eligible for inclusion, but those with restricted ocular disease or who had received previous immunosuppressive therapy were excluded. The primary outcome measures were the maintenance dose of prednisolone, the number of treatment failures (i.e., failure to achieve remission defined as the absence of symptoms or symptoms that were sufficiently mild that they did not interfere with normal activities), and the duration of the initial remission. Patients were followed for 3 years. After allowance for deaths and withdrawals, there were 10 patients in the prednisolone group and eight in the combination treatment group. Median prednisolone dose was significantly reduced at 36 months, the difference having first become apparent after 15 months of treatment. There were also significantly more treatment failures amongst the patients who received only prednisolone. With respect to the third primary outcome measure, the duration of remission was significantly longer in the group who received prednisolone and azathioprine.

Although the sizes of these studies were limited, the results support the conclusion that the addition of azathioprine to a steroid regimen has the effect of reducing the dose of steroid required, reducing the number of relapses, and prolonging the duration of clinical remissions. The efficacy of azathioprine relative to prednisone as a single agent remains unclear.

Is There a Role for Cyclosporine in the Treatment of Myasthenia Gravis?

Cyclosporine is an immunosuppressive agent that acts predominantly by inhibiting T-lymphocyte–dependent immune responses. Its efficacy in MG has been evaluated in two randomized, double-blind, placebo-controlled trials. In the first study,[11] patients with recent-onset moderate to severe generalized MG who had not undergone thymectomy or received other immunosuppressive therapy were eligible for inclusion if their symptoms were not controlled by antiacetylcholinesterase medications. Twenty patients were randomized to receive either cyclosporine or placebo and were followed for a period of 12 months. Efficacy was assessed primarily by changes in strength (using a quantitative scoring system; see Appendix 20 [Quantified Myasthenia Gravis Strength Score]). At both 6 and 12 months, the cyclosporine-treated patients fared significantly better than the placebo group with respect to muscle strength score. This improvement was evident as early as 2 weeks after the start of therapy, and the mean time to maximal improvement in the cyclosporine group was 3.6 months. It should be noted, however, that only four of 10 patients completed the cyclosporine protocol, three patients in the cyclosporine group received prednisone after a protocol violation or drug failure, and six of nine patients in the placebo group received some form of immunosuppressive therapy (prednisone, methotrexate, cyclosporine, or plasma exchange) after treatment failure or protocol violation. Significant side effects in the cyclosporine group included nephrotoxicity in three of 10 patients who required withdrawal from the study. Risk factors for nephrotoxicity included age older than 50 years, preexisting hypertension, or baseline impairment of renal function. In summary, therefore, this study suggested a beneficial effect of cyclosporine, but the number of patients treated was small, the dropout rate was high, and nephrotoxicity was an important side effect.

The second study[12] included patients with generalized MG, irrespective of whether they were still receiving corticosteroids or had received azathioprine or undergone thymectomy in the past. Twenty patients were randomized to receive cyclosporine and 19 to receive placebo. The proportion of patients who had received previous immunosuppressive therapy and concurrent steroid doses was similar between the two groups. The dose of cyclosporine was also reduced from 6 mg/kg per day as a single daily dose in the prior study to 5 mg/kg per day in two divided doses. The primary measures of efficacy were the changes in strength (using a quantitative scoring system) and the percentage of reduction in steroid dose required. Based on the mean time to maximal benefit of 3.6 months in the prior study, the duration of this study was 6 months. Cyclosporine-treated patients demonstrated a significantly greater increase in strength, but there was no difference in the percentage of reduction in steroid dose at 6 months. Although not a prespecified endpoint, the percentage of reduction in steroid dose became more significant between 12 and 24 months. Overall, a sustained improvement was noted in 8 of 20 (40%) cyclosporine-treated patients and only 2 of 19 (11%) who received placebo. Using the lower dose in a divided schedule with trough levels of 300–500 ng/ml, there was no clinically significant nephrotoxicity within the first 6 months, although this subsequently developed in 10% of patients over 12–24 months of follow-up.

These studies demonstrate that cyclosporine is effective in the treatment of MG and that a meaningful reduction in steroid dose may be achieved by 12 months. However, the utility of cyclosporine compared to azathioprine as a steroid-sparing agent remains unclear. Concern has been raised about the potential long-term toxicity of both agents. Prolonged use of azathioprine may be associated with an increased risk of secondary malignancy, but this risk appears small. The risk of nephrotoxicity with prolonged use of cyclosporine appears to be clinically more significant.

Is There a Role for Plasmapheresis or Intravenous Immunoglobulin in the Treatment of Myasthenia Gravis?

As for many of the other treatments used in patients with MG, plasmapheresis and intravenous immunoglobulin (IVIg) have become well established as therapeutic options even though they have never been studied in large prospective controlled trials.

For plasmapheresis, the closest approximations are the studies by Kornfeld and colleagues. In a letter to the editor of *The Lancet*,[13] they described their experience with 12 patients who had severe MG unresponsive to other forms of immunosuppression. Six patients were assigned to receive plasma exchange and six to receive placebo. None of the controls but all of the plasma-exchanged patients responded. Five of the control patients subsequently underwent plasmapheresis, with a good clinical response observed in three patients. The overall response rate to plasmapheresis, therefore, was 75%, and clinical remission after plasmapheresis typically lasted 3–13 weeks.

In a subsequent study,[14] patients with severe generalized MG, and unresponsive to other forms of therapy were randomized either to receive plasmapheresis (nine patients) or be part of the control group (seven patients). Four of the control patients became extremely ill and were crossed over to the plasmapheresis group. After 40 days, only two of the controls had shown signs of improvement, and all were crossed over to receive plasmapheresis. All of the initial nine patients randomized to plasmapheresis improved. Moreover, three of the patients initially randomized to the control group also responded to plasmapheresis after having been crossed over. The overall response rate, therefore, was 75%. A slightly greater response rate was observed amongst those with thymoma (82%) compared to those without (60%). The addition of azathioprine to those receiving plasmapheresis facilitated extension of the interval between exchanges to approximately 5 weeks. Those who only received plasmapheresis required exchanges every 2 weeks.

Yeh et al.[15] recently reported their experience with double-filtration plasmapheresis in 45 patients with severe MG who were unresponsive to other forms of therapy. Patients were evaluated clinically with an 18-point score comprising timed measures of outstretched arms and legs, vital capacity, as well as functional grading of facial, chewing, and swallowing muscles. Thirty-eight of 45 patients (84%) achieved significant clinical improvement. There was a trend towards greater improvement in patients with more severe disease.

Gajdos et al.[16] compared plasma exchange and IVIg in a prospective randomized trial. Eighty-seven patients with an exacerbation of MG were randomized to receive plasma exchange for 3 days (41 patients) or IVIg (46 patients), with the latter group randomized to receive IVIg for 3 or 5 days (23 patients each). The primary endpoint was the absolute variation of a myasthenia muscular score (see Appendix 21 [Myasthenia Muscular Score]) ranging from 0 to 100 (normal) that included assessment of strength of limb, trunk, and cranial nerve musculature between randomization and day 15. Improvements in the myasthenia muscular score were similar between the two treatment groups. Overall response rates were 66% in the 3-day plasma exchange group, 61% in the 3-day IVIg group, and 39% in the 5-day IVIg group. Median response time was estimated at 9 and 15 days in the plasma exchange and IVIg treatment groups, respectively. The lower incidence of side effects amongst the IVIg-treated patients as well as the absence of a real difference in outcome between the two treatment groups led the authors to suggest IVIg as a safe and effective alternative to plasma exchange.

Rønager et al. performed a randomized, investigator-blinded crossover study comparing the clinical efficacy of plasmapheresis and IVIg in patients with stable moderate to severe generalized MG.[17] All patients had received immunosuppressive therapy with azathioprine or prednisone in the preceding months. Eight patients were randomized to IVIg followed by plasma exchange and a 16-week observation period; four patients received plasma exchange followed by IVIg. Clinical evaluation was performed using the quantified MG score. Patients who received plasma exchange showed improvement 1 week after initiation of therapy, but IVIg-treated patients did not. At 4 weeks' follow-up, comparable improvement was noted in both treatment groups.

For patients with chronic severe generalized MG, therefore, the response rate to plasmapheresis is approximately 66–80%. These and other results are summarized in Table 15-2. Rønager and colleagues found that plasmapheresis and IVIg were of similar efficacy except that the onset of benefit was quicker after plasmapheresis.

What Is the Role of Thymectomy in Patients with Nonthymomatous Myasthenia Gravis?

Thymectomy is widely held to be part of the standard care for patients with MG, even though this conclusion has not been established in clinical trials.

TABLE 15-2
Effects of Plasmapheresis in Myasthenia Gravis

Frequency of response (%)	66[a]–84[b]
Duration of response (wks)	3–13[c]
Median latency to onset of response (days)	9[a]

[a]Data from P Gajdos, S Chevret, B Clair, et al. Clinical trial of plasma exchange and high-dose intravenous immunoglobulin in myasthenia gravis. Myasthenia Gravis Clinical Study Group. *Ann Neurol* 1997;41:789–796.
[b]Data from JH Yeh, HC Chiu. Double filtration plasmapheresis in myasthenia gravis—analysis of clinical efficacy and prognostic parameters. *Acta Neurol Scand* 1999;100:305–309.
[c]Data from P Kornfeld, EP Ambinder, AE Papatestas, et al. Plasmapheresis in myasthenia gravis: controlled study. *Lancet* 1979;2:629.

The theoretical rationale for removal of the thymus rests on the recognition that the thymus plays a central role in the pathogenesis of MG as a site of specific autoantibody production.

A recent evidence-based review by Gronseth and Barohn found that patients who had undergone thymectomy were more likely to achieve medication-free remission and to become asymptomatic or less symptomatic on medication than those who did not undergo thymectomy. They note, however, that this observation must be tempered by the recognition of important confounding differences in baseline characteristics of prognostic significance in all of the available studies. In view of the widespread acceptance of thymectomy, their conclusion was remarkably conservative: "We cannot determine from the available studies whether the observed association between thymectomy and improved MG outcome was a result of a thymectomy benefit or was merely a result of the multiple differences in baseline characteristics between the surgical and nonsurgical groups. Based on these findings, we conclude that the benefit of thymectomy in nonthymomatous autoimmune MG has not been established conclusively."[18]

In the absence of evidence either way, Lanska[19] surveyed 56 neurologists with an interest and expertise in MG. Most advocated thymectomy for patients with thymoma based on the potential for local invasion and the possibility of an improvement in myasthenic symptoms. The most controversy existed regarding patients with generalized MG without evidence of a thymoma. Variables such as age of the patient, severity of the disease, response to medication, and duration of the disease were used to individualize treatment decisions.

Notwithstanding the absence of evidence regarding the fundamental question of whether thymectomy is beneficial, a number of other controversies surrounding thymectomy have emerged. Which surgical technique, transcervical or trans-sternal, is superior? What is the appropriate timing of thymectomy? Are there particular subgroups of patients with MG who are liable to derive greater benefits from thymectomy? Not surprisingly, there are no clear answers to these questions, and in the absence of a carefully designed controlled trial, therapeutic benefit will remain unproven, and specific indications and contraindications for thymectomy will be based on individual preference.

Should Patients with Ocular Myasthenia Gravis Receive Immunosuppressive Therapy?

A commonly voiced opinion is that limited ocular MG does not warrant immunosuppressive therapy. The argument, at least in part, is based on the contention that symptoms of ocular MG are seldom disabling or severe enough to warrant the risk of toxicity associated with long-term steroid (or other immunosuppressive drug) use. However, it is also recognized that a significant proportion (perhaps 40–50%) of patients with ocular MG progress to develop generalized disease. Acetylcholinesterase inhibitors only offer symptomatic relief and clearly do not influence the underlying disease process. Some, therefore, have suggested that patients with ocular MG should not be denied immunosuppressive therapy. This argument is based, in part, on the recognition that purely ocular symptoms may be very disabling and on the acknowledgment of the need to treat the disease and not just its symptoms. There are no prospective controlled studies that shed light on this controversy. Kupersmith and colleagues,[20] however, performed a retrospective chart review to identify 32 patients who were treated with high-dose daily prednisone that was then gradually tapered to an alternate-day low-dose regimen or withdrawn completely. They observed that 66.0% of patients had resolution of extraocular muscle weakness and only 9.4% of patients progressed to generalized MG over the 2-year duration of the study. This compared favorably to the previously reported rates of 44–53% progression to generalized disease. A transient deterioration in symptoms was not observed in this group of patients, notwithstanding the initiation of therapy with high-dose daily prednisone.

Thus, although it is true that there are no randomized controlled data to support the use of steroids (or other immunosuppressive therapy) in patients with ocular MG, the same is true of the use of these agents in patients with generalized disease. The decision to treat patients with ocular MG with steroids, therefore, will remain an individualized one until a randomized controlled trial is performed.

Summary

- Steroids, azathioprine, cyclosporine, plasmapheresis, IVIg, and thymectomy have each become accepted therapies, notwithstanding the relative lack of data from prospective controlled trials.

- The response rate to corticosteroids (with remission or improvement) varies from 70% to 94%.
- The response rate to plasmapheresis in patients who have not responded to other forms of immunosuppressive therapy has varied from 66% to 84%.
- IVIg may be as effective as plasmapheresis, although the effects may take slightly longer to become apparent.
- Azathioprine is an effective adjunctive therapy, facilitating either a reduction in the dose of corticosteroid required or an increase in the interval between plasma exchanges.
- Cyclosporine is probably as effective as azathioprine, but long-term therapy is associated with a significant risk of nephrotoxicity.
- The benefits of thymectomy remain unproven. In particular, there are very little controlled data to guide decisions about the timing of thymectomy or whether to employ the transcervical or transsternal approach.
- Data from a retrospective series suggest that steroid treatment of patients with ocular MG may reduce the likelihood of progression to generalized disease.

References

1. Howard FM, Duane DD, Lambert EH, Daube JR. Alternate-day prednisone: preliminary report of a double-blind controlled study. *Ann N Y Acad Sci* 1976;274:596–607.
2. Sghirlanzoni A, Peluchetti D, Mantegazza R, et al. Myasthenia gravis: prolonged treatment with steroids. *Neurology* 1984;34:170–174.
3. Pascuzzi RM, Coslett HB, Johns TR. Long-term corticosteroid treatment of myasthenia gravis: report of 116 patients. *Ann Neurol* 1984;15:291–298.
4. Evoli A, Batocchi AP, Palmisani MT, et al. Long-term results of corticosteroid therapy in patients with myasthenia gravis. *Eur Neurol* 1992;32:37–43.
5. Seybold ME, Drachman DB. Gradually increasing doses of prednisone in myasthenia gravis. Reducing the hazards of Treatment. *N Engl J Med* 1974; 290:81–84.
6. Arsura E, Brunner NG, Namba T, Grob D. High-dose intravenous methylprednisolone in myasthenia gravis. *Arch Neurol* 1985;42:1149–1153.
7. Lindberg C, Andersen O, Lefvert AK. Treatment of myasthenia gravis with methylprednisolone pulse: a double blind study. *Acta Neurol Scand* 1998;97:370–373.
8. A randomized clinical trial comparing prednisone and azathioprine in myasthenia gravis. Results of the second interim analysis. Myasthenia Gravis Clinical Study Group. *J Neurol Neurosurg Psychiatry* 1993;56:1157–1163.

9. Bromberg MB, Wald JJ, Forshew DA, et al. Randomized trial of azathioprine or prednisone for initial immunosuppressive treatment of myasthenia gravis. *J Neurol Sci* 1997;150:59–62.

10. Palace J, Newsom-Davis J, Lecky B. A randomized double-blind trial of prednisolone alone or with azathioprine in myasthenia gravis. Myasthenia Gravis Study Group. *Neurology* 1998; 50:1778–1783.

11. Tindall RS, Rollins JA, Phillips JT, et al. Preliminary results of a double-blind, randomized, placebo-controlled trial of cyclosporin in myasthenia gravis. *N Engl J Med* 1987;316:719–724.

12. Tindall RS, Phillips JT, Rollins JA, et al. A clinical therapeutic trial of cyclosporine in myasthenia gravis. *Ann N Y Acad Sci* 1993;681:539–551.

13. Kornfeld P, Ambinder EP, Papatestas AE, et al. Plasmapheresis in myasthenia gravis: controlled study. *Lancet* 1979;2:629.

14. Kornfeld P, Ambinder EP, Mittag T, et al. Plasmapheresis in refractory generalized myasthenia gravis. *Arch Neurol* 1981;38:478–481.

15. Yeh JH and Chiu HC. Double filtration plasmapheresis in myasthenia gravis—analysis of clinical efficacy and prognostic parameters. *Acta Neurol Scand* 1999;100:305–309.

16. Gajdos P, Chevret S, Clair B, et al. Clinical trial of plasma exchange and high-dose intravenous immunoglobulin in myasthenia gravis. Myasthenia Gravis Clinical Study Group. *Ann Neurol* 1997;41:789–796.

17. Rønager J, Ravnborg M, Hermansen I, Vorstrup S. Immunoglobulin treatment versus plasma exchange in patients with chronic moderate to severe myasthenia gravis. *Artif Organs* 2001;25:967–973.

18. Gronseth GS, Barohn RJ. Practice parameter: thymectomy for autoimmune myasthenia gravis (an evidence-based review): report of the Quality Standards Subcommittee of the American Academy of Neurology. *Neurology* 2000;55:7–15.

19. Lanska DJ. Indications for thymectomy in myasthenia gravis. *Neurology* 1990;40:1828–1829.

20. Kupersmith MJ, Moster M, Bhuiyan S, et al. Beneficial effects of corticosteroids on ocular myasthenia gravis. *Arch Neurol* 1996;53:802–804.

CHAPTER 16

Bell's Palsy

Introduction

Bell's palsy is the term used to describe facial neuropathy of unknown cause. It is a common condition with an incidence of approximately 20 per 100,000 population. Men and women are equally affected and there is no seasonal predilection. A variety of treatments have been proposed, ranging from oral steroids to surgical decompression. Uncontroversial measures are to protect the cornea from drying and ulceration, as well as facial physical therapy to reduce the likelihood of developing contractures. Some controversy, however, has surrounded the appropriate use of steroids and acyclovir. To assess the efficacy of any therapeutic intervention and to make recommendations to patients about the advisability of a potentially toxic treatment, it is useful to have an idea of the natural history of untreated Bell's palsy. What is the natural history of untreated Bell's palsy? How does treatment with steroids, with or without acyclovir, impact on the disability that may result from Bell's palsy? These and other questions are the focus of this chapter.

What Is the Natural History of Untreated Bell's Palsy?

In their population-based study, Hauser et al.[1] identified 121 cases of idiopathic facial paralysis and invited these patients to return for a follow-up evaluation. With the exception of one patient who had received steroids and one who had undergone surgical decompression, physical therapy and nicotinic acid were the only treatment modalities employed. At follow-up examination (completed successfully in 85 of 121 patients), seven clinical features were evaluated (synkinesis, mouth weakness, forehead weakness, orbicularis oculi weakness, platysma weakness, contracture of the angle of the mouth, and contracture of the orbicularis oculi) and the degree of abnormality was scored. Patients were then assigned to four categories based on the severity of residua. Twenty-four percent of patients had full recovery, 48% had residua described as generally not noticeable in casual social interactions, 14% had sequelae detectable only by a close observer, and another 14% had residua that were generally obvious.

Peitersen[2] reviewed the Copenhagen experience with 1,011 patients with untreated Bell's palsy. Overall, 71% of patients recovered normal function of facial muscles. Although not directly comparable to Hauser's study[1] because different outcome measures were used, the rates of effectively full recovery are similar if the first two groups of patients in the Hauser study are combined (72% with none or no casually detectable residua).

The majority of instances of Bell's palsy represent a monophasic illness. In a small proportion of patients, however, the facial weakness may recur. In Peitersen's series,[2] 6.8% of 1,011 patients had a history of Bell's palsy. Adour et al.[3] recorded a history of recurrent Bell's palsy in 9.3% of their 446 patients.

Which Clinical Features Have Prognostic Importance with Regard to Recovery in Bell's Palsy?

In their study of the natural history of Bell's palsy, Hauser et al.[1] attempted to define features of the acute illness that correlated with the degree of permanent residua. They reported that older age, increased tearing, and longer latency from onset to either first signs of improvement or maximal improvement were predictive of a worse prognosis, but the primary data to support these claims were not provided. The study by Peitersen[2] also addressed this issue and found age and interval at the beginning of recovery to be important factors. Although the overall rate of complete recovery was 71%, the outcome was most favorable in children (with 90% making a full recovery) and worst in patients older than 60 years (with only 37% of patients achieving complete recovery). Although the overall rate of residua was 29%, permanent sequelae were detected in only 12% of patients who showed signs of improvement within the first week of the onset of symptoms. The respective proportions of patients with permanent sequelae for those who began to improve after 2 weeks, 3 weeks, and 4 months were 16%, 39%, and 100%. This study also indicated that the likelihood of incomplete recovery was greater amongst patients with loss of the stapedial reflex or those with decreased tearing (in contrast to the suggestion by Hauser et al. that increased lacrimation represented a poor prognostic factor).

The study by Adour et al.[3] of 446 patients revealed similar results even though only half of these patients were untreated (262 of the 446 patients had been treated with prednisone). As a measure of final outcome, they developed the Facial Paralysis Recovery Profile (FPRP; see Appendix 6 [Facial Paralysis Recovery Profile]) and evaluated the presence or absence of complications such as synkinesis and facial contractures. Consistent with other studies, they found older age to portend a poorer prognosis. The mean FPRP score was 9.47 and 8.75 among those younger and older than 60 years, respectively, and the prevalence of contractures or synkinesis was 50% in those older than 60 years compared to only 11% in the younger age group. Hyperacusis and decreased tearing were again identified as poor prognostic factors. Decreased tearing (according to subjective report and confirmed by the Schirmer's test) was associated with a higher incidence of clinically complete paralysis, occurring in 45% and 26%, respectively, of those with and without clinically complete paralysis. Similarly, hyperacusis was reported in 44% of those with clinically

TABLE 16-1
Factors Associated with a Poor Prognosis for Recovery in Bell's Palsy

Older age[1-3]
Clinically complete paralysis at some stage during the illness[4,5]
Longer latency from onset to signs of initial improvement[2]
Hyperacusis[2,3]
Decreased tearing[2,3]

complete paralysis compared to 23% of those without. The inference is that clinically complete paralysis at some stage during the illness correlates with a greater likelihood of muscle denervation and the risk of permanent sequelae, but it should be noted that these data rely on inference rather than observation. Hyperacusis, however, was present amongst 20% of those who developed contractures and synkinesis, compared to only 7.8% of those who did not. These results, therefore, do lend support to the findings of Peitersen.[2]

In the study of the natural history of untreated Bell's palsy, Peitersen[2] hints at the idea that prognosis is worse amongst those with complete rather than incomplete facial paralysis, but the data are not reported in a way that clearly demonstrates this impression. In their prospective randomized study of steroids in 51 patients with Bell's palsy, May et al.[4] observed that recovery was complete in all patients who presented with partial loss of facial function that did not progress, as compared to a complete recovery rate of only 50% among those who presented with complete facial paralysis. The prognosis for recovery was intermediate amongst those with partial loss of function at presentation that increased in severity or progressed to complete paralysis over a period of a few weeks. In their series of 1,048 patients with Bell's palsy, Adour et al.[5] similarly observed a worse outcome amongst those with complete paralysis. They note that of the patients who presented with complete paralysis, 37% of the untreated and 71% of the steroid-treated patients had a complete recovery.

Finally, Adour et al.[3] remark that outcome was worse amongst those with a history of hypertension and diabetes but provide no data from the study to support this claim. In the randomized, double-blind study of steroids performed by May et al.[4] that included a total of 51 patients, there were only two patients with diabetes and 10 with hypertension. These numbers were too small for meaningful statistical analysis. The factors that have most consistently been found to be associated with a poor prognosis are summarized in Table 16-1.

What Is the Evidence That Steroids Should Be Used to Treat Patients with Bell's Palsy?

The efficacy of steroids in the treatment of patients with Bell's palsy has been the subject of a number of studies. These have varied widely in terms

TABLE 16-2
Utility of Steroids in the Treatment of Bell's Palsy

Study	No.	Study Design	Favorable Outcome (%)		Relative Risk*
			Control	Steroids	
Taverner[6]	26	Randomized, placebo-controlled	67	72	1.07
May[4]	51	Randomized, placebo-controlled	65	60	0.92
Brown[7]	82	Placebo-controlled	73	87	1.20
Austin[8]	107	Randomized, placebo-controlled	83	100	1.20

*Relative risk >1 indicates benefit from steroids.

of the sample size, adequacy of randomization, nature of steroid regimen employed, latency from symptom onset to initiation of treatment, duration of follow-up, outcome measure used, and the presence or absence of observer blinding. The four studies deemed to be of the greatest quality have been selected for review, and their findings are summarized below.

Taverner[6] randomized 26 patients to treatment with either hydrocortisone or placebo (Table 16-2). Patients with Bell's palsy who could start treatment within 10 days of the onset of symptoms were eligible for inclusion in this study. Patients were examined clinically and with electromyography at the time of randomization and at subsequent intervals. The presence or absence of volitional motor units on electromyography was used to classify patients as having either partial or complete paralysis. The development of denervation as evidenced by fibrillations on electromyography was used to define outcome as a failure. The mean (range) time from onset of the facial palsy to the start of treatment was 4.5 (1–9) days in the cortisone-treated patients and 3.6 (1–8) days in the control group. There were four failures and eight successes in the control group, compared to four failures and 10 successes in the treated group. Sixty-seven percent of untreated patients, therefore, were regarded as having a favorable outcome, compared to 72% of those who were treated with steroids. The relative risk of a good outcome for those treated with steroids, therefore, was 1.07. Possible reasons for failure to demonstrate a beneficial effect of steroids include the small sample size and the prolonged latency from symptom onset to the initiation of treatment.

May et al.[4] included 51 patients in a prospective randomized, controlled, and double-blind study (see Table 16-2). Patients were randomized to treatment with prednisone (a total of 410 mg in tapering doses over 10 days) and vitamins or only vitamins. Patients with recurrent or bilateral paralysis were excluded, as were those with loss of lacrimation (because of its purported poorer prognostic significance). Only those presenting within 2 days of the

onset of symptoms were eligible for inclusion in the study. The degree of ultimate facial motor recovery was determined 6 months after symptom onset by
physicians blinded to treatment category. Patients with no differences between
the affected and normal sides of the face and no evidence of aberrant reinnervation were classified as having a *complete* recovery; those with incomplete
return of facial motor function and very mild complications of reinnervation
were regarded as having a *fair* recovery; and those with obviously incomplete
return of facial motor function and complications of aberrant reinnervation
were classified as having a *poor* outcome. There were no significant differences
between the steroid- and vitamin-treated patients in terms of those with complete, fair, or poor outcomes, with complete recovery in approximately 63%,
fair recovery in approximately 17%, and poor recovery in 20%. This was a
well-conducted study, but its major limitations were its small sample size and
insufficient power to detect a beneficial effect of steroids.

Brown[7] reported his experience with the treatment of 174 patients
with Bell's palsy (see Table 16-2). Patients were divided into two groups
based on whether the facial palsy was complete or incomplete. The 82
patients with incomplete facial palsy were alternately assigned to treatment with steroids (prednisone 400 mg divided over 10 days) or supportive
measures, and outcome was assessed in a blinded fashion. Those with complete facial palsy were matched for a variety of clinical features and then
assigned to treatment with either steroids or surgical decompression. The
majority of patients were assigned treatment within the first 2 days of
symptom onset, but a small number were only seen on the third day.
Patients were evaluated at 3, 6, and 12 months and outcome classified as
complete (no observable differences between the affected and the normal
sides of the face), *fair* (slight to moderate facial weakness and synkinesis),
or *poor* (severe facial weakness and synkinesis). Consider first the outcomes
amongst the patients with incomplete facial palsy. Of the 41 patients who
received supportive treatment alone, only 30 (73%) were deemed to have
achieved a complete recovery, compared to 36 (87%) of those patients
treated with steroids. The 73% rate of complete recovery is consistent with
natural history studies of untreated patients, and the greater recovery rate
amongst those treated with steroids yields a relative risk (for improved outcome) of 1.2. An interesting observation was made during the analysis of
the 41 patients with complete facial palsy who received steroids. Twenty
(49%) were judged to have a complete recovery. Eighteen of these 20
patients received their steroids on the first day of symptom onset, whereas
the other two patients received steroids on day 2 of their illness. These
results suggest that the efficacy of steroid therapy is maximized by early
initiation of treatment. The qualities of this study lie in its larger size and
completeness of follow-up, but it is deficient in its not being randomized.

Austin et al.[8] also conducted a randomized, double-blind, placebo-
controlled trial of prednisone in the treatment of patients with Bell's palsy (see
Table 16-2). Patients were eligible for inclusion if symptoms had begun within

the preceding 5 days. One hundred seven patients were randomized, but follow-up data were available for only 76 patients (71%). This high dropout rate is the major limiting aspect of this study. Time to recovery, facial paralysis grade at onset versus grade at recovery, and the presence of permanent sequelae (synkinesis, hemifacial spasm, and crocodile tears) were among the primary measures of outcome that were employed. Facial nerve function was evaluated according to the House-Brackmann grading system (see Appendix 13 [House-Brackmann Facial Nerve Grading System]). Good recovery was judged to occur when the patient reached a facial nerve paralysis of at least grade II (slight weakness noticeable only on close inspection; may have slight synkinesis). The prednisone group had a mean time to improvement of 51.4 days, compared to 69.3 days in the placebo group (not significant). All the prednisone-treated patients achieved a recovery grade of I (complete) or II, compared to 83% of the placebo-treated patients. The respective rates of complete recovery were 53% and 33% for the steroid- and placebo-treated patients. Although there were no differences between the two treatment groups in terms of the development of synkinesis or crocodile tears, hemifacial spasm occurred significantly less frequently in the prednisone-treated group.

The results of these studies, each with their own limitations, are conflicting, with some reporting a beneficial effect of steroids and others not. The results of these and other studies of steroids in the treatment of Bell's palsy were recently summarized in a meta-analysis.[9] The authors of this review concur with the conclusion drawn here—that there is insufficient quality evidence to conclusively answer the question of whether steroids should unequivocally be used in patients with Bell's palsy. Nevertheless, given the available data with a number of studies demonstrating improved outcome associated with steroid treatment, particularly when initiated early, a recommendation in favor of steroid use can be made. This recommendation is made with knowledge of the limitations of the available data.

Is There Evidence to Support the Use of Acyclovir in the Treatment of Bell's Palsy?

There are two key studies that have addressed the question of whether there is evidence to support the use of acyclovir in the treatment of Bell's palsy. In the first, the combination of prednisone and acyclovir was compared to treatment with only prednisone.[5] The second study compared acyclovir alone to prednisone.[10]

Adour et al.[5] randomized 119 patients with Bell's palsy, presenting within 3 days of symptom onset, to treatment with either acyclovir (400 mg five times per day) or placebo. All patients also received prednisone (1 mg/kg) administered in two divided doses. Ninety-nine patients completed the study, 53 of whom received the combination of acyclovir and prednisone and 46 of whom received placebo and prednisone. The two treatment groups were comparable, with complete facial paralysis developing in approximately 20% of each group. Final outcome was determined by blinded observers using the FPRP and Facial Paralysis Recovery Index (FRPI) (the FPRP adjusted for the presence of the complications of aberrant reinnervation). FPRP scores of 10 (complete recovery) were observed in 92% of the acyclovir-prednisone–treated patients compared to 76% of the prednisone-treated group. FPRI scores of 10 (complete recovery) were noted in 87% and 72% of the acyclovir-prednisone and prednisone groups, respectively. This study, therefore, supports the use of acyclovir and prednisone in patients presenting within 3 days of symptom onset, but an unequivocal recommendation cannot be made because of the relatively high proportion of patients (17%) who were lost to follow-up.

De Diego et al.[10] examined 113 patients with Bell's palsy who presented within 4 days of the onset of symptoms. Twelve patients were lost to follow-up, leaving a total of 101 patients for whom complete clinical data were available. Fifty-four patients were randomized to receive acyclovir (800 mg three times per day for 10 days) and 47 to receive prednisone (1 mg/kg for 10 days and then tapered over 6 days). Facial nerve function was assessed using the House-Brackmann facial nerve grading scale and the FPRP. Primary outcome measures included grade of recovery and the presence or absence of sequelae. Normal recovery was defined as House-Brackmann grade II or a score of greater than or equal to 8 on the FPRP. Ninety-four percent of the prednisone-treated patients and 78% of the acyclovir-treated patients achieved a House-Brackmann grade of II. Similarly, 94% of the prednisone-treated patients scored at least 8 on the FPRP, compared to 83% of the acyclovir-treated patients. These differences were statistically significant. There were no significant differences between the two treatment groups in terms of the occurrence of sequelae that developed in approximately 24% of patients. Outcome in this study was not assessed in a blinded manner.

The available data, therefore, suggest that acyclovir alone is inferior to prednisone in the treatment of Bell's palsy, but there is some support for the use of acyclovir as adjunctive therapy (together with steroids). The evidence, however, is limited, and the optimal dose and duration of therapy are unclear.

Summary

- Complete recovery can be expected in approximately 70% of untreated patients with Bell's palsy.
- Bell's palsy is usually a monophasic illness but may be recurrent in 7–9% of cases.
- Older age and greater severity of paralysis, evidenced by paralysis being complete at presentation or a longer latency to initial signs of recovery, are predictive of a worse outcome with a greater likelihood of permanent sequelae.

- There is some disagreement regarding which, if any, of the clinical symptoms or signs at presentation are predictive of a poor prognosis. Hyperacusis is the one symptom that consistently appears to be associated with a worse outcome.
- It has been suggested that prognosis is adversely affected by the presence of underlying diabetes or hypertension, but there are insufficient data to substantiate or dismiss this claim.
- There is insufficient quality evidence to conclusively answer the question of whether steroids should unequivocally be used in patients with Bell's palsy. Given the available data with a number of studies demonstrating improved outcome associated with steroid treatment, particularly when initiated early, a recommendation in favor of steroid use can be made.
- Although the available data are not conclusive, they do provide some support for the use of acyclovir as adjunctive therapy (together with steroids) in the treatment of Bell's palsy. The evidence is limited, and the optimal dose and duration of therapy are unclear.

References

1. Hauser WA, Karnes WE, Annis J, Kurland LT. Incidence and prognosis of Bell's palsy in the population of Rochester, Minnesota. *Mayo Clin Proc* 1971;46:258–264.
2. Peitersen E. The natural history of Bell's palsy. *Am J Otol* 1982;4:107–111.
3. Adour KK, Wingerd J. Idiopathic facial paralysis (Bell's palsy): factors affecting severity and outcome in 446 patients. *Neurology* 1974;24:1112–1116.
4. May M, Wette R, Hardin WB, et al. The use of steroids in Bell's palsy: a prospective controlled study. *Laryngoscope* 1976;86:1111–1122.
5. Adour K, Ruboyianes JM, Von Doersten PG, et al. Bell's palsy treatment with acyclovir and prednisone compared with prednisone alone: a double-blind, randomized, controlled trial. *Ann Otol Rhinol Laryngol* 1996;105:371–378.
6. Taverner D. Treatment of Bell's palsy. *Lancet* 1971;2:168.
7. Brown JS. Bell's palsy: a 5 year review of 174 consecutive cases: an attempted double-blind study. *Laryngoscope* 1982;92:1369–1373.
8. Austin JR, Peskind SP, Austin SG, Rice DH. Idiopathic facial nerve paralysis: a randomized double blind controlled study of placebo versus prednisone. *Laryngoscope* 1993;103:1326–1333.
9. Grogan PM, Gronseth GS. Practice parameter: steroids, acyclovir, and surgery for Bell's palsy (an evidence-based review). Report of the Quality Standards Subcommittee of the American Academy of Neurology. *Neurology* 2001;56:830–836.
10. De Diego JI, Prim MP, De Sarriá MJ, et al. Idiopathic facial paralysis: a randomized, prospective, and controlled study using single-dose prednisone versus acyclovir three times daily. *Laryngoscope* 1998;108:573–575.

CHAPTER 17

Cervical Spondylosis

Introduction

Cervical spondylosis is a disorder characterized by degenerative disk disease, the formation of spondylotic ridges and osteophytes, facet and uncovertebral joint arthritis, ossification of the posterior longitudinal ligament, redundancy of the ligamentum flavum, and vertebral body listhesis. Injury to nerve roots or the spinal cord may occur either directly via mechanical trauma or compression, or indirectly via arterial insufficiency or venous stasis.

The clinical manifestations of cervical spondylotic myelopathy include weakness and spasticity due to motor long-tract dysfunction, sensory impairment due primarily to dorsal column involvement, and bladder dysfunction. Cervical spondylosis may also manifest only with neck and head pain or with signs and symptoms attributable to cervical radiculopathy. The syndrome of cervical spondylotic myelopathy must be distinguished from these related clinical entities.

What is the natural history of cervical spondylosis, and can it be altered by surgery? Are there particular circumstances that should dictate either surgical intervention or conservative measures? Is surgery more or less indicated if symptoms are due to cervical root or spinal cord compression? These questions are the focus of this chapter.

What Is the Natural History of Cervical Spondylosis?

To put into perspective the results of treatment, either conservative or surgical, it is important to know the natural history of cervical spondylosis. Ideally, it is necessary to know the natural history of both cervical spondylotic radiculopathy and myelopathy. With respect to cervical spondylotic myelopathy, there are no reliable data. The study by Lees and Turner[1] is often cited as a description of the natural history of cervical spondylosis. However, it is clear that some of the patients in their study underwent various forms of therapy, but a distinction was not made between those who were treated and those who were not. Therefore, their conclusion that cervical spondylotic myelopathy is a disease with a lengthy clinical course marked by long periods of nonprogressive disability should be regarded with some caution. Clarke and Robinson[2] described their experience with

26 untreated patients amongst their larger series of patients with cervical spondylotic myelopathy. They found that progression was common, albeit gradual, and that improvement was rare and concluded that prognosis was generally poor. With respect to cervical spondylotic radiculopathy, longitudinal studies suggest that symptoms may resolve with time. In the population-based study of residents of Rochester, Minnesota,[3] 90.5% of patients with cervical radiculopathy were asymptomatic or only mildly affected after a mean follow-up period of almost 6 years. This figure includes those patients who were treated surgically, but these were a minority (26%) of the whole group.

What Are the Options for the Treatment of Cervical Spondylosis?

In broad terms, the options for the treatment of cervical spondylosis are either conservative or surgical. Conservative treatment encompasses immobilization with a cervical collar (usually a soft collar), use of analgesics or muscle relaxants, and physical therapy. Surgery may be performed either by the anterior or the posterior approach and may involve either single or multiple cervical segments. Anterior cervical discectomy and fusion implies removal of the offending disk and osteophytes with fusion via either a bony graft or instrumentation (e.g., cage or plate). The alternative is a vertebrectomy (also known as *corpectomy*) in which the relevant vertebral body is removed. The posterior approach involves either a laminectomy or some form of a laminoplasty. Although the former involves removal of the lamina, the latter is a technique that aims to enlarge the spinal canal by preserving and elevating the lamina roof over the dura, and it typically has less potential than laminectomy to cause spinal instability.

Is There Any Evidence to Favor Surgery over Conservative Measures for Cervical Spondylotic Myelopathy?

The vast majority of the literature on the treatment of cervical spondylotic myelopathy is retrospective and uncontrolled. There are only two prospective studies comparing conservative and surgical therapy,[4,5] and only one of these was randomized.[4] In addition, there is a single prospective study of the results of surgical management.[6] Finally, there are three retrospective studies that reported the results of both conservative and surgical therapy.[7–9]

Kadanka et al.[4] recruited 48 patients with clinical signs and symptoms of mild to moderate cervical spondylotic myelopathy with a modified Japanese Orthopedic Association score (see Appendix 16 [Modified Japanese Orthopedic Association Scale)) greater than 12. Patients with other neurologic diseases and those with previous cervical spine surgery were excluded. Patients were randomized into two groups that underwent either conservative or surgical therapy, and follow-up was planned for 2 years. Three types of surgical procedures were used—anterior decompression was performed in 13 (nine of which included an osseous graft), corpectomy in five, and laminoplasty in three. Conservative treatment comprised soft collar, anti-inflammatory drugs, intermittent bedrest, and active discouragement of high-risk physical activities. These measures were also used in patients who underwent surgery. Efficacy was measured by change in the modified Japanese Orthopedic Association score, a quantitative video-assisted assessment of activities of daily living (ADL), a timed 10-m walk, and a self-evaluation questionnaire. Outcome was reported on the basis of an intention-to-treat analysis.

No differences in modified Japanese Orthopedic Association score were observed at 6, 12, and 24 months. There were no significant differences in ADL scores within the conservatively managed group at 6-, 12-, or 24-month follow-up compared to baseline, but significant decline was observed in surgically treated patients. There were no differences between the two groups in the timed 10-m walk. Finally, there was no change in subjective evaluation in the conservatively treated group, but surgically treated patients reported deterioration between 6 and 12 months' and between 6 and 24 months' follow-up.

The authors concluded that there were no significant differences in the objective outcome measures of patients with mild to moderate forms of cervical spondylotic myelopathy, irrespective of whether they were treated conservatively or surgically. Based on the patient population included in this study, no comment could be made about the role of surgery in patients with more severe or rapidly progressive forms of cervical spondylotic myelopathy. Problems with this study include the relatively small sample size, the questionable method of randomization (coin toss), and the absence of a discussion about the power of the study.

Sampath et al.[5] reported the outcome in 62 patients with cervical spondylotic myelopathy, half of whom were treated surgically and half with conservative measures. Inclusion and exclusion criteria did not specify the severity of the disease. Conservative therapy included pharmacologic agents, bedrest, cervical traction, neck bracing, and spinal injections. Surgery was performed either via the posterior approach (foraminotomy or laminotomy and laminectomy), the anterior approach (anterior cervical discectomy), or a combination of the two. A variety of outcome measures were used, including an assessment of neurologic symptoms (seven-point scale), functional status (four-point scale), patient satisfaction, severity of pain (six-point scale), and a measure of independence with ADL (six-point scale). All of these measures were made on the basis of subjective patient report rather than objective measurement. The results are summarized in Table 17-1, with recorded values indicating the change in score from baseline.

TABLE 17-1
Outcome of Patients with Cervical Spondylotic Myelopathy

	Conservative	*Surgery*	p *Value*
Pain (0–5)[a]	–0.61	–0.98	<0.05
Neurologic symptoms (0–6)[a]	+0.42	–0.54	NS
Functional status (0–3)[b]	+0.27	+0.48	<0.05
Activities of daily living (0–5)[a]	+0.63	No change	NS

NS = not significant.
[a]Low scores indicate better performance; – = improving status.
[b]High score indicates better performance; + = improving status.

Comparisons were not made directly between the two groups (because patients were not randomized to receive only the one treatment or the other). Results indicated as significant by $p < 0.05$ represent a significant change between pre- and postoperative periods. The mean follow-up was 11.2 months (with a range of 8–13 months), and follow-up data were available for 43 of 62 patients (69%), which represents a 31% dropout rate that was fairly evenly distributed between the two treatment groups.

This study was limited by subjects not being randomized to the two treatment groups, by the high dropout rate, and by the use of purely subjective measures of outcome. Moreover, the outcome measures used are not clearly measures of myelopathic symptoms. Finally, the magnitude of benefit derived from surgery is small and, although statistically significant, is not clearly clinically significant.

Mann and colleagues[6] conducted a prospective study of 50 patients with advanced cervical spondylotic myelopathy who were treated surgically. They included only patients with gross clinical evidence of spinal compression, but further specification was not provided. They used a five-point clinical grading system to monitor clinical outcome. Surgery comprised a multilevel anterior discectomy with fusion (modified Cloward's procedure) when disks measured more than 4 mm, combined with simple discectomy for disks measuring 2–4 mm. Patients were followed for 2–5 years. All patients showed progressive improvement, mostly during the first year. The major limitation of this study, of course, was the absence of a control group.

Finally, there are the three retrospective studies that compared surgical and conservative treatment. Each of these studies was of limited quality, and the duration of follow-up was not specified in any. The study by Nurick[8] was the only one to employ a clinical grading system with clear definition of what constituted an improvement or deterioration (see Appendix 23 [Nurick's Clinical Grading of Cervical Spondylotic Myelopathy]). The results of these three studies are summarized in Table 17-2.

TABLE 17-2
Retrospective Studies of Surgical and Conservative Therapy of Cervical
Spondylotic Myelopathy

Study	Improved		Unchanged		Worse	
	Surgical	*Medical*	*Surgical*	*Medical*	*Surgical*	*Medical*
Nurick[8]	8% (n = 3)	7% (n = 3)	64% (n = 29)	81% (n = 29)	28% (n = 12)	12% (n = 4)
Campbell[7]	58% (n = 7)	77% (n = 10)	25% (n = 3)	23% (n = 3)	17% (n = 2)	0%
Arnasson[9]	62% (n = 21)	0%	29% (n = 10)	100% (n = 4)	9% (n = 3)	0%

The sample size in each of these studies was small. The results are variable with improvement ranging from 8% to 62% in the surgically treated group and 0% to 77% in the medically treated group. The rate of deterioration ranged from 9% to 28% in the surgically treated group and was approximately 12% in the medically treated group. Finally, there have been refinements and improvements in surgical technique since publication of these studies.

In conclusion, therefore, data from the only prospective randomized study[4] indicate that surgery offers no benefit over conservative therapy in patients with myelopathy of a mild to moderate degree. The study by Sampath and colleagues[5] that included patients with myelopathy of any severity is difficult to interpret because of its various limitations, and it did not provide clear evidence of benefit from surgery. Finally, data from the three retrospective series[7–9] that compare patients treated conservatively and surgically do not indicate any clear benefit of one approach to treatment over the other.

Is There Any Evidence to Favor Surgery over Conservative Measures for Cervical Spondylotic Radiculopathy?

Quality literature on the optimal management of radiculopathy due to cervical spondylosis is even more sparse than that on the subject of cervical myelopathy. There are no prospective randomized studies and only a single prospective study that was not randomized.[10] This study was part of the Cervical Spine Research Society study, the results of which, for patients with myelopathy, have already been described. The outcome measures used were the same as those reported previously and included an assessment of neurologic symptoms (seven-point scale), functional status (four-point scale),

TABLE 17-3
Outcome of Patients with Cervical Spondylotic Radiculopathy

	Conservative	*Surgery*
Pain (0–5)[a]	−1.04 (p <0.001)	−1.6 (p <0.01)
Neurologic symptoms (0–6)[a]	−0.28	−0.64 (p <0.01)
Functional status (0–3)[b]	+0.3 (p <0.01)	+0.57 (p <0.01)
Activities of daily living (0–5)[a]	+0.11	−0.56 (p <0.01)

[a]Low scores indicate better performance; – = improving status.
[b]High score indicates better performance; + = improving status.

patient satisfaction, severity of pain (six-point scale), and a measure of independence with ADLs (six-point scale). All of these measures were made on the basis of subjective patient report rather than objective measurement.

This study included 246 patients with isolated cervical radiculopathy; follow-up data (mean of 11.2 months) are only available for 155 (63%) patients. Of these 155 patients, 104 (67%) were treated medically and 51 (33%) surgically. The primary surgical treatment consisted of neural decompression using a posterior approach with foraminotomy or laminectomy, anterior cervical discectomy, or both. The results are summarized in Table 17-3, with reported values indicating the change in score from baseline.

In general, therefore, the outcome measures were more favorable in the surgically treated group. However, as with the Cervical Spine Research Society study of cervical myelopathy, this study was similarly limited by subjects not being randomized, a high dropout rate, and the use of purely subjective measures of outcome. The lack of randomization precludes direct comparisons being made between the two treatment groups. The short duration of follow-up may also have generated a bias in favor of the surgical group, because with increasing time, spondylosis may develop adjacent to the level previously subjected to surgery.

In view of the relatively benign prognosis of cervical radiculopathy[3] and in the absence of clear data to indicate otherwise, surgical intervention should be undertaken with caution and perhaps reserved for patients with unremitting and progressive symptoms in whom medical therapy has failed.

Summary

- With conservative management, the outcome of cervical spondylotic radiculopathy is generally benign.
- There are no prospective, randomized, controlled trials of surgery versus conservative therapy in patients with cervical radiculopathy, but in view of what is known about the natural history of the dis-

ease, surgery should not be performed unless there is no improvement with time and conservative therapy.

- The natural history of untreated cervical spondylotic myelopathy is unknown, with conflicting prognosis reported in different studies.
- There are data from a single prospective randomized study indicating that patients with mild to moderate cervical spondylotic myelopathy do not benefit more from surgery than from conservative measures.
- Whether patients with more severe forms of cervical spondylotic myelopathy would benefit from surgery remains an unanswered question.

References

1. Lees F, Turner JW. Natural history and prognosis of cervical spondylosis. *BMJ* 1963;2:1607–1610.
2. Clarke E, Robinson PK. Cervical myelopathy: a complication of cervical spondylosis. *Brain* 1956;79:483–510.
3. Radhakrishnan K, Litchy WH, O'Fallon M, Kurland LT. Epidemiology of cervical radiculopathy—a population-based study from Rochester, Minnesota, 1976 through 1990. *Brain* 1994;117:325–335.
4. Kadanka Z, Bednarik J, Vohanka S, et al. Conservative treatment versus surgery in spondylotic cervical myelopathy: a prospective randomized study. *Eur Spine J* 2000;9:538–544.
5. Sampath P, Bendebba M, Davis JD, Ducker TB. Outcome of patients treated for cervical myelopathy. A prospective, multicenter study with independent clinical review. *Spine* 2000;25:670–676.
6. Mann KS, Khosla VK, Gulati DR. Cervical spondylotic myelopathy treated by single-stage multilevel anterior decompression. A prospective study. *J Neurosurg* 1984;60:81–87.
7. Campbell AMG, Phillips DG. Cervical disk lesions with neurological disorder. *BMJ* 1960;481–485.
8. Nurick S. The natural history and the results of surgical treatment of the spinal cord disorder associated with cervical spondylosis. *Brain* 1972;95:101–108.
9. Arnasson O, Carlsson CA, Pellettieri L. Surgical and conservative treatment of cervical spondylotic radiculopathy and myelopathy. *Acta Neurochir (Wien)* 1987:84:48–53.
10. Sampath P, Bendebba M, Davis JD, Ducker T. Outcome in patients with cervical radiculopathy. Prospective multicenter study with independent clinical review. *Spine* 1999:24:591–597.

CHAPTER 18

Amyotrophic Lateral Sclerosis

Introduction

The term *amyotrophic lateral sclerosis* (ALS) is often used interchangeably with *motor neuron disease*. Strictly speaking, however, *motor neuron disease* is a broader term that encompasses a range of neurodegenerative disorders characterized by loss of motor neurons. When the dominant symptoms are related to speech and swallowing, the term *progressive bulbar atrophy* is used. *Progressive muscular atrophy* refers to an isolated lower motor neuron (LMN) syndrome, and the designation *primary lateral sclerosis* is used when signs of upper motor neuron (UMN) dysfunction predominate. ALS manifests clinically with a combination of UMN and LMN signs and symptoms and is characterized pathologically by loss of motor neurons in the spinal cord, brainstem, and cerebral cortex.

ALS is an uncommon disease with an incidence in the range of 1.0–2.5 cases per 100,000 population. Incidence increases with age and there is a slight male preponderance. The etiology remains unknown and treatment is largely supportive. The recent introduction of the glutamate antagonist riluzole, however, has prompted much controversy, and an evaluation of the two placebo-controlled trials of riluzole is the major focus of this chapter. Consideration, however, is also given to issues relevant to the diagnosis and natural history of the disease.

What Are the El Escorial Criteria, and How Useful Are They in Clinical Practice?

Perceiving a need for precise diagnostic criteria for ALS, the World Federation of Neurology convened a workshop at El Escorial (in Spain) that led to the publication of the El Escorial criteria for the diagnosis of ALS.[1,2] According to these criteria, the diagnosis of ALS requires

A—The presence of
- Evidence of LMN degeneration (by clinical, electrophysiologic, or neuropathologic examination)

- Evidence of UMN degeneration (by clinical examination)
- Progressive spread of symptoms or signs within a region or to other regions (as determined by history or examination)

B—The absence of

- Electrophysiologic and pathologic evidence of other disease processes that might explain the signs of LMN or UMN degeneration
- Neuroimaging evidence of other disease processes that might explain the observed clinical and electrophysiologic signs

These criteria recognize four regions of the central nervous system—bulbar, cervical, thoracic, and lumbosacral. Progression of signs within a region and, even more importantly, progression of signs to involve other regions, is a crucial feature for the clinical diagnosis of ALS. The clinical diagnosis may be made with varying degrees of certainty. Recognized categories include clinically definite ALS, clinically probable ALS (with or without laboratory support), clinically possible ALS, and clinically suspected ALS. Clinically definite ALS requires the presence of UMN and LMN dysfunction in three of the four regions of the central nervous system. Involvement of only two regions satisfies criteria for clinically probable ALS.

The role of electrophysiologic studies in the diagnosis of ALS is to confirm LMN dysfunction in clinically affected regions, to detect electrophysiologic evidence of LMN dysfunction in clinically uninvolved regions, and to exclude other pathophysiologic processes. No neuroimaging tests are required to positively support the diagnosis of ALS but should be used to exclude other conditions that might cause UMN or LMN signs.

These criteria were devised primarily for research purposes, leaving unanswered the question of how well they perform in the clinical arena. Traynor et al.[3] conducted a prospective population-based study of the natural history of ALS in Ireland, using the El Escorial criteria to examine their utility. They identified 383 patients of whom 131 (34%) had definite ALS, 87 (23%) probable ALS, 136 (36%) possible ALS, and 29 (8%) suspected ALS at the time of initial diagnosis. Patients were followed prospectively, and there was a general trend towards increasing diagnostic confidence with time. At the time of death, 179 (71%) had definite ALS, 49 (19%) had probable ALS, 32 (9%) possible, and three (1%) suspected ALS. Median survival times and mortality rates were similar across the different diagnostic categories, and the El Escorial category at diagnosis did not emerge as an independent predictor of prognosis. These data suggest that the El Escorial criteria have high specificity but low sensitivity, especially in the early stages of the disease when the potential benefit from therapeutic intervention is likely to be greatest.

What Is the Natural History of Amyotrophic Lateral Sclerosis, and Are There Factors That Predict Prognosis?

Although ALS is a progressive and fatal disease with a mean survival of 3–4 years after diagnosis, the course may be quite variable and it is, therefore, difficult to predict the rate of progression and the expected survival for an individual patient. This has generated a number of studies that have attempted to identify variables that might help to predict the course of the disease for a particular patient. Age of onset has most consistently been identified as an important prognostic variable, with younger age of onset predicting a slower progression of disease with a longer median survival.[4–8] In the study by Norris et al.,[7] for example, the median survival correlated inversely with age of onset of symptoms (Table 18-1).

There is less consensus regarding the matter of whether the site of disease onset (limb vs. bulbar) has prognostic significance. The studies by Norris et al.,[7] Preux et al.,[6] and Chancellor et al.[8] identified bulbar onset as a predictor of a more aggressive disease with shorter mean survival. Caroscio et al.[4] and Eisen et al.,[5] however, did not confirm this finding. Eisen and colleagues, for example, found that the predictive value of bulbar onset of symptoms could be entirely accounted for by the older age of onset of patients with this form of the disease. Bulbar onset of disease, therefore, was a contingent variable rather than being of primary prognostic significance. This issue remains controversial.

What Is the Strength of the Evidence Supporting the Use of Riluzole?

The efficacy of riluzole in the treatment of patients with ALS has been examined in two prospective, placebo-controlled trials. In the first study by Bensimon et al.,[9] 155 patients with probable or definite ALS were randomized to receive either placebo (n = 78) or 100 mg riluzole per day (n = 77).

TABLE 18-1
Effect of Age on Survival in Amyotrophic Lateral Sclerosis

Age of Onset (Yrs)	Median Survival (Mos)
25–44	71.5
45–54	35.0
55–74	32.5

TABLE 18-2
Effect of Riluzole on Survival in Amyotrophic Lateral Sclerosis

| | *Tracheostomy-Free Survival at 1 Yr* | | |
	Riluzole	*Placebo*	p *Value*
Total population	74% (57/77)	58% (45/78)	0.014
Bulbar onset	73% (11/15)	35% (6/17)	0.014
Limb onset	74% (46/62)	64% (39/61)	0.17

Randomization was stratified according to the site of onset of disease. The study included 32 patients with bulbar onset disease and 123 with limb onset of symptoms. The primary outcome measures were tracheostomy-free survival and functional status after 12 months of treatment. Survival data at 21 months were also reported. No patients were lost to follow-up. The results of the primary efficacy analysis are summarized in Table 18-2.

For the combined population of bulbar- and limb onset disease, there was a statistically significant difference in survival between the riluzole-treated and placebo-treated groups. This survival advantage, however, barely reached significance by 21 months of follow-up, with tracheostomy-free survival rates of 37% and 49% for the placebo- and riluzole-treated patients, respectively ($p = 0.046$). Separate analyses of the bulbar and limb onset groups showed that the 12-month survival advantage conferred by riluzole was entirely due to the improved survival in the bulbar onset group. There was no significant difference in the endpoint of tracheostomy-free survival at 1 year in the subgroup of patients with limb onset disease.

The second prespecified endpoint was the rate of change in functional status. Limb and bulbar function were evaluated with modified Norris scales (see Appendix 26 [Norris Scale for Amyotrophic Lateral Sclerosis]), and muscle function was assessed by clinical examination of 22 muscle groups using the Medical Research Council five-point grading system. For each functional score, the rate of deterioration was slower in the riluzole-treated group than in the placebo-treated group, but only the rate of deterioration of the muscle-testing score was statistically significant.

Overall, these results suggest that riluzole is beneficial in those patients with bulbar onset disease and that the therapeutic effect diminishes with time. Caution should be exercised in the interpretation of these results given the relatively small number of patients with bulbar onset disease. Moreover, the reason for the discrepant results between the limb- and bulbar onset patients was not explained.

TABLE 18-3
Dose-Response Effect of Riluzole on Survival in Amyotrophic Lateral Sclerosis

	Tracheostomy-Free Survival at 18 Mos (%)
Placebo	50.4
Riluzole 50 mg	55.3
Riluzole 100 mg	56.8
Riluzole 200 mg	57.8

The design of the second large trial of riluzole was similar to the first; however, it incorporated a dose-ranging design as well as a longer period of follow-up and included a larger number of patients.[10] Patients were stratified according to limb or bulbar onset, and the design was double-blind and placebo-controlled. A total of 959 patients were enrolled (295 with bulbar onset and 664 with limb onset) and randomized to receive placebo or 50 mg, 100 mg, or 200 mg of riluzole. Tracheostomy-free survival (at 18 months) was again chosen as the primary outcome measure. The results are summarized in Table 18-3.

The relative risks of tracheostomy-free survival were calculated both before (log-rank test) and after (Cox method) adjustment for prognostic factors, and although the 18-month time interval had been prespecified, relative risk for survival at 12 months was also reported. The calculated relative risks are tabulated (Table 18-4; *p* values are emboldened for the results that are statistically significant). Values less than 1 indicate a lower risk of death or tracheostomy.

The justification for the separate analyses after adjustment for prognostic factors was based on the demonstration of significantly different sur-

TABLE 18-4
Relative Risk of Survival in Amyotrophic Lateral Sclerosis for Patients
Treated with Riluzole

Riluzole Dose	*No Adjustment for Prognostic Variables*		*After Adjustment for Prognostic Variables*	
	12 Mos	*18 Mos*	*12 Mos*	*18 Mos*
50 mg	0.76 ($p = 0.089$)	0.85 ($p = 0.25$)	0.72 (**$p = 0.04$**)	0.76 (**$p = 0.04$**)
100 mg	0.66 (**$p = 0.019$**)	0.79 ($p = 0.076$)	0.57 (**$p = 0.001$**)	0.65 (**$p = 0.002$**)
200 mg	0.69 (**$p = 0.021$**)	0.79 ($p = 0.075$)	0.57 (**$p = 0.0007$**)	0.61 (**$p = 0.0004$**)

Note: *p* values in boldface indicate statistically significant results.

vival curves for high- and low-risk patients. The study population was divided into high- and low-risk groups according to the median value of the overall prognostic score (that was calculated from the factors identified by the Cox model for survival). In contrast to the previous study, there was no significant difference in the treatment effect between the groups with different sites of disease onset (limb vs. bulbar).

These results were taken by the authors to indicate a dose-dependent beneficial effect of riluzole on tracheostomy-free survival among patients with ALS. It should be noted, however, that in the analysis before adjustment for prognostic variables, the beneficial effect of riluzole was apparent at 12 but not 18 months. Greater likelihood of tracheostomy-free survival was apparent at both 12 and 18 months in the analysis that adjusted for the variables found to independently affect prognosis. Changes in a variety of functional scores (muscle strength as well as limb and bulbar scores) were among the prespecified secondary outcome measures, but significant differences were not observed between the riluzole-treated and placebo-treated groups on these measures of efficacy.

Summary

- The El Escorial criteria were established by the World Federation of Neurology to serve as guidelines for the purposes of clinical research and therapeutic trials; these rely on the progressive spread of signs of both UMN and LMN dysfunction within and between different regions of the nervous system.
- There is some evidence that the El Escorial criteria have high specificity but low sensitivity, especially in the early stages of the disease.
- Age of onset is the most important variable predicting survival in ALS, with younger age of onset being characterized by a longer median survival; it remains controversial whether limb onset disease (rather than bulbar onset) implies a better prognosis.
- The efficacy of riluzole has been examined in two prospective double-blind, placebo-controlled trials, each of which used tracheostomy-free survival as the primary measure of efficacy.
- The first study suggested that riluzole imparted a beneficial effect for bulbar- but not limb onset disease.
- The second (larger) study demonstrated a beneficial effect of riluzole on tracheostomy-free survival at 12 months but not at 18 months. After correction for factors found to be of prognostic importance, the beneficial effects of riluzole became more apparent with reduced relative risks of death for the riluzole-treated patients at both 12 and 18 months.

References

1. Brooks BR. El Escorial World Federation of Neurology Criteria for the diagnosis of amyotrophic lateral sclerosis. Subcommittee on motor neuron disease/amyotrophic lateral sclerosis of the World Federation of Neurology Research Group on neuromuscular diseases and the El Escorial "Clinical Limits of Amyotrophic Lateral Sclerosis" Workshop Contributors. *J Neurol Sci* 1994;124(Suppl):96–107.
2. http://www.wfnals.org/Articles/elescorial1998criteria.htm. Accessed July 10, 2002.
3. Traynor BJ, Codd MB, Corr B, et al. Clinical features of amyotrophic lateral sclerosis according to the El Escorial and Airlie House Diagnostic Criteria. A population-based study. *Arch Neurol* 2000;57:1171–1176.
4. Caroscio JT, Mulvihill MN, Sterling R, Abrams B. Amyotrophic lateral sclerosis—its natural history. *Neurol Clin* 1987;5:1–8.
5. Eisen A, Schulzer M, MacNeil M, et al. Duration of amyotrophic lateral sclerosis is age dependent. *Muscle Nerve* 1993;16:27–32.
6. Preux PM, Couratier P, Boutros-Toni F, et al. Survival prediction in sporadic amyotrophic lateral sclerosis. Age and clinical form at onset are independent risk factors. *Neuroepidemiology* 1996;15:153–160.
7. Norris F, Shepherd R, Denys E, et al. Onset, natural history and outcome in idiopathic adult motor neuron disease. *J Neurol Sci* 1993;118:48–55.
8. Chancellor AM, Slattery MJ, Fraser H, et al. The prognosis of adult-onset motor neuron disease: a prospective study based on the Scottish motor neuron disease register. *J Neurol* 1993;240:339–346.
9. Bensimon G, Lacomblez L, Meininger V. A controlled trial of riluzole in amyotrophic lateral sclerosis. ALS/Riluzole Study Group. *N Engl J Med* 1994;330:585–591.
10. Lacomblez L, Bensimon G, Leigh PN, et al. Dose-ranging study of riluzole in amyotrophic lateral sclerosis. Amyotrophic Lateral Sclerosis/Riluzole Study Group II. *Lancet* 1996;347:1425–1431.

CHAPTER 19

Spinal Cord Injury and Compression

Introduction

Traumatic spinal cord injury is a common problem and frequently affects young people, imposing enormous personal and financial costs. Compression of the spinal cord by metastatic cancer is even more common, with estimates of approximately 5% of patients with metastatic cancer developing spinal cord compression. The former has been the subject of a series of large prospective studies that have led to the widespread acceptance of intravenous methylprednisolone in the acute management of patients with traumatic spinal cord injury. The evidence supporting any form of treatment of metastatic spinal cord compression is far less robust. Do the available studies really support the use of steroids in the management of spinal cord injury? Should steroids be used in the treatment of metastatic spinal cord compression, and if so, in what sorts of dosages? What is the relative utility of steroids, radiotherapy, and surgery in the management of these patients? These questions are the focus of this chapter.

Does the Evidence Support the Use of Steroids for the Treatment of Acute Spinal Cord Injury?

The second National Acute Spinal Cord Injury Study (NASCIS-2)[1] was the first prospective, placebo-controlled trial that examined the efficacy and safety of high-dose methylprednisolone for the treatment of acute spinal cord injury. Patients with acute spinal cord injury who presented within 12 hours of the injury were eligible for inclusion. Those with acute traumatic lesions of the cauda equina were excluded. Four hundred eighty-seven patients were randomized to receive one of three treatment regimens—methylprednisolone (administered as a bolus of 30 mg/kg followed by a maintenance dose of 5.4 mg/kg per hour), naloxone (given as a bolus of 5.4 mg/kg and a maintenance dose of 4 mg/kg per hour), or placebo. The overwhelming majority of patients also underwent surgery. Neurologic evaluation was performed at 6 weeks and 6 months, and the primary endpoint was a change in neurologic function between the baseline and follow-up examinations. Although not specified in advance, analysis of the results was stratified according to the latency until receipt of the loading dose (within the first 8 hours and beyond 8 hours). Considering only those patients treated within 8 hours, there was a significantly greater improvement in motor and sensory function at 6 weeks that persisted at 6 months amongst those who received methylprednisolone. No beneficial effects were observed amongst those treated with naloxone, and patients treated with either drug beyond 8 hours similarly demonstrated no improvement. On the basis of these results, steroids have become a routine part of the medical management of patients with traumatic spinal cord injury.

There are, however, reasons to question whether the results of this study really provide evidence that methylprednisolone should be used in the treatment of acute spinal cord injury. It should be recalled that the positive outcomes observed in the 8-hour latency to treatment subgroup were not observed for the entire study population. This issue is particularly important given that the decision to conduct separate analyses based on the stratification of patients who presented within or beyond 8 hours of the spinal cord injury was made post hoc. Stratification by time to treatment could lead to multiple potential subgroups depending on the time intervals chosen, and with only 20 subgroups, significant results could be obtained in one by chance alone. It is also relevant to note that the neurologic outcome was worse (although not reaching statistical significance) amongst those patients treated with methylprednisolone more than 8 hours after the injury, suggesting that steroid treatment may be detrimental to some spinal cord injury patients.

A more detailed analysis of the motor and sensory indices used in this study also raises concerns. Patients were assigned to one of five motor groups (quadriplegic, quadriparetic, paraplegic, paraparetic, and normal) and one of five sensory groups (absent soft touch and pinprick sensation at or above T1, absent soft touch and pinprick sensation below T1, diminished soft touch and pinprick sensation at or above T1, diminished soft touch and pinprick sensation below T1, and normal). Combining the motor and sensory groups, there are, therefore, 25 possible subgroups. The results of NASCIS-2 were reported in various combinations of motor and sensory subgroups (e.g., plegic patients with total sensory loss below the level of injury). The plethora of available subgroups for analysis and the failure to identify specific endpoints in advance raises doubts about the veracity of these results. Finally, even if the results of NASCIS-2 are accepted, it should also be recalled that patients with cauda equina injury were excluded; thus, the results are not applicable to patients with paraplegia due to lesions below the conus medullaris.

The follow-up NASCIS-3 study[2] was designed to evaluate whether a 48-hour maintenance dose of methylprednisolone would lead to a greater degree of recovery than the 24-hour protocol employed in the NASCIS-2 study. Patients with a spinal cord injury and randomized within 8 hours of the onset of the injury were eligible for inclusion. All patients received a bolus of open-label methylprednisolone (20–40 mg/kg) and were then randomized to one of three treatment groups—methylprednisolone infused continuously over 48 hours at 5.4 mg/kg per hour, the same dose of methylprednisolone infused over 24 hours, or intravenous infusions every 6 hours of tirilazad mesylate. There was no placebo group. Neurologic evaluation was performed at 6 weeks and 6 months according to the protocol employed in NASCIS-2 with the additional use of the Functional Independence Measure (see Appendix 8 [Functional Independence Measure])—a scoring system that incorporates measures of self-care, sphincter control, mobility, locomotion, communication, and social cognition. A total of 499 patients were randomized to one of the three treatment groups, and the primary endpoint was a change in neurologic function between baseline and follow-up examinations. Compared to those who received 24 hours of methylprednisolone, those treated with 48 hours of methylprednisolone demonstrated a nonsignificant trend towards improved motor and sensory function as well as Functional Independence Measure scores. Marginally significant improvements in motor scores and Functional Independence Measure subscores were observed for patients in the 48-hour methylprednisolone group who were treated between 3 and 8 hours after the injury. These minor differences should be interpreted with caution given that the benefits were not observed for the group as a whole and in view of the notable differences in the baseline motor scores of the two treatment groups (normal motor function in 24.7% of the 24-hour methylprednisolone-treated group and 13.9% in the 48-hour methylprednisolone-treated group). Nonsignificant differences in the rates of severe complications were also observed with severe sepsis occurring in 2.6% and 0.6% of the 48-hour and 24-hour treatment groups, respectively.

In summary, therefore, the results of the NASCIS-2 and NASCIS-3 studies have been widely accepted as providing the rationale for treatment, with methylprednisolone of patients presenting within 8 hours of the onset of acute spinal cord injury. The foregoing analysis, however, raises questions about whether the NASCIS trials have convincingly demonstrated benefit from high-dose methylprednisolone treatment. Although these insights are unlikely to lead to a change in prescribing practice, it is helpful to recognize the limitations of the available data, especially in the context of individuals who may be at greater risk for the infectious complications that occur more commonly in those treated with high-dose steroids.

Is There a Role for Steroids in the Treatment of Metastatic Spinal Cord Compression?

The treatment of metastatic spinal cord compression with steroids alone has not been the subject of prospective study. There is, however, a single prospective, randomized study that investigated the use of steroids as an adjunct to radiotherapy.

Sørensen et al.[3] conducted a single-blind, randomized trial in which they compared high-dose dexamethasone therapy with no steroids as an adjunct to radiotherapy for the treatment of metastatic spinal cord compression. Patients randomized to treatment with steroids received an intravenous bolus of 96 mg dexamethasone, followed by 96 mg per day for 3 days (usually administered orally) and a 10-day steroid taper. The study population comprised 57 patients, 27 of whom received dexamethasone. The underlying malignancy was breast cancer in the majority of patients. Using an intention-to-treat analysis, the effect of therapy was assessed in terms of gait function with successful treatment defined as retained ability to walk in ambulatory patients and walking ability regained in nonambulatory patients. At 3 months, treatment was successful in 22 of 27 patients (81%) who received dexamethasone compared to 19 of 30 patients (63%) who did not. This difference was maintained at 6 months, with 16 (59%) of dexamethasone-treated patients ambulatory, compared to 10 (33%) of those who did not receive steroids. Significant side effects occurred in three patients who received high-dose dexamethasone. Subgroup analysis of only those patients with breast cancer revealed an even more marked beneficial effect of steroid treatment for this group of patients.

This study, therefore, provides evidence for the use of high-dose dexamethasone in the management of these patients. There are retrospective series in which lower doses of steroids were used and the reported outcomes were similar, but these studies were uncontrolled; high- and medium-dose steroids have not been compared head-to-head.

What Is the Evidence Supporting the Use of Radiotherapy in the Treatment of Metastatic Epidural Spinal Cord Compression?

Most studies that have examined the effects of radiotherapy have been retrospective. There is a single, uncontrolled, prospective study. Kim et al.[4] reported their experience with 65 patients with metastatic spinal cord compression who were treated with the combination of steroids and radiotherapy. Before the initiation of therapy, patients were divided into five categories based on motor function—normal, ambulatory, nonambulatory but able to offer resistance to gravity, nonambulatory and unable to resist gravity, and paraplegic. The acquisition or retention of the ability to ambulate was accepted as a marker of treatment success. All patients who were ambulatory before irradiation remained stable, 35% of those who were nonambulatory recovered the ability to walk, and only one paraplegic patient (7%) became ambulant after treatment. The radiosensitivity of the underlying tumor was the other factor predictive of a good response to treatment. Although this was not a randomized or even a controlled study, it does indicate that pretreatment locomotor function is an important predictor of ambulatory outcome and that a significant minority of nonambulatory patients may recover the ability to walk after treatment with the combination of steroids and irradiation.

What Is the Relative Utility of Radiotherapy and Surgery in the Management of Metastatic Extradural Spinal Cord Compression?

Surgery and radiotherapy for the treatment of metastatic spinal cord compression have never been compared head-to-head in a prospective randomized study. Current practice, therefore, is based on retrospective uncontrolled data.

Gilbert et al.[5] retrospectively reported their experience with 235 patients with metastatic spinal cord compression to compare the results of decompressive laminectomy followed by radiotherapy with those of radiotherapy alone. This study cohort comprised two series of patients treated at different times. All patients had clinical and myelographic evidence of metastatic epidural spinal cord compression. In the earlier series, most patients received prednisone, 60 mg per day (although there was some variation in the choice of steroid agent and dose), and in the later series, all patients received dexamethasone 16 mg per day in divided doses. Definitive therapy, initiated as soon as possible after the diagnosis was established, comprised either radiotherapy alone or the combination of decompressive laminectomy and postoperative radiotherapy. The decision to operate or irradiate was based on the clinical judgment of the treating physician, and no effort was made to control or randomize patients to the different treatment groups. Before treatment, patients were divided into three groups—those who were ambulatory (with or without leg weakness), those who were not ambulatory but able to move their legs, and those who were paraplegic and unable to elevate their legs against gravity. Of the 235 patients, 65 underwent surgical decompression followed by irradiation and 170 were treated with radiotherapy alone. Successful treatment was defined as the ability to walk at the time of hospital discharge. For each treatment group as a whole, there were no outcome differences (46% of the surgical group and 49% of the radiotherapy group were ambulatory at the time of discharge). The results of subgroup analysis for patients in the different clinical groups similarly revealed no significant differences.

Further subgroup analysis based on the relative radiosensitivity of the underlying tumor similarly revealed no differences in outcome between the two treatment groups. The durability of the response to therapy was also comparable between the two treatment groups, with 75% and 79% of the successfully treated surgical and radiotherapy groups respectively remaining ambulatory at 6 months. As a result of studies like these, as well as the recognition of the high rate of spinal instability after laminectomy, this surgical procedure has largely been abandoned as a form of treatment for metastatic spinal cord compression.

More recently, however, there has emerged the suggestion that more aggressive surgery aimed at gross total tumor resection combined with spinal stabilization may represent a useful form of therapy. Sundaresan et al.[6] retrospectively reported their experience with aggressive surgery for patients with metastatic spinal cord compression. Indications for surgery included presentation with metastatic spinal cord compression but no histologic diagnosis, spinal instability, relapse after irradiation, and the presence of a radio-resistant tumor or a solitary metastasis. The surgical procedure was tailored to each individual patient with the intention of performing a gross total resection and spinal reconstruction. Fifty percent of the 110 patients included in this study underwent prior treatment (surgery or radiotherapy) but had clinical and radiographic evidence of tumor progression. Postoperative radiotherapy was administered to 20 of the 51 patients who had not previously been irradiated; results are not reported separately for those who did and did not receive radiotherapy.

Preoperatively, patients were divided into those who were ambulatory and those who were not. Postoperatively, patients were considered improved if they became or remained ambulatory at the time of hospital discharge. Overall, 90 patients (82%) were improved, including 32 patients (67%) who were initially nonambulatory. Complications occurred in 53 patients (48%), the most common of which included wound breakdown, stabilization failure, and infection. The high rate of success, reported by these authors, does compare favorably with the results observed in prior studies of steroid, radiotherapy, and surgical treatment; however, the lack of follow-up data (i.e., results reported at the time of hospital discharge) and the absence of an internal control group make it difficult to interpret these results. Thus, although laminectomy has been abandoned for the treatment of metastatic spinal cord compression, it may be that these newer and more aggressive operative procedures will offer advantages over radiotherapy and steroids. The efficacy of these newer operative interventions, however, remains to be proven in prospective controlled trials.

Finally, as noted in a recent systematic review of the treatment of metastatic spinal cord compression by Loblaw and Laperriere,[7] surgical intervention is frequently recommended for bony compression or spinal instability. This recommendation is based on "expert opinion" that has been rendered despite the absence of quality data that outcome is improved by surgery for bony compression, spinal instability, or salvage after progression following radiotherapy. Under these circumstances, laminectomy alone is insufficient, and a more extensive surgical procedure that encompasses vertebrectomy or spinal reconstruction is necessary.

In conclusion, therefore, recommendations regarding the treatment of metastatic spinal cord compression surgically or with radiotherapy can only be made on the basis of inadequate data. Laminectomy seems to offer little benefit and may even be harmful given the frequency with which it results in spinal instability. Data from retrospective uncontrolled trials suggest that more aggressive operative intervention with spinal reconstruction

TABLE 19-1
Successful Outcome of Patients with Metastatic Spinal Cord Compression

Study	Design	XRT	XRT + Steroids	XRT + Laminectomy	XRT + Spinal Reconstruction
			Treatment		
Sørenson[3]	Prospective randomized	90%[a]/ 18%[b]	100%[a]/ 50%[b]	—	—
Kim[4]	Prospective uncontrolled	—	100%[a]/ 26%[b]	—	—
Gilbert[5]	Retrospective case series	79%[a]/ 34%[b]	—	64%[a]/37%[b]	—
Sundaresan[6]	Retrospective case series	—	—	—	94%[a]/67%[b]

XRT = radiotherapy.
[a]Ambulatory at baseline.
[b]Not ambulatory at baseline.

after gross total resection of the tumor (with or without irradiation) may offer an advantage over radiotherapy alone. The recommendation that spinal instability and bony compression of the spinal cord are indications for surgery is based on expert opinion rather than on evidence.

Summary

- NASCIS-2 was the key prospective randomized, placebo-controlled trial that tested the utility of intravenous methylprednisolone in the treatment of patients with traumatic spinal cord injury. Although this study is not without flaws, it has been widely accepted as providing the evidence for the efficacy and safety of steroids when administered within 8 hours of the spinal cord injury.
- There are limited quality data regarding the appropriate use of steroids, radiotherapy, and surgery in patients with metastatic spinal cord compression, with only a single, prospective, controlled trial in which high-dose dexamethasone treatment was compared to no-steroids treatment as an adjunct to radiotherapy.
- The results of studies examining the effects of radiotherapy, steroids, or surgery in various conditions are summarized in Table 19-1.

Data shown are the percentages of patients with a successful outcome, defined as regained or retained ambulatory capacity.

References

1. Bracken MB, Shepard MJ, Collins WF, et al. A randomized, controlled trial of methylprednisolone or naloxone in the treatment of acute spinal-cord injury. Results of the second National Acute Spinal Cord Injury Study. *N Engl J Med* 1990;322:1405–1411.
2. Bracken MB, Shepard MJ, Holford TR, et al. Administration of methylprednisolone for 24 or 48 hours or tirilazad mesylate for 48 hours in the treatment of acute spinal cord injury. Results of the third Acute Spinal Cord Injury Randomized Controlled Trial. National Acute Spinal Cord Injury Study. *JAMA* 1997;277:1597–1604.
3. Sørensen S, Helweg-Larsen S, Mouridsen H, Hansen HH. Effect of high-dose dexamethasone in carcinomatous metastatic spinal cord compression treated with radiotherapy: a randomised trial. *Eur J Cancer* 1994;30A:22–27.
4. Kim RY, Spencer SA, Meredith RF, et al. Extradural spinal cord compression: analysis of factors determining functional prognosis—prospective study. *Radiology* 1990;176:279–282.
5. Gilbert RW, Kim JH, Posner JB. Epidural spinal cord compression from metastatic tumor: diagnosis and treatment. *Ann Neurol* 1978;3:40–51.
6. Sundaresan N, Sachdev VP, Holland JF, et al. Surgical treatment of spinal cord compression from epidural metastasis. *J Clin Oncol* 1995;13:2330–2335.
7. Loblaw DA, Laperriere NJ. Emergency treatment of malignant extradural spinal cord compression: an evidence-based guideline. *J Clin Oncol* 1998;16: 1613–1624.

CHAPTER 20

Parkinson's Disease

Introduction

Idiopathic Parkinson's disease (PD) is a chronic degenerative disorder defined clinically and neuropathologically. The clinical features include bradykinesia, rigidity, tremor, and postural instability as well as a response to levodopa (L-dopa) replacement therapy. Pathologically, PD is defined by the presence of Lewy bodies and the progressive death of neuromelanin-containing dopaminergic neurons of the substantia nigra pars compacta. L-Dopa remains the mainstay of therapy, and although the motor symptoms of PD may improve dramatically with L-dopa treatment, the underlying neurodegenerative process is not arrested. With time, the motor symptoms become more profound and often less responsive to L-dopa therapy. Long-standing disease and use of L-dopa are accompanied by the development of late motor complications, including dyskinesias (chorea, dystonia) and motor fluctuations ("wearing off" and "on-off" phenomena). These are responsible for significant morbidity later in the course of the disease. There is uncertainty as to whether the duration and dosage of L-dopa is primarily responsible for these motor complications or whether they occur simply because of increasing severity of the disease. This has prompted a longstanding controversy regarding the optimal timing of the initiation of L-dopa and whether this should be delayed in favor of the early use of dopamine agonists. A discussion of this issue is the major focus of this chapter. Attention, however, is also devoted to the evidence that amantadine may be effective in the treatment of dyskinesias and to the question of whether selegiline is neuroprotective. These and other issues are the focus of this chapter.

What Is the Relationship between Essential Tremor and Parkinson's Disease?

Several different forms of tremor occur in PD. Most typical is the rest tremor that is activated by mental stress and at least temporarily suppressed when the extremity is voluntarily activated. The usual frequency is 4–6 Hz. It is also recognized that patients with PD may have a prominent action tremor. Essential tremor (ET), on the other hand, is characterized by a combination of postural and kinetic tremors. Rest tremor may rarely occur in elderly patients with advanced disease, but this is usually a postural tremor that is caused by incomplete muscle relaxation. A general question that has emerged is whether there is a relationship between ET and PD. More specifically, there is some suggestion that the prevalence of PD may be increased amongst the population with ET. Reasons for this controversy include the absence of a biological marker that is pathognomonic of ET and the lack of uniformly agreed on diagnostic criteria.

In their retrospective study, Geraghty et al.[1] evaluated 130 patients with ET. The diagnosis was based on the presence of a tremor with at least two of three specified features: (1) a typical flexion-extension postural hand tremor or a characteristic head tremor, (2) an improvement associated with the use of alcohol or propranolol, and (3) a family history of ET. Of these 130 patients, 25 also met criteria for PD based on the presence of at least three of the cardinal signs of PD (tremor at rest, bradykinesia, rigidity, and postural instability). Onset of ET preceded the symptoms of PD in all patients. The observed concurrence of PD in 19% of patients with ET is well in excess of the expected approximate 1% prevalence of PD in the general population. In considering only those patients with ET duration of at least 5 years, the prevalence of PD remained in excess of that expected in the general population, suggesting that the observed prevalence was not simply due to a misclassification of a parkinsonian tremor as an ET. Other epidemiologic studies have not revealed an increased prevalence of PD amongst patients with ET. For example, in their retrospective review of 266 patients with ET, Rajput et al.[2] found that only 2% of patients with ET also carried the diagnosis of PD.

In an effort to resolve this controversy, Koller et al.[3] prospectively evaluated 678 patients with ET who were seen at a movement disorder clinic. ET was diagnosed by the presence of bilateral postural tremor (with or without kinetic tremor) involving the hands and forearms or tremor of the head that was visible and persistent and not due to another etiology such as drugs, trauma, or psychogenicity. They observed a prevalence of PD of 6.1%. The prevalence of PD in the general population aged between 60 and 69 (similar in age to those in this study) is estimated to be between 0.1% and 1.0%. This would suggest that PD does occur more commonly among patients with ET than in the general population.

Is Deprenyl Neuroprotective in Parkinson's Disease?

The Deprenyl and Tocopherol Antioxidative Therapy of Parkinsonism (DATATOP) study was designed to determine whether long-term therapy with deprenyl (selegiline) or tocopherol would extend the length of time before advancing disability required the initiation of L-dopa therapy.[4,5] This study enrolled 800 untreated patients with idiopathic PD and randomized them to receive one of four treatment regimens—tocopherol/placebo, deprenyl/placebo, deprenyl/tocopherol, or placebo. The "primary endpoint of the trial occurred when, in the judgment of the enrolling investigator, a subject reached a level of functional disability sufficient to warrant the initiation of leveodopa [*sic*] therapy." At the outset, it was planned to follow all patients for 24 months. Following an interim analysis (with mean duration of follow-up of 12 months), however, it was decided to withdraw treatment from those who had not yet reached the endpoint and to evaluate them after 1–2 months of no therapy.

Tocopherol treatment did not reduce the probability of reaching the endpoint. However, the probability of reaching the endpoint of the study was significantly lower amongst those subjects randomized to receive deprenyl, compared to those who received no deprenyl. Based on Kaplan-Meier plots, the projected median lengths of time to reach the endpoint were 719 days for the subjects who received deprenyl and 454 days for those who did not, representing an approximate difference of almost 9 months. Moreover, there was an improvement in the Unified Parkinson's Disease Rating Scale (UPDRS; see Appendix 30 [Unified Parkinson's Disease Rating Scale]) scores after the initiation of deprenyl and a worsening of the UPDRS motor scores during the 2 months after withdrawal. These findings suggested that the observed benefit of deprenyl in delaying disability was at least in part related to a symptomatic amelioration of parkinsonian symptoms. This effect had not been expected based on prior studies; thus, the ability of this study to answer the question that it set out to resolve was impaired.

The question is whether deprenyl delayed the need for L-dopa therapy solely because of this effect or whether it also exerted some neuroprotective effect in delaying the progression of the disease. A change in the study protocol after the interim analysis was effected to address this question. The 367 patients who had not reached the endpoint at the time of the interim analysis were withdrawn from experimental treatments and evaluated approximately 1–2 months later. During this 2-month period, four subjects reached the study endpoint, and 52 patients were judged to have had an increase in the severity of their PD and were administered deprenyl. There were no differences, however, among the different treatment groups in terms of the need for symptomatic therapy, suggesting that deprenyl had not altered the natural history of the disease (i.e., had not exerted a neuroprotective effect). In a separate analysis, the average rate of decline in all UPDRS variables was found to be significantly slower among subjects receiving deprenyl compared to those who were not. Moreover, for the subjects who did not reach the study endpoint, the rate of decline in UPDRS (calculated from baseline to the evaluation that occurred 2 months after the withdrawal of treatment) was significantly slower for those who had been originally randomized to receive deprenyl. To further explore the possibility of a neuroprotective effect, the patients who were withdrawn from therapy (and who did not reach the study endpoint) were given open-label deprenyl for a further 18 months.[6] Over the course of this extended follow-up period, the subjects who had originally been randomized to receive deprenyl tended to reach the endpoint of disability (requiring the addition of L-dopa) faster than the subjects who had originally been assigned to receive no deprenyl. These results, therefore, confirm the initial impression that the early beneficial effects of deprenyl were due to its symptomatic antiparkinsonian action rather than to a neuroprotective effect.

Some controversy, however, persists. Olanow et al.[7] performed a second prospective double-blind, placebo-controlled study to evaluate the effect of deprenyl on the progression of mild PD. They randomized 101 patients to one of four treatment groups—deprenyl/carbidopa–L-dopa (Sinemet), placebo/ Sinemet, deprenyl/bromocriptine, or placebo/bromocriptine. Patients were evaluated before the initiation of treatment and at 14 months (2 months after the withdrawal of deprenyl). The primary endpoint was defined as the change in UPDRS score between baseline and the final follow-up visit. In the primary analysis of patients who received deprenyl compared to those who did not (irrespective of whether in addition they received Sinemet or bromocriptine), there was a significant difference between the mean increase (deterioration) in UPDRS score (0.4 in the deprenyl-treated group and 5.8 in the placebo-treated group; $p < 0.001$). Moreover, within the group that also received Sinemet, the mean increase in UPDRS score between baseline and the final visit was significantly less among those who received deprenyl compared to those who did not. A similar trend was noted amongst the bromocriptine-treated patients. The authors interpreted these results to indicate that deprenyl delays deterioration in the signs and symptoms of PD in patients with mild to moderate disease.

Does Early Dopamine Agonist Rather Than Levodopa Therapy Reduce the Severity or Likelihood of Developing Motor Response Fluctuations and Dyskinesias?

It is accepted that the use of L-dopa in patients with PD is associated with the appearance of motor fluctuations and dyskinesias. The efficacy of dopamine agonists in providing symptomatic relief of parkinsonian symptoms, even if to a lesser extent than L-dopa, raises the question of whether the early treatment of PD with dopamine agonists could prevent or delay the appearance of motor fluctuations or dyskinesias. Some authors have claimed that the early use of dopamine agonist therapy is associated with a lower likelihood of developing these complications. The literature relevant to this controversy is extensive and characterized by a paucity of quality data as well as substantial dogma. It is, therefore, useful to review the data on which this claim has been based. In reviewing the evidence, it is useful to make a distinction between the possible effect of L-dopa on the development of overall disability on the one hand, and the emergence of motor fluctuations and dyskinesias on the other. Overall disability increases during late-stage PD in part because of motor fluctuations, but also in part because of decreased responsivity to L-dopa. Although related, these two endpoints (overall disability and motor fluctuations or dyskinesias) are not identical, and the inability to draw a clear conceptual distinction between them is part of the reason for the confusion that surrounds this literature.

The study by Rinne[8] is one of those cited in support of the concept that early dopamine agonist rather than L-dopa therapy leads to a reduced risk of late motor fluctuations and dyskinesias in PD. This was a retrospective study of 76 patients naïve to L-dopa who were treated initially with bromocriptine. Of the original 76 patients, however, 42 obtained an inadequate response to bromocriptine; therefore, L-dopa was added within the first 3–6 months. A further five patients required the addition of L-dopa after approximately 4 years. These were designated as the *early* and *late combination* therapy groups comprising 25 and 5 patients, respectively. A comparison was made between the occurrence of motor complications among these bromocriptine-treated patients and those that developed in a historical control group comprising 196 patients treated ab initio with L-dopa (and a decarboxylase inhibitor). Although there were no late motor complications amongst those who received bromocriptine alone, the antiparkinsonian effect was, at best, moderate and decreased with time. Late motor complications were reported to have developed significantly less frequently in the combined bromocriptine and L-dopa group compared to the L-dopa alone group. Caution should be exercised, however, in drawing conclusions, given the retrospective nature of this study, the absence of an appropriate control group, and the high dropout rate from the bromocriptine group. Furthermore, although the patients treated with the combination of bromocriptine and L-dopa were reported to have achieved ". . . significant improvement in parkinsonian disability equal to that achieved with leveodopa [*sic*] alone," no data are provided to substantiate this claim.

The Sydney Multicentre Study of PD was a prospective randomized study designed to compare the efficacy and side effects of low-dose L-dopa/carbidopa with low-dose bromocriptine in the treatment of PD.[9] One hundred twenty-six patients were randomized to receive either bromocriptine or low-dose L-dopa/carbidopa. The two groups were similar with respect to average age, the duration of disease before the initiation of treatment, and the degree of disability. The outcome analysis was complicated by the complex changes that were made to the antiparkinsonian drug regimen over the course of the study. Of the initial 64 patients in the bromocriptine group, only 32 remained on bromocriptine alone at 1 year; this number fell to zero after 5 years. Of 64 patients in the low-dose L-dopa–treated group, 56 remained on L-dopa therapy alone at 1 year; this number fell to 31 at 5 years. The outcome, in terms of the frequency of dyskinesia, was reported primarily on the basis of initial treatment assignment. Thus, dyskinesia developed in 35 of 64 patients randomized to receive L-dopa, compared to only 17 of 62 initially randomized to receive low-dose bromocriptine treatment. On the basis of these results, the authors concluded that ". . . patients randomized to bromocriptine did not develop dyskinesia or troublesome end of dose failure until levodopa-carbidopa was added. The prevalence of dyskinesia in this group was lower than in patients given levodopa-carbidopa alone." This conclusion, however, is misleading in part because the overwhelming majority of patients assigned to receive bromocriptine were either switched to L-dopa or treated with a combination of bromocriptine and L-dopa. Moreover, these patients were ultimately receiving higher doses of L-dopa compared to those originally assigned to receive it. In truth, therefore, it is exceedingly difficult to ascertain a clear relationship between the use of L-dopa and the development of dyskinesias. Certainly, however, it is misleading to point to the lower incidence of dyskinesias amongst those initially randomized to receive treatment with bromocriptine alone.

Lesser et al.[10] retrospectively reviewed their experience with 131 patients with idiopathic PD who were treated with L-dopa (with or without the addition of a dopa-decarboxylase inhibitor). During the course of follow-up, involuntary abnormal movements were the most common side effect (approximately 37%), with slow wearing-off occurring in 20% and sudden on-off phenomena in 14% of patients. Patients with these motor fluctuations had been started on L-dopa at a younger age and had taken the drug for a longer period. The authors ascribed the greater disability amongst patients treated with L-dopa for longer to the drug itself. However, the data do not permit this effect to be disentangled from the confounding issue of whether L-dopa had been started earlier (and, hence, maintained for longer) because of more rapid progression of disease. In this case, the more rapid progression of the disease rather than the L-dopa could be responsible for the greater disability observed. Moreover, the study was a retrospective one, there was no (even historical) control group, and the occurrence of motor fluctuations or dyskinesias was not clearly specified as the endpoint of interest. Instead, the authors describe outcome in terms of activities of daily living (ADL) scores that presumably represented a composite of motor and cognitive dysfunction due to the underlying parkinsonian state as well as the functional impact of the motor fluctuations. Notwithstanding these limitations, the authors deemed it appropriate to comment that ". . . our findings support the concept that utilization of levodopa therapy should be delayed until a patient becomes significantly impaired in occupation or social situations."

Notwithstanding the limitations of these studies, they do suggest that the incidence of dyskinesias and motor fluctuations may be lower amongst those patients treated with bromocriptine compared to those treated with

L-dopa. It is true that one possible explanation for this finding (if indeed it is a valid one) is that the difference is due to a drug effect. An alternative explanation, however, is that those patients remaining on bromocriptine monotherapy represent a cohort with milder and more slowly progressive disease. If this is the case, then the lower incidence of dyskinesias or motor fluctuations may be related to disease severity and not primarily to the treatment regimen. The available data do not permit a reliable distinction to be made between these two competing hypotheses.

In addition to the extensive, but poor quality, literature supporting the concept that early dopamine agonist therapy reduces the risk of late motor complications, there is a body of literature of similar size and quality that does not support this claim.[11-15] In the study by Markham and Diamond,[11] 58 patients were divided into three groups based on the duration of disease before the initiation of L-dopa therapy. Not surprisingly, the only significant difference between the groups was the degree of disability. In an effort to determine whether it is the duration of disease or of L-dopa therapy that primarily determines disability, they performed an analysis in which total duration of disease was held constant; however, the duration of L-dopa therapy varied. Under these circumstances, disability scores were similar, suggesting that disease duration was the critical determinant of disability rather than the duration of L-dopa therapy. These findings are relevant to the dilemma raised by Lesser's study.[10] Moreover, they found no relationship between the incidence and severity of dyskinesia and the duration of either disease or treatment.

The study of Blin et al.[12] was designed to answer the question of whether early initiation of L-dopa increased the risk of the early onset of abnormal involuntary movements and, if so, whether they were caused by the drug or whether they represented a latent consequence of underlying brain lesions that were somehow triggered by the drug. This retrospective study was performed in two parts. Amongst the 185 patients included in part 1, they observed the appearance of abnormal involuntary movements in 133 patients (72%) and found a correlation with longer duration of L-dopa therapy but not with pre–L-dopa duration of disease or the average daily dose of L-dopa. Part 2 of the study, involving 72 patients, was designed to disentangle the reason for the early emergence of abnormal involuntary movements amongst those exposed to L-dopa for longer periods. They observed that abnormal involuntary movements appeared early when L-dopa was started soon after the diagnosis of PD was made and that these movements were delayed when L-dopa therapy was started late. However, they also observed a negative correlation between the time before the initiation of L-dopa therapy and the interval from the initiation of L-dopa to the appearance of abnormal involuntary movements. Expressed another way, the duration of L-dopa therapy was actually shorter amongst those who developed abnormal involuntary movements early in the course of the disease. This finding was taken as evidence that it was the more rapid progression of the disease (rather than the early use of L-dopa) that was responsible for the appearance of abnormal involuntary movements.

Weiner et al.[16] conducted a double-blind, randomized parallel group study to compare the effects of L-dopa monotherapy, bromocriptine monotherapy, and early combination therapy, with particular attention to the development of late complications. They enrolled 25 previously untreated patients with idiopathic PD and randomized them to one of three treatment groups—bromocriptine monotherapy (eight patients), L-dopa monotherapy (10 patients), and a combination of the two drugs (seven patients). Two patients from group 1 and one patient from group 2 were lost to follow-up and not included in the final analysis. Patients were followed for 4 years, and the appearance of motor fluctuations were considered significant if severe enough to interfere with ADL. Treatment efficacy, based on motor examination, was greatest in the L-dopa group and worse in the bromocriptine monotherapy group, but no differences were observed in terms of independence with ADL. The bromocriptine monotherapy patients had fewer motor fluctuations, dystonia, and chorea but had the highest incidence of freezing. There were no significant differences between the L-dopa monotherapy and the combination therapy groups. Considering all motor complications (motor fluctuations, freezing, dystonia, and chorea), there were no significant differences between the three treatment groups. Although this was a prospective study, the sample sizes were small and the dropout rate relatively high (approximately 10%). Caution, therefore, should be exercised in the interpretation of these results.

From the data presented, it should be clear that the issue of whether early dopamine agonist therapy is associated with a lesser likelihood of developing late motor complications remains unresolved. The opponents and proponents of this theory each have studies to cite, but the results of these studies are conflicting and all are limited in some significant respect.

In addition to this slightly older literature, there are three recent studies that compared L-dopa therapy with one of the newer dopamine agonists. The first, published in 1998, was a multicenter randomized, double-blind study designed to assess whether initial therapy with cabergoline alone or in combination with L-dopa might prevent or delay the development of long-term motor complications.[17] This study recruited 412 patients with newly or recently diagnosed PD who had not previously been treated with L-dopa, selegiline, or dopamine agonist therapy. Patients were randomized to receive either cabergoline (0.25–4.00 mg per day) or L-dopa (100–600 mg per day) titrated over a maximum of 24 weeks to the optimum dose for each patient (defined as a well tolerated dose at which no further improvement was obtained compared with the previous dose level). Treatment was then continued at this dose for up to 3–5 years. Open-label L-dopa could be added in both treatment arms when indicated by deteriorating motor disability. Thirty-five percent of the cabergoline-treated patients and 52% of the L-dopa–treated group required the addition of open-label L-dopa. The mean cumulative exposure to L-dopa in the cabergoline-treated and L-dopa–treated groups was 303 g and 637 g, respectively, per patient. The primary endpoint of the study was the onset of motor complications. This endpoint was reached in 22% of patients treated with cabergoline (four on cabergoline monotherapy and 43 on combination therapy), compared to 34% of patients treated with L-dopa (17 on a stable dose of L-dopa and 53 receiving additional L-dopa; p <0.02). However, the risk of developing motor complications was the same when the combination-therapy patients were compared to those on a stable dose of L-dopa. Moreover, analysis of treatment efficacy, as determined by mean percentage decrease versus baseline in UPDRS factor III (parkinsonian disability) scores, revealed slightly greater disability amongst the cabergoline-treated patients. The authors concluded that initial treatment with a dopamine agonist in patients with early PD significantly reduces the risk of developing motor complications compared with L-dopa treatment.

Rascol et al.[18] performed a prospective, randomized, double-blind study to compare the risk of dyskinesia in early PD among patients treated with ropinirole to that among patients treated with L-dopa (combined with a decarboxylase inhibitor). The dose of study medication was titrated as required, with the maximal doses allowed being 24 mg ropinirole per day and 1,200 mg L-dopa per day. Patients whose symptoms were inadequately controlled by adjustment of the study medication were given supplementary L-dopa in an open-label fashion. The primary outcome measure was the incidence of dyskinesia. Of the 268 patients who entered the trial, 179 were randomized to receive ropinirole and 89 to L-dopa, but only 85 (47%) and 45 (51%) patients in the respective treatment groups completed the study. The primary analysis was performed on an intention-to-treat basis, which is to say that the incidence of dyskinesia was determined amongst those randomized to each treatment group, irrespective of whether they completed the study. Overall, dyskinesia developed in 36 of the 179 patients (20%) in the ropinirole-treated group and in 40 of the 89 patients (45%) of the L-dopa–treated patients. Before the addition of supplementary L-dopa, dyskinesias appeared in nine of 179 patients (5%) in the ropinirole group and 32 of 89 (36%) in the L-dopa group. At face value, these findings support the notion that the early use of a dopamine agonist (ropinirole) has the effect of reducing the likelihood of developing dyskinesias. However, it should be recognized that, in general, the ropinirole-treated patients were under-treated with respect to motor function scores, and that of those completing the study, only 29 in the ropinirole-treated group (34%) and 29 in the L-dopa–treated group (64%) did so without requiring supplemental L-dopa therapy. These observations raise the possibility that dyskinesias are indeed due to L-dopa therapy but that the incidence of dyskinesia in the ropinirole-treated group was lower because these patients were undertreated. The temptation to draw this conclusion, however, should be tempered by the recognition that this was a double-blind study and that there existed the possibility for supplemental L-dopa therapy if perceived necessary by the patient or physician. This would suggest that although the ropinirole groups were undertreated, as measured formally by motor function scores, this deficiency was not apparent to the patients or their treating physicians during the course of the study.

The Parkinsonian Study Group[19] conducted a multicenter randomized trial comparing initial treatment of early PD with pramipexole or L-dopa. Patients with idiopathic PD of up to 7 years' duration who required dopaminergic therapy at the time of enrollment were eligible for inclusion. Patients who had taken L-dopa or dopamine agonist therapy within the preceding 2 months were excluded. Eligible patients were randomized one to one to receive either pramipexole (maximum of 4.5 mg per day) or L-dopa (maximum 600 mg per day) for the duration of a 10-week dose escalation period followed by a 21-month maintenance period. Those with emerging disability despite maximal therapy could be treated with open-label L-dopa/carbidopa as required. Fifty-three percent of the pramipexole group and 39% of the L-dopa group required supplemental L-dopa. The primary outcome variable was prespecified as the time from randomization until the first occurrence of one of three dopaminergic complications (wearing off, dyskinesia, and on-off fluctuations). The study included 301 patients, none of whom were lost to follow-up. On an intention-to-treat analysis, the primary endpoint was reached in 28% of the pramipexole group and 51% of the L-dopa group by the end of the study ($p < 0.001$). The improved outcome, in terms of motor complications, was borne at the cost of a lesser improvement in motor and ADL UPDRS scores in the pramipexole group compared to the L-dopa group. Adverse events (somnolence, hallucinations, and edema) were also significantly more common in the pramipexole group. The investigators concluded that initial therapy with pramipexole rather than L-dopa is associated with an absolute risk reduction of 23% (and a relative risk reduction of 55%) in the likelihood of developing late motor complications over a 2-year period. They acknowledge that this beneficial effect is obtained at the cost of less improvement in UPDRS scores, but they note (as in the ropinirole study) that the patients and their blinded investigators had judged their illness to be satisfactorily controlled.

These three studies of cabergoline, ropinirole, and pramipexole are similar in design and outcome as well as in terms of their shortcomings. All three studies indicate that dopamine agonist therapy (in conjunction with lower-dose L-dopa) is associated with a lower incidence of motor fluctuations and dyskinesias when compared to therapy with higher doses of L-dopa. In each of the studies, this benefit was achieved at the cost of poorer symptomatic control of the underlying PD, but this was an effect not evident to the patients or investigators involved in the study. It is important to recognize that these studies do not establish that *early* dopamine agonist therapy is required to achieve the result of fewer motor complications. For example, the possibility that a similarly lower complication rate could have been achieved by reducing the dose of L-dopa, with or without the late addition of a dopamine agonist, remains untested.

One final concern that relates to all of these studies is their publication bias. Each study was funded by the respective pharmaceutical agency with an obvious interest in the study results. Although this does not necessarily invalidate the studies, it should raise some concern and lead to extra caution in extrapolation and generalization from these results.

Is Amantadine Effective in the Treatment of Levodopa-Induced Dyskinesia?

The pathogenesis of motor complications in PD remains incompletely understood, but increased activity of N-methyl-D-aspartate glutamate receptors on striatal efferent neurons (as a consequence of chronic nonphysiologic dopaminergic stimulation) is thought to contribute. The recent recognition that amantadine exerts an antagonistic effect at N-methyl-D-aspartate receptors prompted the initiation of a study of the effects of amantadine on L-dopa–induced dyskinesias and motor fluctuations. Metman et al.[20] performed the first double-blind, placebo-controlled trial. Eighteen patients with advanced PD (mean duration of disease 13 years) treated with long-term L-dopa (mean duration of therapy 12 years) who had developed motor fluctuations or peak-dose "on" dyskinesias, were randomized to receive either placebo or amantadine in a 6-week double-blind, crossover study. At the end of each 3-week study arm, the subjects were admitted and received an intravenous L-dopa infusion that had been previously titrated to the lowest dose producing the maximal antiparkinsonian effect. During the last 2 hours of the infusion when steady-state conditions had been achieved, parkinsonian symptoms and choreiform dyskinesias were evaluated. Fourteen patients completed both arms of the study, with the average amantadine dose being 350 mg per day. Dyskinesia scores during the steady-state L-dopa infusion were 60% lower among the patients treated with amantadine, and the dyskinesia reduction was not associated with increased parkinsonism. In a 1-year follow-up study,[21] these investigators re-evaluated 17 of the original 18 patients, 13 of whom had continued to receive amantadine over the course of the preceding year. Amantadine was withdrawn 7–10 days before the study and then readministered in a double-blind fashion. The four patients who had not received amantadine over the course of the preceding year were administered a placebo in a double-blind fashion. As in the original study, the patients were then admitted for intravenous L-dopa infusion and their dyskinetic and parkinsonian symptoms evaluated. Dyskinesia scores remained 56% lower among the amantadine-treated patients compared to those in the placebo arm of the original study; an effect comparable to the 60% reduction observed in the initial study. This beneficial antidyskinetic effect was not obtained at the expense of increased parkinsonism. These authors, therefore, concluded that the effects of amantadine in reducing L-dopa–induced dyskinesias persisted after 1 year of therapy.

What Is the Evidence Supporting the Use of Catechol Methyltransferase Inhibitors in Patients with Parkinson's Disease?

Although L-dopa remains the mainstay of symptomatic treatment of patients with PD, prolonged use is associated with the development of wearing-off phenomena caused by wide fluctuations in plasma L-dopa concentrations. Catechol methyltransferase (COMT) is the enzyme responsible for the metabolism of L-dopa. COMT inhibition prolongs the elimination half-life of L-dopa and provides a rational approach to producing a more prolonged and stable plasma L-dopa concentration. Tolcapone (Tasmar) and entacapone (Comtan) are the two COMT inhibitors licensed for clinical practice. Most studies have focused on their use in those patients with wearing-off phenomena, but there are some data to support their use in those patients with stable PD.

The Parkinson Study Group[22] performed a randomized, double-blind, placebo-controlled trial of entacapone for the treatment of wearing-off phenomena in patients with L-dopa–treated PD. Patients with idiopathic PD (Hoehn and Yahr stages 1.5–4.0 in the "off" state; see Appendix 12 [Hoehn and Yahr Parkinson's Disease Disability Scale]) who were responsive to L-dopa and had motor fluctuations paralleling their L-dopa dosing were eligible for inclusion. After a period of stable L-dopa/carbidopa dosing, patients were randomized to receive either placebo or entacapone. Entacapone was administered at a dose of 200 mg, taken together with each dose of L-dopa. During the first 8 weeks after the introduction of entacapone, the dose of L-dopa/carbidopa was adjusted to obtain an optimal clinical response. The primary outcome variable was the percent of "on" time while awake, as determined from the home diaries of patients during the 3 days preceding a scheduled visit. "On" time was defined as the subject being relatively free of parkinsonian symptoms (e.g., mobile or capable of moving with relative ease and independence). A total of 205 patients were entered into the study; 10 patients in the placebo-treated group and 13 in the entacapone-treated group withdrew before completing the trial.

The mean percent "on" time was significantly higher at 8, 16, and 24 weeks for the entacapone-treated group compared to the placebo-treated group. The overall treatment effect was approximately 5% or approximately 1 hour per day. This effect of increasing "on" time was more prominent in subjects with less than 55% "on" time at baseline. The effect on "on" time was also more prominent toward the end of the day. With regard to secondary outcome measures, entacapone had a nominally significant beneficial effect on the UPDRS score, reflected mainly in the motor and ADL subscales. The average total daily dose of L-dopa was also approximately 100 mg lower in the entacapone-treated group. These beneficial effects were rapidly reversible on withdrawal of entacapone at the end of the 24- to 26-week study period. The authors concluded that these results demonstrate that entacapone is effective in increasing "on" time in L-dopa–treated patients who experience motor fluctuations.

The efficacy of tolcapone in reducing motor fluctuations and decreasing "off" time has been demonstrated in a series of randomized, double-blind, placebo-controlled trials.[23-26] The design of these studies was similar. They recruited patients with predictable end-of-dose motor fluctuations in response to L-dopa therapy and randomized them to receive either placebo or tolcapone. Mobility was rated as "on," "intermediate," or "off" either by patients or physicians, and the proportion of "on" and "off" time was normalized as percentages of a standardized waking day (although this varied from 10 to 16 hours in the different studies). In general, the primary outcome measure of efficacy was a change in "on" or "off" time. Secondary outcome measures have included the degree of reduction of daily L-dopa dose and performance on the UPDRS motor subscale score.

In the study by Kurth et al.,[23] patients meeting eligibility criteria were administered their first daily dose of Sinemet (plus placebo) and then underwent a 10-hour assessment during which the on-off rating scale and UPDRS motor examination were repeated at 30-minute intervals. Patients were then randomized to receive placebo or one of three doses of tolcapone. At the conclusion of the study, subjects underwent a repeat 10-hour evaluation. Data are available for the 151 patients who completed the 6-week study period. Mean percent "off" time showed a significant decline at all doses of tolcapone compared to placebo between baseline and week 6. Change in "off" time as a percent of the 10-hour day was decreased by approximately 1.5 hours (40% of baseline "off" time) in all tolcapone groups. Tolcapone treatment resulted in a significant increase in "on" time for all three dosages when compared to the placebo group (approximately 16–17% of a 10-hour day). For all tolcapone groups compared to placebo, there was also a significant improvement in UPDRS motor subscale scores.

Baas et al.[24] randomized 177 patients to receive either placebo or one of two doses of tolcapone (100 mg or 200 mg three times daily). Efficacy and tolerability were assessed at multiple time points up to and including month 12. The primary outcome measure, however, was the change in the proportion of "on" and "off" time between baseline and month 3. Changes in on-off time were expressed as a percentage of a standardized 16-hour day. "On" time increased by approximately 21%, with both 100-mg and 200-mg doses of tolcapone. "Off" time decreased by 31% and 26%, with 100-mg and 200-mg tolcapone doses, respectively. The beneficial effects observed in the 200-mg tolcapone-treated group were persistent at the 9-month evaluation. With regard to secondary outcome measures, the daily dose of L-dopa was reduced to 109 mg and 122 mg in the lower-dose and higher-dose tolcapone groups, respectively. The UPDRS motor subscale score was significantly improved in the 200-mg tolcapone-treated group. Significant improvements in both tolcapone-treated groups were also noted on the investigators' global assessment scale.

The double-blind, placebo-controlled trial by Rajput et al.[25] randomized 202 patients with predictable wearing-off motor fluctuations in response to the L-dopa therapy to receive either placebo or one of two doses of tolcapone. "On" and "off" times were defined as the principal measures of efficacy. At the end of 3 months, patients in the higher-dose tolcapone-treated group (200 mg three times per day) had a mean 3.25-hour reduction in daily "off" time. The average daily dose of L-dopa was also reduced in both tolcapone-treated groups.

These studies suggest that tolcapone is more effective than entacapone in reducing "off" time or increasing "on" time. Although both drugs belong to the class of COMT inhibitors, they have a number of pharmacologic differences. Tolcapone, for example, has a greater bioavailability, area under the curve, and COMT enzyme affinity than does entacapone, which results in a greater percent and duration inhibition of COMT. Tolcapone, therefore, prolongs the half-life of L-dopa to a greater extent than entacapone; this is reflected in the different dosing schedules of the two drugs. Tolcapone is administered three times per day, although it is necessary to administer entacapone with each dose of L-dopa.

Notwithstanding these differences, the two drugs have never been compared head-to-head in a randomized, controlled fashion. The closest approximation is the uncontrolled study by Factor et al.[27] The authors of this study were involved in double-blind, placebo-controlled trials of both tolcapone and entacapone that were followed by open-label extension phases. They followed 14 patients enrolled in the tolcapone study and 11 in the entacapone study during these open-label extensions to compare the long-term efficacy and safety of these two drugs. There were significant differences between the two groups in relation to changes in duration of "off" time. At both 6 and 12 months, the tolcapone-treated group had a significantly greater decrease in the duration of "off" time compared to the entacapone-treated group. The entacapone-treated group also required a larger dose of L-dopa from 6 months onwards, whereas the dose of L-dopa remained lower in the tolcapone-treated group throughout the 36-month duration of the study. Caution, however, should be exercised when interpreting these results in view of the differences between the two treatment groups at baseline. For example, the UPDRS motor score and the score for duration of "off" time were significantly worse at baseline in the tolcapone-treated group, and the average daily dose of L-dopa was higher in the tolcapone-treated group.

Finally, there is the double-blind, placebo-controlled study by Waters et al.[28] of tolcapone in PD patients without wearing-off motor fluctuations. A total of 298 patients were randomly assigned to receive placebo or tolcapone (100 mg or 200 mg three times per day). The primary efficacy variable was the UPDRS ADL subscale score. Both groups of tolcapone-treated patients showed significant reductions in this score (i.e., improved functioning), compared to placebo-treated patients. This beneficial effect was detectable after 1–2 weeks of treatment and persisted at the 12-month assessment. The effect was also greatest in those patients with the most severe impairment at baseline. The benefit of tolcapone was also evident on the secondary efficacy variables, including improvement in UPDRS motor subscale scores, reduced daily dosage of L-dopa, lower risk of the development of motor fluctuations during the course of the study, and reduction in impairment as determined by the Sickness Impact Profile.

The results of these studies, therefore, suggest that the COMT inhibitors have a role in the management of patients with stable PD as well as patients with more advanced disease and wearing-off motor fluctuations. Although the quality of the comparative data is poor, the available evidence suggests that tolcapone is more effective than entacapone. This has certainly been the informal impression of those working in the field.

Summary

- There is conflicting epidemiologic evidence regarding whether the prevalence of PD is increased amongst patients with ET. The one prospective study suggests that the risk is increased.
- Selegiline offers limited symptomatic antiparkinsonian therapy, and the results of the Deprenyl and Tocopherol Antioxidative Therapy of Parkinsonism (DATATOP) study do not indicate a neuroprotective effect.
- The early literature addressing the nature of the association between L-dopa therapy and the emergence of motor fluctuations is largely retrospective, and of limited quality, and contradictory.
- There are three recent trials comparing the early use of a dopamine agonist (cabergoline, ropinirole, and pramipexole) to the early use of L-dopa in the treatment of PD. The results of all three are similar, with a lower frequency of motor complications emerging in the dopamine agonist–treated patients but at the expense of less well-treated parkinsonian symptoms. These studies also do not address the possibility that similarly low rates of motor complications might be possible with the combination of lower-dose L-dopa and a dopamine agonist, even if initiated later in the course of the disease. That is to say, the case for the *early* use of dopamine agonist in the treatment of PD has not yet been made.
- Amantadine, perhaps via its antagonistic effect on N-methyl-D-aspartate receptors, has recently been shown (in a randomized, double-blind, placebo-controlled trial) to be effective in reducing the severity of motor fluctuations and peak-dose dyskinesias.

- There is a role for the COMT inhibitors in the management of patients with stable PD as well as patients with more advanced disease and wearing-off motor fluctuations.
- The quality of the comparative data is poor, but the available evidence suggests that tolcapone is more effective than entacapone.

References

1. Geraghty JJ, Jankovic J, Zetusky WJ. Association between essential tremor and Parkinson's disease. *Ann Neurol* 1985;17:329–333.
2. Rajput AH, Offord KP, Beard CM, Kurland LT. Essential tremor in Rochester, Minnesota: a 45-year study. *J Neurol Neurosurg Psychiatry* 1984;47:466–470.
3. Koller WC, Busenbark K, Miner K. The relationship of essential tremor to other movement disorders: report of 678 patients. Essential Tremor Study Group. *Ann Neurol* 1994;35:717–723.
4. Effect of deprenyl on the progression of disability in early Parkinson's disease. The Parkinson Study Group. *N Engl J Med* 1989;321:1364–1371.
5. Effects of tocopherol and deprenyl on the progression of disability in early Parkinson's disease. The Parkinson Study Group. *N Engl J Med* 1993;328:176–183.
6. Impact of deprenyl and tocopherol treatment on Parkinson's disease in DATATOP subjects not requiring levodopa. The Parkinson Study Group. *Ann Neurol* 1996;39:29–36.
7. Olanow CW, Hauser RA, Gauger L, et al. The effect of deprenyl and levodopa on the progression of Parkinson's disease. *Ann Neurol* 1995;38:771–777.
8. Rinne UK. Early combination of bromocriptine and levodopa in the treatment of Parkinson's disease: a 5-year follow-up. *Neurology* 1987;37:826–828.
9. Hely MA, Morris JG, Reid WG, et al. The Sydney Multicentre Study of Parkinson's disease: a randomised, prospective five year study comparing low dose bromocriptine with low dose levodopa-carbidopa. *J Neurol Neurosurg Psychiatry* 1994;57:903–910.
10. Lesser RP, Fahn S, Snider SR, et al. Analysis of the clinical problems in parkinsonism and the complications of long-term levodopa therapy. *Neurology* 1979;29:1253–1260.
11. Markham CH, Diamond SG. Evidence to support early levodopa therapy in Parkinson disease. *Neurology* 1981;31:125–131.
12. Blin J, Bonnet A, Agid Y. Does levodopa aggravate Parkinson's disease? *Neurology* 1988;38:1410–1416.
13. Roos RA, Vredevoogd CB, van der Velde EA. Response fluctuations in Parkinson's disease. *Neurology* 1990;40:1344–1346.
14. Caraceni T, Scigliano G, Musicco M. The occurrence of motor fluctuations in parkinsonian patients treated long term with levodopa: role of early treatment and disease progression. *Neurology* 1991;41:380–384.
15. Cedarbaum JM, Gandy SE, McDowell FH. "Early" initiation of levodopa treat-

ment does not promote the development of motor response fluctuations, dyskinesias, or dementia in Parkinson's disease. *Neurology* 1991;41:622–629.

16. Weiner WJ, Factor SA, Sanchez-Ramos JR, et al. Early combination therapy (bromocriptine and levodopa) does not prevent motor fluctuations in Parkinson's disease. *Neurology* 1993;43:21–27.

17. Rinne UK, Bracco F, Chouza C, et al. Early treatment of Parkinson's disease with cabergoline delays the onset of motor complications: results of a double-blind levodopa controlled trial. The PKDS009 Study Group. *Drugs* 1998;55(Suppl 1):23–30.

18. Rascol O, Brooks DJ, Korczyn AD, et al. A five-year study of the incidence of dyskinesia in patients with early Parkinson's disease who were treated with ropinirole or levodopa. The 056 Study Group. *N Engl J Med* 2000;342:1484–1491.

19. Pramipexole vs levodopa as initial treatment for Parkinson disease: a randomized controlled trial. Parkinson Study Group. *JAMA* 2000;284:1931–1938.

20. Metman LV, Del Dotto P, van den Munckhof P, et al. Amantadine as treatment for dyskinesias and motor fluctuations in Parkinson's disease. *Neurology* 1998;50:1323–1326.

21. Metman LV, Del Dotto P, LePoole K, et al. Amantadine for levodopa-induced dyskinesias: a 1-year follow-up study. *Arch Neurol* 1999;56:1383–1386.

22. Entacapone improves motor fluctuations in levodopa-treated Parkinson's disease patients. Parkinson Study Group. *Ann Neurol* 1997;42:747–755.

23. Kurth MC, Adler CH, Hilaire MS, et al. Tolcapone improves motor function and reduces levodopa requirements in patients with Parkinson's disease experiencing motor fluctuations: a multicenter, double-blind, randomized, placebo-controlled trial. Tolcapone Fluctuator Study Group I. *Neurology* 1997;48:81–87.

24. Baas H, Beiske AG, Ghika J, et al. Catechol-O-methyltransferase inhibition with tolcapone reduces the "wearing off" phenomenon and levodopa requirements in fluctuating parkinsonian patients. *J Neurol Neurosurg Psychiatry* 1997;63:421–428.

25. Rajput AH, Martin W, Saint-Hilaire MH, et al. Tolcapone improves motor function in parkinsonian patients with the "wearing-off" phenomenon: a double-blind, placebo-controlled, multicenter trial. *Neurology* 1997;49:1066–1071.

26. Adler CH, Singer C, O'Brien C, et al. Randomized, placebo-controlled study of tolcapone in patients with fluctuating Parkinson disease treated with levodopa-carbidopa. Tolcapone Fluctuator Study Group III. *Arch Neurol* 1998;55:1089–1095.

27. Factor SA, Molho ES, Feustel PJ, et al. Long-term comparative experience with tolcapone and entacapone in advanced Parkinson's disease. *Clin Neuropharmacol* 2001;24:295–299.

28. Waters CH, Kurth M, Bailey P, et al. Tolcapone in stable Parkinson's disease: efficacy and safety of long-term treatment. Tolcapone Stable Study Group. *Neurology* 1997;49:665–671.

CHAPTER 21

Headache

Introduction

Headache is one of the most common symptoms with which patients present to neurologists. Some patients seek reassurance that they do not harbor a brain tumor; others are simply in search of a diagnosis or better symptomatic treatment. A perennial problem relates to the question of which patients with nonacute headache should undergo some form of neuroimaging. Is computerized tomography (CT) adequate, or is it necessary to perform magnetic resonance imaging (MRI)?

Migraine is the most common primary headache and is both underdiagnosed and undertreated. The management of patients with migraine has been revolutionized by the development of triptans for the abortive treatment of migraine attacks. There are concerns, however, based in part on theory and scattered reports, that triptans may not be safe in those at risk for coronary artery disease (CAD). Who is at risk and how should this determination be made? Are there patients with complex migraine in whom neurologic deficits are prominent or persistent? Are triptans safely used in these patients? Are patients with migraine at increased risk for stroke? These and other questions are the subjects of this chapter.

Should Patients with Nonacute Headache Undergo Some Form of Neuroimaging?

The perennial question of whether patients with nonacute headache should undergo some form of neuroimaging has been the subject of many reports, most of which have been retrospective. There are many reasons to consider neuroimaging in patients who present with headache. These might include the alleviation of patient anxiety regarding possible causes of headache or the physicians' perceived need to obtain a CT or MRI to avoid litigation. Although these may be legitimate reasons, the concern here relates to the importance of imaging in identifying underlying disease processes that are responsible for the headaches and that, if treated, would lead to improved health outcome. It is helpful to consider separately those studies that have examined patients with migraine and those patients with other types of headaches.

The largest series of patients with migraine was that reported by Cuetter and Aita.[1] All 435 patients had migraine with aura, were aged between 17 and 52 years, and had a normal neurologic examination. Enhanced CT was normal in all but one patient, in whom a small choroid plexus papilloma in the fourth ventricle was identified. This patient's headaches persisted unchanged after surgical removal of the tumor, suggesting that the tumor may have been an incidental finding unrelated to the headaches. Kuhn and Shekar[2] evaluated 74 patients with migraine of 2 years' duration with both CT and MRI. The only clinically significant finding was that of an occipital infarct (seen on CT and MRI) in one patient with a homonymous hemianopia. Igarashi et al.[3] examined 91 patients with migraine, 40% of whom demonstrated multiple foci of T2 hyperintensity in the white matter. These abnormalities were thought to be the consequence of frequent migraines, and no other structural lesions were identified. In patients with migraine, therefore, the diagnostic yield of neuroimaging appears to be very low. This may be particularly true for migraine with aura, perhaps because the diagnosis can be made with a greater degree of certainty.

A systematic review by Frishberg[4] in 1994 that included all reports of neuroimaging in patients with headache or migraine supports this conclusion. Smaller studies (describing fewer than 18 patients) were excluded in order not to introduce a reporting bias. The results of neurologic examination were normal in all of the patients included in this review. The results of these studies were pooled irrespective of whether CT (with or without contrast) or MRI was employed. This systematic review included a total of 2,377 patients, and the significant abnormalities detected included brain tumor, arteriovenous malformation (AVM), subdural hematoma, and hydrocephalus. Amongst the 897 patients with migraine who were included in this study, there were only three brain tumors identified and a single AVM. One of the tumors was incidental and one was associated with seizures in addition to migraine. Similarly, in the patient with the AVM, seizures were also present. In summary, therefore, the likelihood of detecting clinically significant lesions amongst patients with migraine and no other neurologic signs or symptoms is exceedingly low. These results are further reinforced by the findings of the U.S. Headache Consortium's[5] meta-analysis in which the prevalence of significant abnormalities was approximately 0.2%. It is relevant to note that this figure is lower than the 0.8% incidence of AVMs reported in unselected autopsy series.

The results of studies that have investigated the diagnostic yield of neuroimaging among patients with unspecified headache are a little different. The largest series of such patients was that reported by Laffey et al.[6] in which head CT was performed on 595 patients in whom headache was the only symptom. Tumor was identified in seven patients (1%), hydrocephalus in five (0.8%), and AVM in three (0.5%). However, this publication did not provide data regarding the presence or absence of abnormal neurologic findings on examination, and so it is unclear whether other factors might have pointed to the presence of an underlying structural brain lesion. Baker reported the experience of the Mayo Clinic,[7] where 505 patients with headache as their only symptom underwent CT. Tumor was identified in 13 (3.0%), subdural hemorrhage in four (0.8%), aneurysm in three (0.6%), and hydrocephalus in two (0.4%). The high frequency of abnormal findings on CT in this study is at variance with other studies and may have been due to the population being highly selected (i.e., most of the patients were referred by Mayo Clinic neurologists). However, no historical data are provided to determine whether there were other features that might have accounted for the high rate of abnormal scans. The results of a study of CT in patients with headache in a community-based health maintenance organization were quite different.[8] This study included 89 patients in whom headache was the only symptom and no clinically significant abnormalities were detected on CT. Sargent et al.[9] retrospectively reported the results of nonenhanced CT scan in 177 patients with headache (including patients with migraine and other types of headaches). No clinically significant abnormalities were detected. A prospective study by Mitchell et al.[10] of 347 patients with the chief complaint of headache reported seven clinically significant abnormalities. In those patients without other symptoms or abnormal findings on neurologic examination, only one instance of a tumor (0.3%) was identified.

Of the 1,825 patients with unspecified headaches in Frishberg's systematic review,[4] there were 21 tumors (1.0%), three AVMs (0.2%), five subdural hematomas (0.3%), and eight cases of hydrocephalus (0.4%), yielding an overall incidence of significant findings of approximately 2%. It is worth noting (as described in detail above) that the frequencies of abnormalities varied tremendously between the series from major referral centers[6,7] and those from community-based practices.[8–10] In the U.S. Headache Consortium's systematic review,[5] the frequencies of significant abnormalities were similarly more variable (ranging from 0.0% to 6.7%) than in patients with migraine.

Based on these findings, the U.S. Headache Consortium recommended that neuroimaging is not usually warranted for patients with migraine and normal neurologic examination. This conclusion was tempered by the statement that the threshold for neuroimaging should be lower in patients with atypical headache features or in patients who do not fulfill the strict criteria for the definition of migraine. They believed that the data were insufficient to make a recommendation for patients with other forms of headache. Not surprisingly, the finding of an abnormality on neurologic examination significantly increased the likelihood of finding intracranial pathology; the Consortium, therefore, also recommended that patients with unexplained abnormal findings on neurologic examination should undergo neuroimaging. The available data, as outlined above, support these recommendations.

Do Patients with Cluster Headache Require Neuroimaging?

The question of whether patients with cluster headache require neuroimaging is difficult; it has not been the subject of a large study. Before even trying to answer the question, however, it is necessary to clarify a few concepts. There are two varieties of cluster headache, episodic and chronic. Periodicity is the main feature of episodic cluster headache (ECH), with the cluster period (that period during which a series of headaches occurs) lasting 2–3 months. Cluster periods typically occur every 1–2 years. In chronic cluster headache (CCH), headache attacks continue for more than 1 year without remission or with remission lasting less than 14 days. In both ECH and CCH, each headache usually lasts 15–180 minutes and attacks occur at a frequency of one to eight times per day.[11] The headaches are accompanied by autonomic symptoms that can be attributed to sympathetic paresis and relative parasympathetic overaction. These include lacrimation, conjunctival injection, nasal stuffiness, rhinorrhea, ptosis, and meiosis. Onset is typically in the third decade of life, and men are affected more often than women.

Two syndromes that should be distinguished from cluster headache are chronic paroxysmal hemicrania and Raeder's syndrome. *Chronic paroxysmal hemicrania* is a syndrome characterized by headaches with the same pain characteristics and associated symptoms and signs as cluster headache, but the attacks are shorter and occur more frequently, and the pain is always responsive to indomethacin. This syndrome occurs mostly in women. *Raeder's paratrigeminal neuralgia* is a much less well-defined entity, in large part because of the varied way in which the term has been used. Salvesen[12] has provided a very clear account of the history and evolution of this term. Raeder described a clinical syndrome of unilateral periocular pain associated with ptosis, meiosis, some involvement of the trigeminal nerve, as well as occasional symptoms or signs of oculomotor or abducens nerve involvement. He believed that this combination of symptoms and signs indicated a paratrigeminal lesion and should, therefore, prompt a thorough search for serious pathology. Confusion regarding the significance of the clinical syndrome, however, has arisen because some authors have used it also to refer merely to a painful postganglionic Horner's syndrome. This led to a blurring of the distinction between *Raeder's syndrome* and *cluster headache*. The confusion may be avoided by using the term *Raeder's paratrigeminal neuralgia* to refer only to the syndrome of painful oculosympathetic paresis associated with evidence of trigeminal nerve dysfunction, with or without associated cranial nerve deficits. This clinical syndrome should always prompt aggressive investigation for an underlying lesion.

Returning to the entity of ECH, it is clear from the many published case reports that this syndrome may occasionally be symptomatic of an underlying vascular lesion or tumor. The frequency, however, with which underlying lesions are present in cluster headache is not known. Nevertheless, the diversity of the underlying pathology can be discerned from case reports that have recorded, amongst others, the presence of an upper cervical or parasellar meningioma,[13] pituitary adenoma,[14] nasopharyngeal carcinoma,[15] giant cell arteritis,[16] as well as carotid[17] and vertebral[18] artery aneurysms.

In the absence of data from large prospective series, it is appropriate to rely on expert opinion. Mathew has suggested that symptomatic cluster headache should be suspected when the clinical features are atypical.[19,20] He notes that these atypical features include (1) the absence of the typical periodicity of ECH, (2) the presence of a certain degree of background headache that does not subside between the headache clusters, (3) the presence of neurologic signs other than meiosis and ptosis, and (4) inadequate response to traditional therapies that are usually effective in ECH.

The available evidence and expert opinion, therefore, suggest that caution should be exercised in the diagnosis of cluster headache and the related syndromes. Imaging is not necessary if patients meet the strict criteria for the diagnosis of ECH. Greater caution is required under certain circumstances including the absence of the typical periodicity of ECH (i.e., when the attacks behave more like CCH). A careful neurologic examination is essential, and the presence of any cranial nerve dysfunction other than meiosis and ptosis should prompt an aggressive search for underlying pathology, the range of which may be quite broad.

Are Triptans Safe in Patients Who Are at Risk for Coronary Artery Disease?

Triptans are selective 5-hydroxytryptamine ($5HT_{1B/D}$) receptor agonists. Intracranial blood vessels have a rich supply of $5HT_{1B}$ receptors, the stimulation of which result in vasoconstriction. The principal serotonin receptor in coronary arteries is the $5HT_2$ receptor subtype. The presence, however, of $5HT_{1B}$ receptors in the coronary artery, albeit at a lower density, raises the theoretical possibility of triptan-induced coronary vasoconstriction and myocardial ischemia. Indeed, there are case reports of myocardial infarction after the administration of subcutaneous sumatriptan. Although the preponderance of data relate to the use of sumatriptan, there is general agreement that triptans are contraindicated in patients known to have CAD. A question, however, arises regarding the appropriate use of triptans in people not known to have, but who are at risk for, CAD by virtue of their age or comorbidity.

There are limited data to guide practice. A recent prospective study[21] of 23,339 patients, each of whom treated a mean of 15.4 migraine attacks during the study period, reported the frequency of various complications after the administration of subcutaneous sumatriptan. There were three myocardial infarctions (which occurred at least 3 days after the most recent use of sumatriptan) and six cases of angina pectoris (with the most recent use of sumatriptan reported 1 day before in one patient and 13–246 days later in the remainder). Given that sumatriptan has an elimination half-life of 1.5–2.0 hours and that the drug is effectively eliminated from the circulation within five half-lives (i.e., 10 hours), it is difficult to implicate sumatriptan in the etiology of these ischemic events.

In view of this potential for adverse cardiovascular events, a cardiac evaluation has been recommended for those at risk of unrecognized CAD before the use of triptans. There is, however, no consensus on who is at risk, nor is there any regard for what constitutes an appropriate evaluation. A recent opinion piece[22] provides an excellent encapsulation of these issues. Based on the known prevalence of data of CAD in asymptomatic patients with various risk factors (hypertension, left ventricular hypertrophy, smoking, glucose intolerance, and hypercholesterolemia) and the known sensitivities and specificities of noninvasive cardiac stress tests, it is possible to establish guidelines for rational cardiac evaluation. Using these data, the absence of significant electrocardiogram (ECG) abnormalities (the presence of Q waves, poor R-wave progression, ischemic T-wave or ST-segment changes, or a bundle branch block) in asymptomatic women would suffice to make the presence of CAD sufficiently unlikely to permit the use of a triptan. This recommendation is true even for women with multiple cardiac risk factors given the relatively low prevalence (13–31%) of CAD. Such a recommendation could not be made for asymptomatic men with multiple risk factors given their higher prevalence of CAD (20–49% in the presence of four cardiac risk factors). The same would be true for men with atypical chest pain (prevalence of 67%). This author, therefore, would recommend noninvasive stress testing in women with an abnormal ECG as well as in men with (1) an abnormal ECG, (2) more than four risk factors or atypical chest pain, or (3) either diabetes or peripheral vascular disease.

Are Triptans Contraindicated in Patients with Complicated Migraine?

There are very little data on which to base an answer to the question of whether triptans are contraindicated in patients with complicated migraine. Traditionally, triptans have been considered contraindicated in hemiplegic or basilar migraine based on the concern for potential cerebral vasoconstriction that might aggravate the neurologic deficit. In a recent survey of headache specialists in attendance at a meeting sponsored by the American Headache Society and the American Medical Association, 34% believed that triptans could be used safely in patients with basilar migraine after the resolution of neurologic symptoms and signs, 36% disagreed, and 30% were unsure.[23] In an abstract published at the fifty-third annual meeting of the American Academy of Neurology, Mathew et al.[24] described their experience with triptans in 24 patients with complicated migraine. They found that all four oral triptans (suma-, zomi-, nara-, and riza-) were tolerated with no patient showing signs of neurologic deterioration. Moreover, they noted that the duration of neurologic symptoms was significantly shortened.

Are Patients with Migraine at an Increased Risk for Stroke?

In considering the relationship between migraine and stroke, it is useful to make a distinction between migraine as a background risk factor for stroke and what has been designated *migrainous stroke*. The International Headache Society recognizes the latter entity and requires that three criteria be met: (1) The patient has previously fulfilled criteria for migraine with aura, (2) the present attack is typical of previous attacks, but neurologic deficits are not completely reversible within 7 days or neuroimaging demonstrates ischemic infarction in a relevant area, and (3) other causes of infarction have been excluded by appropriate investigations.

There are two case series that describe the importance of migraine as an acute precipitant of stroke. Rothrock et al.[25] reported their experience with 22 patients whom they regarded as having had a migrainous stroke. They defined *migrainous stroke* as the occurrence of "at least one attack of migraine with associated focal neurologic deficit persisting for more than 30 days and/or brain MRI or CT evidence of acute stroke." Twenty (91%) of the 22 migrainous strokes occurred in women, and the mean age at the time of stroke was 35 years. In the majority, extensive investigation did not reveal a mechanism for the stroke. Three patients were taking oral contraceptives or estrogen replacement at the time of the stroke, mitral valve prolapse was detected in a single patient, and cerebral angiography revealed evidence of vasospasm in only three of the 12 patients in whom it was performed. The authors concluded that there was no single process clearly responsible for migrainous stroke and that the relevance of vasospasm would have to remain conjectural in the majority. Bogousslavsky et al.[26] described their experience with 22 consecutive patients who developed an ischemic stroke in the midst of an attack of migraine with aura. They compared these subjects to two age- and sex-matched control groups— migraineurs with a history of stroke remote from an attack of migraine and patients with a history of a remote stroke but no history of migraine. The study group included 17 women (77%) and five men; the mean age was 32.7 years. Apart from a history of smoking and oral contraceptive use, other risk factors were uncommon. Mitral valve prolapse was detected less frequently in the patients with migrainous stroke, and cerebral angiography was normal in the 19 of 22 patients who consented to the procedure. They found no significant differences between the migrainous stroke and control populations and concluded that migraine itself was the most likely cause of the infarct during migraine attacks. These two studies confirm the impression that ischemic stroke may complicate migraine with aura but do not support vasospasm as the likely etiology. Migrainous stroke is more common in women, a proportion of whom have a history of smoking and oral contraceptive use.

The question of whether migraine represents a background risk factor for subsequent development of stroke has been the subject of a number of retrospective case-control studies as well as a single prospective study. The first case control study that employed the International Headache Society's diagnostic criteria for migraine was performed by Tzourio and colleagues.[27] They recruited 212 patients aged 18–80 who were admitted with the diagnosis of an ischemic stroke. An equal number of controls, selected from patients hospitalized for other reasons, were matched for age, gender, and history of hypertension. Each subject's history of headache was recorded during an interview by a neurologist with a highly structured questionnaire. For the study population as a whole, they found no association between migraine (with or without aura) and ischemic stroke. In a separate analysis, however, in which the study population was stratified according to age (older or younger than 45 years), they found a significant association between migraine and stroke in younger women. These results were of doubtful significance, however, given that they were extracted from a subgroup analysis comprising only 20 pairs of cases and controls. To further investigate this association, Tzourio and colleagues[28] conducted a second case-control study in which they recruited 72 women younger than the age of 45 who were hospitalized with a first acute ischemic stroke. One hundred seventy-three age-matched controls were selected from patients hospitalized for other reasons. All subjects were interviewed by a neurologist about their history of headaches. In the primary analysis, they found a strong association between migraine and ischemic stroke, with 60% of stroke patients reporting a history of migraine compared to only 30% of controls. This association persisted after controlling for age, history of hypertension, and smoking as well as the use of oral contraceptives— factors that differed between the two groups at baseline. Women with migraine had a more than threefold increased risk of ischemic stroke compared to women without migraine, and the increased risk was observed for both migraine with and without aura. These studies, therefore, established the association of an increased risk of ischemic stroke in women younger than 45 years of age with migraine (with or without aura).

Moreover, a recent study suggested that concurrent smoking and use of the oral contraceptives exert a synergistic effect in terms of increasing the risk of ischemic stroke. As part of the World Health Organization Collaborative Study of cardiovascular disease and steroid hormone contraception,

Chang et al.[29] recruited women aged 20–44 years who had had a stroke to determine whether a history of migraine was more frequent than in the control population. Cases and controls were interviewed using a standardized questionnaire to establish a history of migraine. Migraine was reported in 25% of women with ischemic stroke compared to 13% of controls. The risk of ischemic stroke was increased amongst women with migraine regardless of the presence or absence of aura. The risk of stroke was also increased among women with a history of hypertension, oral contraceptive use, or a history of smoking. The coexistence of each of these factors had a synergistic effect on the risk of ischemic stroke in women with migraine (although this effect was only statistically significant for a history of heavy smoking). Compared with women who did not smoke, did not use oral contraceptives, and did not report a history of migraine, the odds ratio for ischemic stroke associated with the use of oral contraceptives in current smokers with a history of migraine was a staggering 34. Although caution should be exercised in the interpretation of this effect given that it was based on data from nine cases and two controls, the data suggest that the risk of ischemic stroke amongst young women with migraine is increased by a history of hypertension, concurrent smoking, and use of oral contraceptives.

Whether migraine also represents an independent risk factor for stroke in men is less clear. The Physician's Health Study was a large randomized, double-blind, placebo-controlled trial of aspirin and beta-carotene in the prevention of cardiovascular disease and cancer, respectively. Data on the prevalence of migraine had been collected from follow-up questionnaires and was used to address the question of whether a personal history of migraine represented an independent risk factor for stroke.[30] The population examined in this study included male physicians aged 40–84 years. The diagnosis of migraine was based on the physician's report (in a questionnaire) that he had a history of migraine even though no instructions were given as to what headaches should be regarded as such. The occurrence of stroke during follow-up, however, was confirmed by independent evaluation. During an average follow-up period of 60 months, there were 19 strokes amongst the 1,479 physicians with migraine (1.30%) and 194 amongst the 20,418 without migraine (0.95%). For ischemic stroke, there was an almost twofold increase in the relative risk of stroke amongst those with a history of migraine. This study, therefore, seems to suggest that men with migraine, irrespective of their age, are also at an increased risk for ischemic stroke. Although the advantages of this study included its large size and prospective design, the major drawback was that the diagnosis of migraine was based purely on subjective report. Moreover, there was insufficient historical data gathered to determine whether the increased risk of stroke occurred amongst those with migraine with or without aura, or both.

The available data, therefore, seem to suggest that young women (younger than 45 years) with migraine are at an increased risk for ischemic stroke and that this risk is increased by concurrent smoking or use of oral contraceptives. Whether men with migraine are similarly at an increased risk remains an unsettled issue. It should be recognized, however, that based on the quality of the available data, there is reason to be cautious in accepting these conclusions. Although the diagnosis of migraine was usually confirmed by a neurologist and care was taken to avoid misdiagnosis of transient ischemic attack as migraine (a misdiagnosis that would inflate the real effect of migraine on the risk of stroke), the case-control studies are retrospective and relatively small in size. They are also inherently affected by factors such as recall and publication bias. On the other hand, although the prospective series were limited by their lack of precise diagnostic criteria, the conclusions do lend support to the case-control data. The consistency of the results across studies of different populations suggests that the association is a real one.

Summary

- In patients with migraine and no other neurologic symptoms or findings on examination, the diagnostic yield of neuroimaging is sufficiently low enough that it need not be performed routinely.
- The data regarding the role of neuroimaging in patients with unspecified headaches are less clear, with estimates of the diagnostic yield varying widely depending on the population under study. On the basis of the available data, it is reasonable to obtain a CT scan or MRI in patients with unspecified headaches who are selected on the basis of their referral to a neurologist for evaluation.
- Imaging is not necessary if patients meet the strict criteria for the diagnosis of ECH. Greater caution is required under certain circumstances, including the absence of the typical periodicity of ECH (i.e., when the attacks behave more like CCH). A careful neurologic examination is essential, and the presence of any cranial nerve dysfunction other than meiosis and ptosis should prompt an aggressive search for underlying pathology.
- Triptans are contraindicated in patients with known CAD.
- There are limited data to guide the use of triptans in patients who may be at risk for underlying CAD.
- The absence of ECG abnormalities in asymptomatic women (even in the face of as many as four cardiac risk factors) should suffice to make the presence of CAD sufficiently unlikely to permit the use of triptans.
- Noninvasive cardiac stress testing before the use of triptans is recommended for men or women with an abnormal ECG and for men with atypical chest pain, more than four risk factors, or with either diabetes or peripheral vascular disease even in the face of a normal ECG.

- There are very limited data that inform on the safety of triptans in patients with complicated migraine. Although they remain formally contraindicated, preliminary reports suggest that they may be used safely.
- Ischemic stroke may complicate migraine with aura, but the mechanism remains unclear.
- Women younger than the age of 45 with migraine are at increased risk for ischemic stroke, particularly with concurrent heavy smoking and the use of oral contraceptives.

References

1. Cuetter AC, Aita JF. CT scanning in classic migraine. *Headache* 1983;23:195.
2. Kuhn MJ, Shekar PC. A comparative study of magnetic resonance imaging and computed tomography in the evaluation of migraine. *Comput Med Imaging Graph* 1990;4:149–152.
3. Igarashi H, Sakai F, Kan S, et al. Magnetic resonance imaging of the brain in patients with migraine. *Cephalalgia* 1991;11:69–74.
4. Frishberg BM. The utility of neuroimaging in the evaluation of headache in patients with normal neurologic examinations. *Neurology* 1994;44:1191–1197.
5. Frishberg BM, Rosenberg JH, Matchar DB, et al. for the US Headache Consortium. Evidence-based guidelines in the primary care setting: neuroimaging in patients with nonacute headache. http://www.aan.com/professionals/practice/pdfs/gl0088.pdf. Accessed July 19, 2002.
6. Laffey PD, Oaks WW, Swami RK, et al. Data supplement/computerized tomography in clinical medicine. Philadelphia: Medical Directions, Inc., 1978.
7. Baker HL Jr. Cranial CT in the investigation of headache: cost-effectiveness for brain tumors. *J Neuroradiol* 1983;10:112–116.
8. Weingarten S, Kleinman M, Elperin L, Larson EB. The effectiveness of cerebral imaging in the diagnosis of chronic headache. *Arch Intern Med* 1992;152:2457–2462.
9. Sargent JD, Lawson RC, Solbach P, Coyne L. Use of CT scans in an out-patient headache population: an evaluation. *Headache* 1979;19:388–390.
10. Mitchell CS, Osborn RE, Grosskreutz SR. Computerized tomography in the headache patients: is routing evaluation really necessary? *Headache* 1993;33:82–86.
11. Classification and diagnostic criteria for headache disorders, cranial neuralgias and facial pain. Headache classification committee for the International Headache Society. *Cephalalgia* 1988;8(Suppl 7):1–96.
12. Salvesen R. Raeder's syndrome. *Cephalalgia* 1999;(Suppl 25):42–45.
13. Hannerz J. A case of parasellar meningioma mimicking cluster headache. *Cephalalgia* 1989;9:265–269.
14. Pora-Etessam J, Ramos-Carrasco A, Berbel-Garcia A, et al. Clusterlike headache as first manifestation of a prolactinoma. *Headache* 2001;41:723–725.

15. Noronha A, Appelbaum J. Symptomatic cluster. *Neurology* 1993;43:1270.
16. Jimenez-Jimenez FJ, Garcia-Albea E, Zurdo M, et al. Giant cell arteritis presenting as cluster headache. *Neurology* 1998;51:1767–1768.
17. Greve E, Mai J. Cluster headache-like headaches: a symptomatic feature? A report of three patients presenting with intracranial pathologic findings. *Cephalalgia* 1988;8:79–82.
18. West P, Todman D. Chronic cluster headache associated with a vertebral artery aneurysm. *Headache* 1991;31:210–212.
19. Mathew NT. Symptomatic cluster. *Neurology* 1993;43:1270.
20. Mathew NT. Cluster headache. *Neurology* 1992;42(Suppl 2):22–31.
21. O'Quinn S, Davis RL, Gutterman DL, et al. Prospective large-scale study of the tolerability of subcutaneous sumatriptan injection for acute treatment of migraine. *Cephalalgia* 1999;19:223–231.
22. Evans RW, Martin V. Expert opinion assessing cardiac risk prior to use of triptans. *Headache* 2000;40:599–602.
23. Evans RW, Lipton RB. Topics in migraine management: a survey of headache specialists highlights some controversies. *Neurologic Clinics* 2001;19:1–21.
24. Mathew NT, Kailasam J, Fischer AS. Oral triptans are effective and well tolerated in migraine with neurological symptoms (basilar, hemiplegic and familial migraine with complex neurological manifestations). *Neurology* 2001;56 (Suppl 3):A218–A219.
25. Rothrock JF, Walicke P, Swenson MR, et al. Migrainous stroke. *Arch Neurol* 1988;45:63–67.
26. Bogousslavsky J, Regli F, Van Melle G, et al. Migraine stroke. *Neurology* 1988;38:223–227.
27. Tzourio C, Iglesias S, Hubert JB, et al. Migraine and risk of ischemic stroke: a case-control study. *BMJ* 1994;307:289–292.
28. Tzourio C, Tehindrazanarivelo A, Iglesias S, et al. Case-control study of migraine and risk of ischaemic stroke in young women. *BMJ* 1995;310;830–833.
29. Chang CL, Donaghy M, Poulter N. Migraine and stroke in young women: case-control study. World Health Organization Collaborative Study of cardiovascular disease and steroid hormone contraception. *BMJ* 1999;318:13–18.
30. Buring JE, Hebert P, Romero J, et al. Migraine and subsequent risk of stroke in the Physicians' Health Study. *Arch Neurol* 1995;52:129–134.

CHAPTER 22

Dementia

Introduction

Dementia increasingly is becoming an important public health issue given that its prevalence rises exponentially with advancing age. The costs—both in terms of the impact on the affected individual as well as the economic burden of caring for the afflicted individual and the income lost by those caring for the demented—are enormous. Alzheimer's disease (AD) and diffuse Lewy body disease (DLBD) are the two most common causes of dementia, and their coexistence may be frequent. The cholinergic hypothesis of AD states that a deficiency of acetylcholine in the brain of affected individuals plays an important role in the deterioration of cognitive functioning. There is also emerging evidence for a severe cholinergic deficit in patients with DLBD.

This has been the rationale for the development of therapies, such as the acetylcholinesterase (AChE) inhibitors, for the treatment of patients with dementia. There are four agents in this class: tetrahydroaminoacridine (Tacrine), donepezil hydrochloride (Aricept), rivastigmine (Exelon), and galantamine (Reminyl). Tacrine has fallen out of favor because of its potential for hepatotoxicity, but the other agents in this class remain popular for the treatment of patients with various forms of dementia or minor cognitive impairment.

What is the evidence, however, that these agents are effective? Are they more or less appropriate amongst patients with dementia of different causes? Is there a role for their use in those with minor cognitive impairment (i.e., those at risk for the development of dementia)? What is the place, if any, of estrogens and nonsteroidal anti-inflammatory drugs (NSAIDs) in the prevention or treatment of AD? These and other questions are the focus of this chapter.

How Good Is the Evidence Supporting the Efficacy of Donepezil in Patients with Alzheimer's Disease?

The safety and efficacy of donepezil were initially evaluated in a 24-week, double-blind, placebo-controlled trial in patients with AD.[1] Otherwise healthy patients older than age 50 years with AD diagnosed according to the National Institute of Neurological and Communicative Disorders and Alzheimer's Disease and Related Disorders Association (NINCDS-ADRDA) were eligible for inclusion. Patients had Mini-Mental State Examination (MMSE) scores of 10–26 and a Clinical Dementia Rating score of 1 (mild dementia) or 2 (moderate dementia) (see Appendix 4 [Clinical Dementia Rating] and Appendix 19 [Mini-Mental State Examination]). The study included 473 patients who were randomized to receive placebo; donepezil, 5 mg per day; or donepezil, 10 mg per day. The prespecified primary outcome measures were the cognitive portion of the Alzheimer's Disease Assessment Scale–Cognitive subscale (ADAS-cog) and the Clinician's Interview-Based Impression of Change (CIBIC-plus) scale (Table 22-1) (see Appendix 1 [Alzheimer's Disease Assessment Scale] and Appendix 5 [Clinician's Interview-Based Impression and Clinical Global Impression of Change]). Measures of outcome were assessed at 6-week intervals. Analyses of efficacy were performed for both the fully evaluable population (i.e., only those patients who completed 24 weeks of double-blind treatment) and the intention-to-treat (ITT) population, which included subjects who were randomized but did not complete the 24-week trial. For the ITT analysis, conclusions were based on the results of the patients' last observation carried forward (LOCF). The investigators found that the results for these two populations were essentially the same because of the low discontinuation rate and so focused on what they regarded as the more conservative ITT analysis.

In fact, the ITT analysis may be less conservative. The reason for this relates to the fact that patients with dementia tend to worsen with time. If, therefore, patients drop out of a treatment arm and the results of the last evaluation are carried forward for the final efficacy analysis (i.e., LOCF), these relatively better scores are carried forward. A high dropout rate from an active treatment arm (as may be the case at higher drug dosages) has the effect of creating an artificially better score than is observed in the placebo arm. In evaluating the results of these trials, therefore, it is essential to be aware of the dropout rates and to focus on the results obtained from those patients who remain within the trial until its conclusion.

The ADAS scale is a 21-item score that includes an 11-item cognitive subscale (ADAS-cog) that evaluates memory, language, orientation, reason, and praxis function. Scores on ADAS-cog subscale range from 0 to 70 (maximal impairment). On average, untreated patients with AD show an increase (cognitive decline) of approximately seven to 11 points per year. It should be recognized, however, that the ADAS-cog subscale lacks linearity in patients with mild or severe disease (i.e., this scale exhibits ceiling and floor effects). Untreated patients with mild or severe disease may only decline by five points (or less) per year. It should also be realized that an improvement of a given number of points may have variable clinical significance depending on the severity of the dementia. For example, an improvement of seven to eight points may mean very little in a severely demented patient but may facilitate independence in a patient with mild dementia.

TABLE 22-1
Study Design of Anticholinesterase Trials in Alzheimer's Disease

Drug (Dose)	Trial Duration	Entry Criteria	Size	Outcome Measure*	Reference
Donepezil:					
5 mg, 10 mg, or placebo	24 wks	MMSE 10–26	473	ADAS-cog and CIBIC-plus	1
5 mg, 10 mg, or placebo	12 wks	MMSE 10–26	468	ADAS-cog and CIBIC-plus	2
5 mg or placebo	24 wks	Able to undergo cognitive testing	60	ADAS-cog and CIBIC-plus	3
Rivastigmine: 1–4 mg, 6–12 mg, or placebo	26 wks	MMSE 10–26	~700	ADAS-cog and CIBIC-plus	4
Galantamine: 24 mg, 32 mg, or placebo	6 mos	MMSE 11–24	~600	ADAS-cog and CIBIC-plus	5

ADAS = Alzheimer's Disease Assessment Scale–Cognitive subscale; CIBIC = Clinician's Interview-Based Impression of Change scale; MMSE = Mini-Mental State Examination.
*For each of these studies, the ADAS-cog and the CIBIC-plus scores are expressed as the mean drug-placebo difference.

In view of these limitations, it may be difficult to evaluate the clinical significance of a change in ADAS-cog scores alone. It is, therefore, generally recommended that a global measure of function or change also be employed in treatment trials. In the study in question,[1] the investigators used the CIBIC-plus scale. This is an interview technique used by a clinician barred from knowledge of the patient's performance on rating scales or neuropsychologic tests. It provides a global measure that reflects appearance, behavior, speech, mood, thought content, insight, cognitive function, and independence with activities of daily living. After the interview, the patient is scored on a seven-point scale in which *1* represents marked improvement, *4* is no change, and *7* represents a marked worsening.

In the study of donepezil by Rogers et al.,[1] the mean ADAS-cog scores at the study endpoint (after 24 weeks of therapy) demonstrated an improvement of 0.67 and 1.06 in the donepezil-treated 5- and 10-mg per day groups, respectively. By contrast, the mean ADAS-cog score in the placebo-treated group had deteriorated by 1.82 points. Mean drug-placebo differences, therefore, were a respective 2.49 and 2.88 for the 5- and 10-mg per day groups, suggesting a dose-response relationship (Table 22-2). These results may also be expressed in terms of the relative percentages of patients who either showed no evidence of cognitive decline or who improved over the course of the study. Approximately 80% of donepezil-treated patients showed no evidence of cognitive deterioration compared to 58% in the placebo-treated group. An improvement of seven points or greater was observed in 25% of the donepezil-treated 10-mg per day group, 15% of the 5-mg per day group, and in only 8% of the placebo-treated group.

On the second primary outcome measure at the end of the 24-week treatment period, mean drug-placebo CIBIC-plus score differences were 0.36 and 0.44 for the 5- and 10-mg per day dosing groups, respectively. Twenty-five percent of the donepezil-treated patients were scored as improved, compared with only 11% of the placebo-treated group (see Table 22-2). The beneficial effects of donepezil were contingent on the continuation of therapy as evidenced by the loss of effect on both ADAS-cog scores and CIBIC-plus scores after the 6-week placebo washout period.

A second study of donepezil in AD was reported by the same authors.[2] The design of this study was similar to that of the first except that the double-blind treatment period lasted only 12 weeks and was followed by a 3-week, single-blind washout period. Almost 500 patients were enrolled and randomized to receive 5 or 10 mg per day donepezil or placebo. The primary outcome measures were again the ADAS-cog scores and CIBIC-plus scores (see Table 22-1). For the ADAS-cog scores, the drug-placebo differences were 2.5 and 3.1 for the 5- and 10-mg per day groups, respectively. The drug-placebo differences for the CIBIC-plus scores were 0.3 and 0.4 for the 5- and 10-mg per day groups, respectively (see Table 22-2). On both outcome measures, therefore, the results were very similar to those reported in the prior study.

A third randomized controlled trial of donepezil in AD[3] was motivated by the concern that patients in the first two studies were highly selected and not necessarily representative of the general population of AD patients. All patients with a diagnosis of probable AD were eligible for inclusion unless there existed a specific contraindication to the use of an AChE inhibitor. Also, the study required that patients be cognitively testable; this, out of necessity, limited the study population to those with mild to moderate dementia. The trial was a 24-week double-blind, placebo-controlled crossover study. After a 6-week single-blind placebo wash-in period, patients were randomized to receive either donepezil 5 mg per day or placebo for 6 weeks. They were then crossed over to the alternate treatment for 6 weeks; this was followed by a 6-week washout period. The primary outcome measure was the ADAS-cog score. The caregiver-related clinical global impression of change was amongst the secondary outcome measures employed (see Table 22-1). Combining within-individual changes during drug and placebo treatment, ADAS-cog scores improved 2.17 points in response to donepezil treatment. These results were comparable to the other two studies of donepezil. As with the prior studies, the beneficial effects of donepezil therapy were lost after the 3-week washout period.

TABLE 22-2
Results of the Anticholinesterase Drug Trials in Alzheimer's Disease[a]

| | ADAS-cog | | | | | | CIBIC-plus | | | | | |
| | Drug-Placebo Difference | | Percentage Improved[b] | | | | Drug-Placebo Difference | | Percentage Improved[c] | | | |
	Low	High	Placebo	Low	High		Low	High	Placebo	Low	High
Donepezil[d]	2.49	2.88	27	38	54		0.36	0.44	11.0	26	25.0
	2.5	3.1	—	—	—		0.3	0.4	18.0	32	38.0
	2.17	—	—	—	—		—	—	—	—	—
Rivastigmine[e]	—	2.58	19	—	29		0.14	0.41	22.0	31	41.0
Galantamine[f]	3.9	3.8	—	—	—		—	—	13.2	20	19.5

ADAS-cog = Alzheimer's Disease Assessment Scale–Cognitive subscale; CIBIC-plus = Clinician's Interview-Based Impression of Change scale.
[a]Results reported are from the *observed case* analysis unless otherwise indicated.
[b]Percentage improved defined on the basis of a 4-point improvement in the ADAS-cog score.
[c]Percentage improved defined on the basis of a CIBIC-plus score of ≤3.
[d]Results reported are from the *intention-to-treat* analysis. For donepezil, low dose is 5 mg and high dose is 10 mg/day.
[e]For rivastigmine, low dose is 1–4 mg and high dose is 6–12 mg/day.
[f]For galantamine, low dose is 24 mg and high dose is 32 mg/day.

Of interest is that no significant effect was observed on the global measure used (the caregiver-related impression of change). The authors believed that this negative result may have resulted from insufficient sample size, with the study not designed or powered to detect such a change. This may be true, but it represents a significant shortcoming of this study given the importance of demonstrating an effect of treatment on at least some measure of global function. The authors interpreted the results of this study as having provided supportive evidence for the beneficial effects of donepezil in patients with AD of mild or moderate severity.

Do the Other Acetylcholinesterase Inhibitors Offer Equivalent Efficacy in Alzheimer's Disease?

The question of whether other acetylcholinesterase inhibitors offer equivalent efficacy in AD is difficult to answer because there are no trials that have directly compared the different agents. However, similar study designs and outcome measures have been employed in the studies of rivastigmine and galantamine, and this facilitates some comparison between the different AChE inhibitors.

Rösler et al. examined the efficacy of rivastigmine in patients with AD in a large double-blind, randomized study.[4] They enrolled patients between the ages of 50 and 85 with probable AD according to the NINCDS-ADRDA criteria, and all subjects had MMSE scores between 10 and 26. Patients with severe and unstable cardiac or pulmonary disease or malignancy or those using other central nervous system–acting drugs were excluded. This was a 26-week, double-blind, placebo-controlled parallel group study with approximately 700 patients randomized equally to receive placebo or either lower-dose (1–4 mg per day) or higher-dose (6–12 mg per day) rivastigmine. The first 12 weeks of the study represented a dose-escalation phase; the second 12 weeks represented a maintenance phase. Efficacy was assessed using the ADAS-cog subscale, CIBIC-plus scale, and progressive deterioration scale (see Table 22-1). At 26 weeks for the observed case analysis, the mean placebo-drug difference in ADAS-cog score for the higher-dose rivastigmine group was 2.58 points—an effect comparable to that observed amongst patients receiving 5 mg per day donepezil. It is relevant to note, however, that one-third of the patients in the higher-dose rivastigmine group discontinued treatment (mostly because of adverse events), and no benefit was observed in the ITT analysis (mean placebo-drug ADAS-cog score difference of 1.6 points for the higher-dose rivastigmine group).

In the ITT analysis, the proportion of patients with a clinically meaningful improvement in ADAS-cog scores (defined as a change of at least four points) at the end of the study was 24% in the higher-dose rivastigmine group and 16% in the placebo group. The comparable results from the one donepezil trial[1] were 27% in the placebo group, 38% for those receiving 5 mg per day, and 54% for those treated with 10 mg per day. This comparison suggests that higher-dose donepezil is more effective than higher-dose rivastigmine, but there is no adequate explanation given for the differences observed in the placebo groups in these two studies.

The efficacy of galantamine has been studied in two prospective placebo-controlled trials. The study by Raskind et al.[5] included patients with probable AD according to NINCDS-ADRDA criteria, MMSE scores of 11–24, and baseline ADAS-cog scores of at least 12. During the initial 6-month, parallel-group, double-blind, placebo-controlled phase, approximately 600 patients were randomized to receive placebo or one of two doses of galantamine (24 or 32 mg per day). The primary efficacy measures were the ADAS-cog scores and CIBIC-plus scores (see Table 22-1). Separate analyses were performed for observed cases (randomized subjects who provided post-baseline data) and the ITT population (in which analysis was performed using the LOCF method). At 6 months, the mean drug-placebo improvement in ADAS-cog scores were 3.9 and 3.8 points for the 24- and 32-mg per day groups, respectively (see Table 22-2). This degree of benefit is greater than that observed in the trials of donepezil and rivastigmine. Mean changes in CIBIC-plus scores were not provided, but 68–70% of patients in the galantamine group were reported as remaining stable or improved (CIBIC-plus score less than or equal to 4) over 6 months, compared to only 55% of patients in the placebo group. It is misleading to compare these results to those reported in the donepezil study,[1] in which 11% of placebo-treated patients were rated as improved (CIBIC-plus score less than or equal to 3) compared to 25% in the donepezil-treated patients. Calculated data for comparison are shown in Table 22-2.

The design of the galantamine study with a 6-month open-label phase after the double-blind treatment phase provides data that raise additional questions. On the outcome measure of ADAS-cog scores, patients who continued to receive galantamine, 24 mg per day, remained significantly better than the other treatment groups, suggesting that prolonged treatment with galantamine produces clinically significant benefits even at 12 months. The observation that patients who received galantamine, 24 mg per day for 12 months, fared significantly better than those who received placebo during the double-blind phase followed by galantamine, 24 mg per day, raises the question of whether there is an advantage to early treatment with galantamine. However, this possibility should be tempered by the recognition that patients treated with galantamine, 32 mg per day, during the double-blind phase followed by 24 mg per day during the open-label phase fared no better than the placebo/galantamine 24-mg-per-day group.

Is There a Role for Acetylcholinesterase Inhibitors in Patients with Diffuse Lewy Body Disease?

The question of whether there is a role for AChE inhibitors in patients with DLBD has been the subject of a single prospective double-blind, placebo-controlled trial. McKeith et al.[6] enrolled 120 patients with probable DLBD of mild to moderate severity (as evidenced by MMSE greater than 9). Patients were randomized to receive either placebo or rivastigmine (titrated to tolerability with a maximum dose of 6 mg twice per day) for 20 weeks, followed by a 3-week washout period. In contrast to the ADAS-cog subscale and CIBIC-plus scale used in the AD trials, these investigators employed novel measures of treatment efficacy. A four-item subscore of the neuropsychiatric inventory (NPI; see Appendix 25 [The Neuropsychiatric Inventory]) comprising the sum of the scores for delusions, hallucinations, apathy, and depression was used as the primary measure of efficacy. This measure was specifically chosen based on the prominence of disturbances in these aspects of behavior in patients with DLBD. The sum of latencies measured from the computerized cognitive assessment tests of memory and attention were used as the second primary outcome measure. For efficacy analyses, patients were classified as ITT, LOCF, or observed cases, and the results of each of these analyses are reported.

The mean change from baseline on NPI-4 at week 20 favored rivastigmine for all three analyses, with the LOCF and observed cases analyses being statistically significant. The proportion of patients who improved significantly (i.e., exhibited at least a 30% improvement from baseline on their NPI-4 scores) varied from 20% to 37% depending on the analysis performed. These results are comparable to the observation that approximately 20% of AD patients treated with AChE inhibitors show a treatment response superior to that exhibited by patients who receive placebo treatment.

For the computerized cognitive assessment test scores, differences between rivastigmine and placebo were significant in all three analyses. No significant differences between the rivastigmine and placebo groups were observed on the Clinical Global Change-plus score, which was chosen as one of the secondary measures of efficacy.

In summary, therefore, this study demonstrated that rivastigmine at daily doses of 6–12 mg produced clinically relevant effects on behavior. Patients who received rivastigmine were less apathetic and anxious and had fewer hallucinations and delusions than those in the placebo group. Global measures of cognitive functioning, including attention and memory, were also markedly improved.

Is There Evidence to Support the Use of Acetylcholinesterase Inhibitors in Patients with Mild Memory or Other Cognitive Impairment?

There are no published studies to date to support the use of AChE inhibitors in patients with early cognitive impairment.

Should Patients with Alzheimer's Disease Be Treated with Vitamin E or Selegiline?

The largest and most influential study of the effects of α-tocopherol (vitamin E) and selegiline in AD is not without controversy.[7] The primary purpose of this study was to determine whether selegiline, vitamin E, or a combination of the two would slow clinical deterioration in patients with AD. The study included 341 patients with probable AD of moderate severity who were randomized to receive selegiline, vitamin E, the combination of the two, or placebo. Subjects were followed for 2 years and the primary outcome measure was the time to the occurrence of any one of a number of endpoints, including death, institutionalization, loss of ability to perform at least two of three activities of daily living, and the progression to severe dementia. Secondary endpoints included measures of cognition and behavior. The placebo and various treatment groups were well matched except for scores on the MMSE, with a trend towards higher scores in the placebo group. Because the higher MMSE scores in the placebo group were associated with a delay in the primary outcome, it was necessary to adjust for this variable in the final analysis.

There were no significant differences in the primary outcome measures between the placebo and various treatment groups. After adjustment for the baseline differences in MMSE scores between the placebo and treatment groups, however, there emerged a significant delay in the primary outcome associated with treatment with vitamin E, selegiline, and the combination of the two. The effect of treatment on each of the individual endpoints (that comprise the primary outcome measure) was also examined. With the exception of the endpoint of institutionalization (which was delayed in the vitamin E group), there were no significant differences between the various treatment and placebo groups. Significant differences were also observed on the secondary outcome measures of activities of daily living and the need for care. No differences, however, were observed on the secondary measures of cognitive function.

These results may be subject to a number of interpretations. It may be, as the authors suggest, that functional and occupational measures of cognitive capacity are better indicators of disease progression than formal tests of cognitive function. Alternatively, however, the outcome of improved function without concomitant improvement in cognition may represent a nonspecific health benefit to which the primary outcome measure was sensitive. It is also pertinent to note that significant results were obtained only after adjustment for the baseline differences between the various groups, and the need for such statistical adjustment to discern a benefit underscores the relative weakness of these results. Nevertheless, on the basis of this study, the American Academy of Neurology has issued guidelines that "vitamin E (1,000 IU twice daily) should be considered in an attempt to slow progression of AD."[8]

Is There a Role for Estrogen in the Prevention or Treatment of Alzheimer's Disease?

The question of whether there is a role for estrogen in the prevention or treatment of AD is really two separate questions, and each has been the subject of independent study. A number of studies have sought to demonstrate an association between the use of estrogen replacement therapy and a reduced risk of AD. Henderson and colleagues[9] undertook a retrospective analysis of elderly women, predicting that a history of estrogen replacement therapy would be found less frequently amongst those with AD than amongst those without dementia. Eligible subjects were consecutively identified as elderly women who agreed to longitudinal follow-up and eventual autopsy. There were 143 women with AD and 92 controls. Estrogen use was determined from the list of current medications recorded at the time of enrollment, but no effort was made to elicit information about the duration of treatment. Estrogens (most commonly Premarin) were used by 10 (7%) of the AD subjects and 17 (18%) of the nondemented controls. After controlling for the effects of age and education, the difference in prevalence of estrogen use was significantly different between the demented and control subjects. These results were taken to support the hypothesis that estrogen replacement in postmenopausal women may reduce the relative risk of developing AD. These results, however, should be interpreted with caution, as the study sample was not population-based, the analysis was retrospective, and no data regarding dose or duration of therapy were recorded. Moreover, there is an alternative explanation for the lower rate of estrogen use amongst patients with AD. It may be that estrogen replacement is simply regarded as being less important for patients with dementia and is, therefore, prescribed less frequently. The nature of this study does not permit this conclusion to be reliably distinguished from the possibility that estrogen replacement therapy is associated with a lower relative risk of AD.

The population-based study by Tang et al.[10] included 1,124 nondemented elderly women for whom information about estrogen use (including duration of therapy) was available. Those with a history of stroke or Parkinson's disease were excluded. These women were followed prospectively for 1–5 years, during which time 167 (14.9%) developed AD. The women who developed AD were generally older and had fewer years of education than those who did not develop AD. There was a tendency for estrogen use to be reported by younger women and those with more years of education. A history of estrogen use was significantly less common amongst women who developed AD than those who did not develop the disease. The relative risk of AD associated with a history of estrogen use was 0.4. Furthermore, there was a significant linear trend in the effect of duration of estrogen use on disease risk. The strengths of this study lie in its being population-based and prospective. In addition, information about the duration of therapy was recorded and a dose-response effect was observed, with the relative risk of AD being lower amongst those who had used estrogen for longer periods of time. One limitation of this study is that estrogen use was more common amongst better-educated women, and the apparent beneficial effect of estrogen may have been confounded by the known association between more education and a lower relative risk of AD.

Similar results were obtained in the Baltimore Longitudinal Study of Aging.[11] This was also a prospective population-based study. After adjustment for the level of education, the relative risk for AD amongst those who received estrogen replacement therapy compared to those who did not was 0.46. However, no effect of the duration of estrogen therapy was observed.

These observational studies, therefore, suggested that the use of estrogen replacement therapy might prevent the development of AD. This observation, however, remains untested in a prospective controlled fashion. A separate but related issue is whether estrogen therapy ameliorates the symptoms or course of AD. This question has been the subject of a number of prospective controlled trials. Henderson et al.[12] undertook a randomized, double-blind, placebo-controlled trial of (unopposed) estrogen therapy in a population of women with mild to moderate AD. The study included 42 women who were randomized to receive either placebo or Premarin (conjugated equine estrogen) for 16 weeks. The primary outcome measure was the ADAS-cog subscale. Eighteen women in each group completed the 16-week trial (with a dropout rate of 14%). There were no significant differences between the treatment and placebo groups on any of the primary or secondary outcome measures at either 4 or 16 weeks.

Mulnard et al.[13] undertook a 12-month double-blind trial in which the subjects were randomized to receive placebo or one of two doses of Premarin (0.625 or 1.250 mg per day). The primary outcome measure was the change in score on the Clinical Global Impression-change (CGI) scale. Of the 120 women randomized, 97 completed the trial (dropout rate of 11%). To assess the overall efficacy of estrogen, the high- and low-dose groups were combined into a single group of 81 women with AD and were compared to the 39 placebo subjects regarding performance on the CGI scale, MMSE, ADAS-cog subscale, and Clinical Dementia Rating at 12 months. There were no significant differences between the estrogen and placebo groups on any of these measures. Similarly, no significant differences were observed on the secondary outcome measures that were sensitive to changes in mood, memory, attention, and activities of daily living. On the basis of these two studies, therefore, it would appear that estrogen neither slows the progressive cognitive decline characteristic of AD nor provides symptomatic relief.

Thus, although presymptomatic estrogen therapy may delay the onset of AD or reduce the relative risk of developing AD, the available data from prospective randomized, placebo-controlled studies do not support the use of estrogen in the treatment of women with AD.

Is There a Role for Nonsteroidal Anti-Inflammatory Drugs in the Prevention or Treatment of Alzheimer's Disease?

There have been two prospective placebo-controlled trials of NSAIDs in patients with AD. In the first, Rogers and colleagues[14] evaluated the effects of indomethacin in patients with AD. They recruited 44 patients with probable AD and MMSE scores greater than or equal to 16 and randomized them to receive placebo or indomethacin (100–150 mg per day) for 6 months. Efficacy of treatment was evaluated by comparing the performance on a battery of cognitive tests including the ADAS, MMSE, the Boston Naming Test, and the Token Test. The results were presented as a percentage change in scores at 6 months compared to baseline. Only 28 of the original 44 patients completed the trial. The percentage change from baseline on the ADAS was +1.4 and –13.3 in the indomethacin and placebo groups, respectively. For all tests combined, the mean percentage changes from baseline were +1.3 and –8.4 for the indomethacin and placebo groups, respectively. These results were found to be statistically significant. The authors concluded that indomethacin appeared to protect patients with mild to moderate AD from the degree of cognitive decline experienced by placebo-treated patients over a period of 6 months.

In the second placebo-controlled trial, Scharf et al.[15] combined the NSAID diclofenac with misoprostol to prevent serious adverse gastrointestinal side effects. Similar to the previous study, the aim of this study was to determine whether treatment with an NSAID might protect patients with AD from the expected cognitive decline over the course of the study period. They recruited 41 patients with mild to moderate AD (MMSE of 11–25) and randomized them to receive either diclofenac/misoprostol or placebo for a period of 25 weeks. Primary outcome measures included the ADAS-cog subscale and the CGI-change scale. Only 12 of 24 patients in the diclofenac/misoprostol group and 15 of 17 in the placebo group completed the study. There were no significant differences between the placebo and the treatment groups on any of the primary or secondary outcome measures. Similar results were obtained with the ITT analysis and in the analysis of only those who completed the 25 weeks of treatment. The power of this study was limited by its small size and high dropout rate. Furthermore, the placebo group did not show the expected decline over the course of the study; this, the authors note, may have explained the failure of this study to show any significant difference between the placebo and treatment groups.

There are, therefore, limited data regarding whether NSAIDs may protect against the expected cognitive decline in patients with mild to moderate AD. The high dropout rates in both of the aforementioned studies underscore the poor tolerability of NSAIDs in elderly patients and suggest that the utility of these agents may be limited.

Although these prospective studies have sought to determine whether NSAIDs protect against the cognitive decline in AD, other studies have investigated whether NSAIDs might protect against the development of AD. The design of these studies is similar to those that examined the effects of estrogen in protecting against the development of AD. Broe et al.,[16] for example, identified 163 patients with dementia and 373 controls in the Sydney Older Persons Study. The study population was stratified into four groups: (1) those with AD and no vascular dementia (VaD), (2) those with VaD (with or without AD), (3) those with other dementias, and (4) a control group. Data on patterns of drug use were collected to determine whether there was an inverse association between the use of NSAIDs and the risk of AD and, if so, whether this effect was dose related. They found that NSAID and aspirin usage was significantly lower in the group of patients with AD, but there was no evidence for a dosage effect. The observation that acetaminophen and corticosteroid usage was similar across all groups was taken as evidence that underreporting and prescription bias were not the reasons for the different patterns of NSAID and aspirin use. They also examined the effects of potential confounding factors, including the use of other drugs (e.g., angiotensin-converting enzyme inhibitors), other diagnoses, and risk factors known or thought to be associated with AD (e.g., age, gender, educational level). These factors did not affect the original odds ratio describing the inverse association between aspirin or NSAID use and AD. It should be noted that the data from this study indicated that use of other antirheumatic drugs and angiotensin-converting enzyme inhibitors was less common amongst patients with AD; however, no explanation was offered for this observation. Also, the study did not gather data on the duration of NSAID use and how it might affect the risk of developing AD.

Most recently, in t' Veld et al.[17] undertook a prospective population-based study to determine whether the use of NSAIDs other than aspirin was associated with a decreased risk of AD. A cohort of 6,989 subjects, screened and found to be free of dementia at baseline, were followed prospectively for up to 8 years. All patients were followed until death, a diagnosis of dementia, or the end of the study period. Information on the type, dose, and duration of NSAID use was gathered prospectively. The diagnosis of dementia was made in 394 patients during the mean follow-up of 6.8 years. Of these, 293 had AD, 56 had VaD, and 45 had other types of dementia. There was no association between the use of oral salicylates (aspirin) and the risk of AD. Use of an NSAID at any time, however, compared to those with no history of NSAID use, was associated with a relative risk of AD of 0.86 (confidence interval 0.66–1.09). The relative risk of AD varied as a function of the duration of NSAID use, but there was no association between NSAID use and the risk of VaD. These results are summarized in Table 22-3.

TABLE 22-3
Relative Risk of Dementia with Increasing Duration of Nonsteroidal
Anti-Inflammatory Drug Use

Duration of Nonsteroidal Anti-Inflammatory Drug Use (Mos)	Cohort Size	No. with Dementia	Relative Risk of Alzheimer's Disease	Relative Risk of Vascular Dementia
No exposure	2,553	210	1.00	1.00
Short term (<1)	2,001	88	0.95	1.25
Intermediate term (1–23)	2,202	93	0.83	1.36
Long term (≥24)	233	3	0.20	0.99

The number of patients with long-term NSAID use was relatively small, with the relative risk calculated on the basis of an even smaller number of patients with dementia. In fact, of the three patients with long-term NSAID use who developed dementia, it is not clear how many developed AD rather than VaD. The small sample size is reflected in the large confidence intervals accompanying the relative risk of 0.20 (0.05–0.83).

On the basis of these results, however, the authors concluded that long-term use of NSAIDs has a beneficial effect on the risk of AD. This finding, however, awaits confirmation in a prospective controlled trial that should also examine the tolerability and safety of long-term NSAID use in an elderly population.

Summary

- AChE inhibitor therapy offers benefit to patients with AD as well as to those with DLBD.
- All three presently available AChE inhibitors have been shown to be effective in AD; only rivastigmine has been evaluated in patients with DLBD.
- For the most part, the different agents appear to have a comparable effect in AD (Table 22-4).
- In patients with mild to moderate dementia, the annual decline in ADAS-cog score is approximately six to eight points. The beneficial symptomatic effect of the AChE inhibitors in improving ADAS-cog scores by two to four points, therefore, corresponds to the magnitude of deterioration that might occur over approximately a 6-month period.
- AChE inhibitors represent symptomatic therapy and do not affect the progression or natural history of dementia, as evidenced by the rapid loss of effect after discontinuation of therapy.

TABLE 22-4
Relative Efficacy of Different Acetylcholinesterase Inhibitors

	Drug-Placebo ADAS-cog Score Difference	Percentage with ADAS-cog Score Improvement >4 Points	Percentage with Improved CIBIC-plus Score
Donepezil			
5 mg/day	2.2–2.5	38	26.0
10 mg/day	2.9–3.1	54	25.0
Rivastigmine	2.6	29	41.0
Galantamine	3.9	—	19.5

ADAS-cog = Alzheimer's Disease Assessment Scale–Cognitive Subscale; CIBIC = Clinician's Interview-Based Impression of Change-plus.

- Rivastigmine is effective in patients with DLBD in terms of reducing behavioral symptoms (depression, apathy, hallucinations, and delusions) and improving general cognitive function. The magnitude of this beneficial effect cannot be compared to that achieved in patients with AD because different measures of treatment efficacy were used in the AD and DLBD treatment trials.
- There are presently no published data that address the question of whether AChE treatment is of benefit to patients with mild cognitive impairment.
- The available data do not support the use of estrogen for the treatment of patients with AD; estrogen may, however, be associated with a lower relative risk of developing AD.
- Data from a prospective observational study suggest that the risk of AD may be lower amongst patients who have used NSAIDs for more than 2 years. The data regarding the utility of NSAIDs in patients with established AD, however, are even more controversial, and firm conclusions await the results of large prospective controlled studies.

References

1. Rogers SL, Farlow MR, Doody RS, et al. A 24-week, double-blind, placebo-controlled trial of donepezil in patients with Alzheimer's disease. Donepezil Study Group. *Neurology* 1998;50:136–145.
2. Rogers SL, Doody RS, Mohs RC, Friedhoff LT. Donepezil improves cognition and global function in Alzheimer disease: a 15-week, double-blind, placebo-controlled study. Donepezil Study Group. *Arch Intern Med* 1998;158:1021–1031.
3. Greenberg SM, Tennis MK, Brown LB, et al. Donepezil therapy in clinical practice: a randomized crossover study. *Arch Neurol* 2000;57:94–99.

4. Rösler M, Anand R, Cicin-Sain A, et al. Efficacy and safety of rivastigmine in patients with Alzheimer's disease: international randomised controlled trial. *BMJ* 1999;318:633–638.

5. Raskind MA, Peskind ER, Wessel T, Yuan W. Galantamine in AD—a 6-month randomized, placebo-controlled trial with a 6-month extension. The Galantamine USA-1 Study Group. *Neurology* 2000;54:2261–2268.

6. McKeith I, Del Ser T, Spano P, et al. Efficacy of rivastigmine in dementia with Lewy bodies: a randomised, double-blind, placebo-controlled international study. *Lancet* 2000;356:2031–2036.

7. Sano M, Ernesto C, Thomas RG, et al. A controlled trial of selegiline, alpha-tocopherol, or both as treatment for Alzheimer's disease. The Alzheimer's Disease Cooperative Study. *N Engl J Med* 1997;336:1216–1222.

8. Doody RS, Stevens JC, Beck C, et al. Practice parameters: management of dementia (an evidence-based review). Report of the Quality Standards Subcommittee of the American Academy of Neurology. *Neurology* 2001;56:1154–1166.

9. Henderson VW, Paganini-Hill A, Emanuel CK, et al. Estrogen replacement therapy in older women: comparisons between Alzheimer's disease cases and non-demented control subjects. *Arch Neurol* 1994;51:896–900.

10. Tang MX, Jacobs D, Stern Y, et al. Effect of estrogen during menopause on risk and age at onset of Alzheimer's disease. *Lancet* 1996;348:429–432.

11. Kawas C, Resnick S, Morrison A, et al. A prospective study of estrogen replacement therapy and the risk of developing Alzheimer's disease: the Baltimore Longitudinal Study of Aging. *Neurology* 1997;48:1517–1521.

12. Henderson VW, Paganini-Hill A, Miller BL, et al. Estrogen for Alzheimer's disease in women: randomized, double-blind, placebo-controlled trial. *Neurology* 2000;54:295–301.

13. Mulnard RA, Cotman CW, Kawas C, et al. Estrogen replacement therapy for treatment of mild to moderate Alzheimer disease: a randomized controlled trial. Alzheimer's Disease Cooperative Study. *JAMA* 2000;283:1007–1015.

14. Rogers J, Kirby LC, Hempelman SR, et al. Clinical trial of indomethacin in Alzheimer's disease. *Neurology* 1993;43:1609–1611.

15. Scharf S, Mander A, Ugoni A, et al. A double-blind, placebo-controlled trial of diclofenac/misoprostol in Alzheimer's disease. *Neurology* 1999;53:197–201.

16. Broe GA, Grayson DA, Creasey HM, et al. Anti-inflammatory drugs protect against Alzheimer disease at low doses. *Arch Neurol* 2000;57:1586–1591.

17. in t' Veld BA, Ruitenberg A, Hofman A, et al. Non-steroidal anti-inflammatory drugs and the risk of Alzheimer's disease. *N Engl J Med* 2001;345:1515–1521.

CHAPTER 23

Seizures and Epilepsy

Introduction

Until relatively recently, only a limited range of anticonvulsant drugs were available for the treatment of seizures and epilepsy. The acceptance and introduction of newly developed antiepileptic drugs has required a demonstration of their safety and efficacy. This is one area in the field of epilepsy research where randomized, controlled trials abound, and there are good-quality data to support the use of these agents. The quality of data supporting many other aspects of clinical epilepsy practice, however, is quite variable. Examples include the questionable efficacy of anticonvulsants in preventing alcohol withdrawal seizures and the risk and predictors of seizure recurrence after an initial seizure. The scope of this chapter is broad. What is the risk of seizure recurrence after a first seizure? What is the evidence supporting the use of the traditional as well as the newer anticonvulsants? What is the comparable efficacy of phenytoin and magnesium sulfate in the prophylaxis and treatment of eclamptic seizures? Are anticonvulsants teratogenic? These and other questions are the focus of this chapter.

What Is the Risk of Seizure Recurrence after a First Seizure?

The question of the risk of seizure recurrence after a first seizure has been the subject of many studies, the majority of which are sufficiently flawed in design to preclude a clear and unequivocal answer. For example, in most studies, a significant proportion of patients received anticonvulsant therapy that is expected to affect the risk of seizure recurrence. The issue of treatment is particularly important, as decisions regarding the initiation of anticonvulsant therapy after a first seizure are based in large part on the expected risk of seizure recurrence. The other problem that confounds many of these studies is the issue of whether the index seizure really does represent the first seizure. A history of seizures may not be obtained if a sufficiently detailed history is not obtained.

In making an effort to estimate the risk of seizure recurrence, it is necessary to carefully define the criteria for definition of the first seizure. The most commonly used criteria used in studies of the risk of seizure recurrence rely on the classification of seizures as *idiopathic, acute sympto-matic,* and *remote symptomatic.* Idiopathic seizures are defined as those occurring in the absence of an acute precipitating central nervous system or systemic insult. Acute symptomatic seizures are defined on the basis of their temporal relationship (within 7 days) to an acute neurologic insult (e.g., stroke or head trauma) or systemic toxic/metabolic event (e.g., hypoglycemia). The designation as a *remote symptomatic seizure* is used with reference to seizures that are thought to be due to a prior central nervous system insult thought to be associated with an increased risk of seizures (e.g., stroke, head trauma, or tumor). More recently, there has been a trend to distinguish cryptogenic seizures, in which there is no known cause from idiopathic seizures when the etiology is presumed to be genetic. The distinction, however, was not made in the studies discussed below in which the term *idiopathic* refers to all seizures of unclear etiology. The importance of accurate etiologic classification lies in the observation that etiology is one of the most important predictors of recurrence. The risk of seizure recurrence, for example, approaches 100% in patients with some of the familial epilepsy syndromes such as juvenile myoclonic epilepsy.

The study by Hauser and colleagues[1] included 244 patients recruited at the time of a first idiopathic or remote symptomatic seizure. Seizure recurrence was defined as a second seizure that was not classified as an acute symptomatic seizure. Approximately 70% of patients received anti-convulsant therapy. The results of this study were not stratified on the basis of whether anticonvulsants were used, and so the data do not inform on the question of the risk of seizure recurrence if untreated. For the entire study population, the rates of seizure recurrence were 16% at 1 year, 21% at 2 years, and 27% at 3 years, with the risks being slightly higher amongst those with remote symptomatic rather than idiopathic seizures (Table 23-1). Amongst those with idiopathic seizures, no significant differences in risk of recurrence were associated with age, gender, seizure type, presentation with status epilepticus, or the presence of abnormal findings on neurologic examination. The risk of recurrence, however, was increased amongst those with generalized spike and slow wave on electroencephalography (EEG) as well as those with a sibling with a history of seizures.

In a similar study, Annegers et al.[2] studied 424 patients with a first seizure classified as either remote symptomatic or idiopathic. Approximately 60% of these patients received anticonvulsant therapy. Overall, the cumulative risk of seizure recurrence was 36% at 1 year. When analyzed separately, patients whose first seizure was classified as remote symptomatic had a 1-year risk of recurrence that was double that of those whose first seizure was classified as idiopathic (56% vs. 26%). Those with partial seizures with an abnormal finding on neurologic examination or any abnormality on EEG were also at increased risk of seizure recurrence (see Table 23-1).

The potential importance of anticonvulsant treatment as a confounding factor in the estimation of the risk of seizure recurrence is evidenced by

TABLE 23-1
Seizure Recurrence

Study	No.	Percentage Treated with Antiepileptic Drug	Seizure Recurrence (%)			Predictors of Recurrence
			1 Yr	2 Yrs	3 Yrs	
Hauser[1]	244	70	16	21	27	Remote sympto-matic; generalized spike and slow wave on EEG; sibling with seizures
Annegers[2]	424	~60	36	—	—	Remote sympto-matic; partial seizures; abnormal neurology examination; any EEG abnormality
Elwes[3]	214	0	62	69	71	—
Hopkins[4]	306	13	37	—	—	Seizure onset between 12:00 AM and 9:00 AM

EEG = electroencephalogram.

the differences in the results of the aforementioned studies, with the data reported by Elwes et al.[3] This study included 214 patients with a first seizure (excluding those with acute symptomatic seizures), none of whom were treated. The cumulative risks of seizure recurrence were 62% at 1 year, 69% at 2 years, and 71% at 3 years. Similarly, in the study by Hopkins et al.[4] of 306 adult patients with a first seizure, only 13% of whom were treated with anticonvulsants, the cumulative risk of seizure recurrence was 37% at 1 year (see Table 23-1). This value is intermediate between the 16% in the Hauser study (70% of patients treated with anticonvulsants) and the 62% in the Elwes study (no patients received anticonvulsants). The study by Hopkins et al. also included a slightly different population in that patients with any first seizure (unless due to a known underlying brain lesion) were included. The only factor in this study that was predictive of seizure recurrence was the time of onset of the seizure between 12:00 AM and 9:00 AM.

The results of these and other studies were summarized in the meta-analysis performed by Berg and Shinnar.[5] They included 13 studies of "first-seizure" that addressed the risk of recurrent unprovoked seizures. Broadly speaking, the studies were of two types: prospective and retrospective. A potential bias of retrospective studies is that patients with recurrent seizures are more likely to remain under the care of a physician, thus biasing the study toward a higher risk of recurrence. This may partially explain the high risk of seizure recurrence reported by Elwes et al. The pooled estimate of the 2-year risk of seizure recurrence was 42%. Although the studies included in this meta-analysis differed in many relevant respects, it was possible to make a few generalizations. The risk of seizure recurrence is increased in those with remote symptomatic seizures and in those with some abnormality on EEG (although the predictive value of specific EEG abnormalities is unclear). When these two factors are combined, the risk of seizure recurrence is greatest in those with remote symptomatic seizures as well as an abnormal EEG. The risk is lowest in those with an idiopathic seizure and a normal EEG. Consensus cannot be reached on the issues of partial onset and the presence of a family history of seizures. For patients with idiopathic seizures, presentation with status epilepticus does not increase the risk of seizure recurrence.

What Is the Evidence for the Efficacy of the Traditional Anticonvulsants?

The Veterans Administration Epilepsy Cooperative Study Group (1985) compared the efficacy and toxicity of phenytoin, carbamazepine, phenobarbital, and primidone in adults with partial or secondarily generalized tonic-clonic seizures in a randomized controlled trial.[6] The aim of this study was to determine which drug provided the best seizure control while producing the least number of intolerable side effects. They randomized 622 patients, but only 421 remained in the study until the predetermined endpoint of drug failure or 2-year follow-up. The 32% attrition rate was comparable amongst patients receiving the different anticonvulsants. Treatment failure was designated to result from a combination of side effects and persistent seizures. For patients with partial seizures, the treatment failure rate was significantly higher amongst patients who received primidone or phenobarbital. For patients with secondarily generalized tonic-clonic seizures, the treatment failure rate was highest amongst patients treated with primidone. The most common reason for treatment failure was the presence of intolerable side effects. Complete control of partial seizures was significantly more common with carbamazepine (65%) compared to phenytoin (34%), which was the next most effective (p <0.05). There were no significant differences between the different anticonvulsants with respect to complete control of tonic-clonic seizures.

A second study by the Veterans Affairs Epilepsy Cooperative Study Group[7] compared the efficacy and toxicity of carbamazepine and valproate for the treatment of complex partial and secondarily generalized tonic-clonic seizures. The design of this study was very similar to that of the first study, with patients randomized to receive either carbamazepine or valproate. If seizures were not controlled, the dose was increased. If adverse events occurred, the dose was reduced. If seizures of unacceptable frequency or severity occurred when the dose was reduced, then treatment was deemed to have failed. A total of 480 patients were entered into the study and 130 (27%) did not complete 12 months of follow-up. A variety of outcome measures were used including (1) the seizure count (derived only from patients who remained in the study for 12 months); (2) the seizure rate (derived from all patients for as long as they remained in the study); (3) seizure control (proportion of patients rendered seizure free); (4) the time to first seizure; and (5) the seizure rating score (a composite measure of side effects and seizure frequency and severity). Carbamazepine and valproate were found to be of comparable efficacy in the treatment of secondarily generalized seizures. However, carbamazepine yielded significantly better results on four of the five outcome measures in patients with complex partial seizures. For both seizure types combined, 34% of patients were seizure free on carbamazepine, compared to 30% of patients treated with valproate. No attempt was made to explain why the proportion of patients treated with carbamazepine was so much lower in the second Veterans Affairs study compared to the first. Overall, treatment failure was most commonly due to seizures in patients taking valproate but also due to intolerable side effects amongst those who received carbamazepine. In conclusion, therefore, this study provided evidence that carbamazepine was a better agent for the treatment of complex partial seizures.

What Is the Evidence for Efficacy of the Newer Anticonvulsants?

Initial studies of the newer anticonvulsants focused on a demonstration of their efficacy as add-on therapy. More recently, however, many of these agents have been shown to be effective as monotherapy. A select few of these studies are summarized below.

Chadwick et al.[8] evaluated the efficacy of different dosages of gabapentin (Neurontin) in a double-blind study of patients with newly diagnosed (and untreated) partial seizures with or without secondary generalization. Patients were randomized to receive one of three doses of gabapentin (300, 900, and 1,800 mg per day). The study included an open-label carbamazepine arm but was not designed to evaluate equivalence between the two drugs. The primary efficacy variable was time to exit the study; patients were required to exit if they experienced a single generalized tonic-clonic seizure, three simple or complex partial seizures, or status epilepticus during the 24-week study period. In the primary analysis, which focused on comparing the different doses of gabapentin, the time to an exit event was longer for patients who received 900 mg or 1,800 mg gabapentin per day than for patients who received 300 mg per day. In secondary analyses, the exit rate was lowest for the carbamazepine group (30%), but the rate of withdrawal because of adverse drug effects was high (24%). Conversely, the exit rate for those receiving gabapentin, 900 mg per day, was higher (40%), but the adverse event withdrawal rate was significantly lower (4%). Overall, the clinically most important outcome measure is the combination of the rate of withdrawal from therapy because of seizures or adverse events. This rate was similar for patients who received carbamazepine and for those who were treated with gabapentin, 1,800 mg per day (54% vs. 57%). This study, therefore, demonstrated that gabapentin at 900 mg per day or 1,800 mg per day is as safe and effective as monotherapy for patients with newly diagnosed partial epilepsy. It is worth noting that, by present-day standards, 1,800 mg per day would be considered an extremely low dose, and the impression is that higher doses afford even better seizure control.

Brodie et al.[9] compared lamotrigine (Lamictal) and carbamazepine for the treatment of new-onset partial or generalized tonic-clonic seizures. A total of 260 patients were randomized to receive either lamotrigine or carbamazepine in a double-blind fashion, with follow-up planned for 48 weeks. Both drugs were introduced gradually and doses increased if seizures continued in the absence of clinically relevant adverse events or if serum drug concentration was in the lower half of the therapeutic range (or lower). Patients were withdrawn from the study in the event of unacceptable seizure control or a severe adverse event or because of serious noncompliance. These terms were not defined in greater detail, and the primary efficacy outcome analysis was not prespecified. There were no significant differences between the two treatment groups in the time to first seizure or in the proportion of patients who remained seizure free during the last 40 and 24 weeks of the study. However, the rate of withdrawal because of adverse side effects was higher in the carbamazepine group, and overall, a greater proportion of patients in the lamotrigine group (65%) compared to the carbamazepine group (51%) completed the study. In summary, therefore, this study did not demonstrate any difference in efficacy between the two drugs, but the drugs did differ in terms of their tolerability, with fewer adverse events reported by patients who received lamotrigine.

Sachdeo et al.[10] performed a randomized double-blind trial of topiramate (Topamax) monotherapy for the treatment of partial seizures with or without secondary generalized tonic-clonic seizures. The trial design included an 8-week baseline phase, 1-week open-label treatment phase (during which all patients received topiramate, 100 mg per day), and a 16-week double-blind treatment phase. The latter comprised a 5-week conversion phase during which patients were randomized to receive either placebo or an increasing dose of topiramate to the study target dose of 1,000 mg per day. Concurrent anticonvulsants were tapered and discontinued during this conversion phase. The 5-week conversion phase was followed by an 11-week monotherapy double-blind treatment phase. Patients completed the study either by finishing the 16-week treatment phase or by meeting one of the predefined exit criteria. These criteria included a doubling of the average monthly baseline seizure frequency, a doubling of the highest 2-day baseline seizure frequency, a single generalized tonic-clonic seizure if none occurred during the baseline phase, prolonged or serial seizures, or status epilepticus. The time to exit the study was considered the primary measure of efficacy. The study included 48 patients, 24 of whom were randomized to receive 1,000 mg of topiramate per day and 24 to receive 100 mg per day. The time to exit was significantly greater for the high-dose group. Moreover, successful treatment (defined as at least a 50% reduction in seizure frequency) was more frequent amongst the high-dose group compared to the low-dose group (54% vs. 17%). Side effects were generally mild and occurred with similar frequency in the high- and low-dose treatment groups. It should be noted that a dose of 1,000 mg per day is substantially higher than that used in everyday practice.

In a prospective open randomized study over a 12-month period, Kälviäinen et al.[11] compared the efficacy and safety of vigabatrin (Sabril) and carbamazepine monotherapy in 100 patients with newly diagnosed epilepsy. Patients were regarded as having not responded to treatment if two generalized or five partial seizures occurred during 1 year. Overall, 60% of patients in both treatment groups were treated successfully (i.e., did not meet criteria for treatment failure or withdraw from the study because of intolerable side effects) for 12 months. However, of the patients who remained in the study for the full 12 months, the proportion who were seizure free was significantly higher amongst those receiving carbamazepine (52%) compared to those treated with vigabatrin (32%). The reasons for treatment failure also differed. Patients receiving vigabatrin stopped therapy because of poor seizure control, whereas those treated with carbamazepine discontinued therapy most often because of intolerable side effects. These results provided evidence of the efficacy and safety of vigabatrin as monotherapy in adult patients with newly diagnosed partial or secondarily generalized epilepsy. It is worth noting that the U.S. Food and Drug Administration does not regard demonstration of equivalence to another drug (rather than superiority over placebo) as sufficient proof of efficacy—the rationale being that equivalence may simply imply lack of effect (or similar inefficacy).

Schachter et al.[12] conducted a double-blind, placebo-controlled trial of oxcarbazepine (Trileptal) monotherapy in patients with refractory partial seizures with or without secondary generalized seizures. They took advantage of the fact that anticonvulsants are withdrawn from patients with refractory seizures who undergo presurgical evaluation. Once patients had been withdrawn from regular anticonvulsant therapy, they were randomized to receive either placebo or oxcarbazepine (1,200 mg twice per day) for a maximum of 10 days. Patients exited the trial by completing the 10-day double-blind treatment phase or by fulfilling one of four exit criteria: four partial seizures, two new-onset secondary generalized seizures, serial seizures, or status epilepticus. The primary efficacy variable was the time to meet the exit criteria. Secondary efficacy variables included the percentage of patients meeting one of the exit criteria and the total partial seizure frequency. A total of 102 patients were randomized, with 51 assigned to receive placebo and 51 to receive oxcarbazepine. For the primary efficacy variable, placebo-treated patients were found to be five times more likely to reach one of the exit criteria than those who were treated with oxcarbazepine. The percentage of patients who met one of the exit criteria was significantly lower for the oxcarbazepine-treated group (47%) compared to the placebo-treated patients (84%). The oxcarbazepine-treated patients had a median total partial seizure frequency of two during the study period compared to 31 amongst the placebo-treated patients. These results demonstrated the efficacy of short-term oxcarbazepine in patients with refractory partial seizures. Adverse effects occurred significantly more frequently amongst the oxcarbazepine-treated group, but these were generally mild to moderate in severity.

The efficacy of levetiracetam (Keppra) as monotherapy has not been tested yet. Cereghino et al.,[13] however, have demonstrated its safety and efficacy as add-on therapy for patients with refractory partial seizures. Patients were randomized in a double-blind fashion to receive placebo or one of two doses of levetiracetam. Weekly seizure frequency during the 14-week study period was the primary efficacy variable. They found that levetiracetam was superior to placebo in reducing the frequency of seizures. The percentage of patients responding with at least a 50% reduction in partial seizure frequency ranged from 11% amongst those receiving placebo to 33% in those treated with levetiracetam 1,000 mg per day and 40% in those receiving levetiracetam 3,000 mg per day. This study, therefore, demonstrated the efficacy of levetiracetam as add-on therapy in adults with refractory partial seizures.

Is Magnesium Sulfate Superior to More Traditional Anticonvulsants in the Prophylaxis and Treatment of Eclamptic Seizures?

Pre-eclampsia is a multisystem disorder associated with hypertension and proteinuria. *Eclampsia* is defined as the occurrence of a seizure in association with this syndrome. The two (related) questions that arise are these: What, if any, is the most appropriate prophylactic anticonvulsant in the context of pre-eclampsia? Which agent is most suitable for the prevention of recurrent eclamptic seizures?

Crowther reported her experience with 51 women with eclampsia who were randomized to treatment with either magnesium sulfate or diazepam.[14] Maternal morbidity (defined as recurrence of convulsions, cardio-respiratory problems, disseminated intravascular coagulation, or acute renal failure) occurred more commonly amongst those who received diazepam (52%) than those who were treated with magnesium sulfate (29%). The frequency of recurrent seizures was similar between the two groups:

21% and 26% in the magnesium sulfate and diazepam groups, respectively. Neonatal outcome was also generally better in the magnesium sulfate group, with a significantly smaller proportion of infants being born with abnormal Apgar scores.

These findings were confirmed in the randomized study conducted by the Eclampsia Trial Collaborative Group.[15] This study included two comparative groups: magnesium sulfate versus diazepam (n = 905) and magnesium sulfate versus phenytoin (n = 775). They included women with eclampsia, and the prespecified primary outcome measures were recurrence of convulsions and maternal death. There were significantly fewer seizures in the magnesium sulfate group (13%; n = 60) compared to the diazepam group (28%; n = 126). Similarly, there were significantly fewer seizures in the magnesium sulfate group (6%; n = 22) compared to the phenytoin group (17%; n = 66). In both arms of the study, maternal mortality was not significantly lower amongst those who received magnesium sulfate.

Finally, Lucas and colleagues[16] designed a randomized, controlled study to compare the use of magnesium sulfate and phenytoin for the prevention of eclampsia (i.e., seizures) in women with pre-eclampsia. Women with hypertension were eligible for inclusion in the study and were randomized to receive either magnesium sulfate (n = 1,089) or phenytoin (n = 1,049). The primary outcome variable was the occurrence of a seizure, and the women who developed eclampsia were treated with magnesium sulfate irrespective of their initial treatment assignment. Seizures occurred significantly more frequently in the women given phenytoin (n = 0.9%; 10) compared to those who received magnesium sulfate (0.0%).

Overall, these studies support the use of magnesium sulfate over diazepam or phenytoin in the prevention and treatment of eclampsia. A word of caution, however, relates to the question of whether adequate doses of phenytoin were used in these studies. The loading dose used in the Eclampsia Trial Collaborative Group study was 1 g, and serum drug levels were not examined. Similarly, in the study by Lucas et al., a loading dose of 1 g phenytoin was used, and drug levels, although within the therapeutic range (i.e., less than 10 µg/ml), were on the low side (less than 12.2 µg/ml) in 8 of the 10 patients in whom seizures occurred. This observation does not invalidate these studies, nor does it detract from the conclusion that magnesium sulfate is a safe and effective form of therapy for women with pre-eclampsia or eclampsia. But it is worth noting that phenytoin might prove equally effective if used in the appropriate dose. At this point, however, this remains a matter of conjecture.

Are Anticonvulsant Drugs Teratogenic?

It is well established that the incidence of congenital malformations is increased in children born to women with epilepsy. Some doubt had persisted, however, regarding whether this increased risk is due to the terato-genic effect of the anticonvulsant drugs, the effect of seizures during the pregnancy, or the effect of genetic abnormalities that caused the mother's epilepsy and are transmitted to the fetus. A recent study by Holmes and colleagues[17] was designed to address this issue. They conducted a cohort study involving three groups of singleton infants—those born to mothers who had taken anticonvulsants (either for epilepsy or other reasons) during pregnancy (n = 316), those born to mothers with epilepsy but who had not used anticonvulsants during the pregnancy (n = 98), and a control group whose mothers neither had epilepsy nor had used anticonvulsants (n = 508). There were no significant differences between the control infants and the infants of mothers with a history of seizures but no anticonvulsant use. The infants exposed to anticonvulsants, however, had a higher incidence of major malformations, microcephaly, growth retardation, and hypoplasia of the midface and fingers (anticonvulsant-associated embryopathy). One or more of these abnormalities was detected in 8.5% of control infants, in 20.6% of infants exposed to a single anticonvulsant, and 28.0% in those exposed to more than one anticonvulsant. Amongst the women who had taken a single anticonvulsant, the most commonly used drugs were pheny-toin (n = 87), phenobarbital (n = 64), carbamazepine (n = 58), and valproic acid (n = 6). These numbers were small, but subgroup analysis did not reveal any significant differences in the incidence of embryopathy between the mothers who used the various anticonvulsants.

One problem with this sort of study is the potential confounding that may occur if the women with epilepsy who used anticonvulsants did so because of more severe epilepsy. It then becomes difficult to disentangle the effect of the anticonvulsant from that of the worse seizure disorder.

Is There a Role for Prophylactic Anticonvulsant Use after Head Injury?

Post-traumatic seizures are a common problem, and the question of whether they might be prevented by prophylactic use of an anticonvulsant has been the subject of a number of studies. Before reviewing some of the data that pertain to this question, it is necessary to establish some concep-tual clarity. The potential benefits of anticonvulsant use after head injury are twofold. First, it is hoped that the anticonvulsant might suppress any seizures that otherwise would have occurred in the absence of treatment. This effect really represents a treatment effect. The second potential bene-fit is a prophylactic one and relates to the question of whether use of an anticonvulsant for a specified time might prevent the subsequent (i.e., after the anticonvulsant has been discontinued) occurrence of seizures.

Many of the studies that have examined these questions have been criticized because of their retrospective nature, their small size, or the use of inadequate dosages of anticonvulsant. Temkin et al.[18] conducted a double-blind, randomized study to clarify the role of phenytoin in preventing post-traumatic seizures. To be eligible for the study, patients must have had a cortical contusion visible on a computerized tomographic scan; a subdural, epidural, or intracerebral hemorrhage; a depressed skull fracture; a penetrating head injury; a depressed level of consciousness; or a seizure within 24 hours of the injury. Eligible patients were randomized to receive either placebo or phenytoin 20 mg/kg administered intravenously; maintenance doses were adjusted by an unblinded investigator to ensure therapeutic drug levels. Patients were maintained in the study for 12 months unless seizures or serious drug reactions occurred or patients were withdrawn from the study (e.g., withdrawal of consent or death). The occurrence of seizures was the primary endpoint of the study, and these were arbitrarily classified as occurring *early* (within 7 days of the administration of phenytoin) or *late* (between 8 days and 1 year). The primary analysis was an intention-to-treat analysis and, therefore, included those assigned to phenytoin who stopped taking it and those assigned to placebo who had early seizures and were crossed over to receive phenytoin. The dropout rate was high. A total of 208 patients were randomized to receive phenytoin and 196 to receive placebo. At the end of the 7 days (the cut off for early seizures), 162 patients continued to take phenytoin and 134 continued with placebo. By the end of 1 year, only 59 patients remained on phenytoin and 67 on placebo.

Within the first 7 days, the phenytoin group had a cumulative seizure rate of 3.6% compared to 14.2% amongst those receiving placebo. By 1 year, the seizure rates were 21.5% and 15.7% in the phenytoin and placebo groups, respectively. Study drugs were discontinued after 1 year, and final follow-up performed at 2 years. At final follow-up, the seizure rate was 27.5% and 21.0% in the phenytoin- and placebo-treated patients, respectively. Only the results within the first 7 days were statistically significant. There was concern that the late efficacy of phenytoin may have been obscured in the primary intention-to-treat analysis by the high proportion of patients who did not receive the assigned therapy. Secondary analysis of only those patients who were treated for 1 full year, however, similarly failed to demonstrate a significant benefit from phenytoin.

This randomized, double-blind study, therefore, provided evidence of the effectiveness of phenytoin in the treatment of post-traumatic seizures during the first week after serious head injury. Perhaps surprisingly, the ongoing use of anticonvulsant therapy was not associated with a reduction in the frequency of late seizures. Moreover, prolonged use of phenytoin did not constitute effective prophylaxis against the development of seizures beyond the period of treatment. These results, therefore, support the use of phenytoin in the immediate posthead injury period but provide no justification for the ongoing use of an anticonvulsant in the absence of seizures that warrant therapy.

Is Anticonvulsant Therapy Effective
for Alcohol-Related Seizures?

Alcohol abuse is one of the common causes of adult-onset seizures. Alcohol may induce seizures or exacerbate underlying epilepsy. Patients who abuse alcohol also have an increased risk of structural abnormalities in the brain (e.g., old subdural hematoma) that may contribute to the prevalence of epilepsy. Finally, alcohol withdrawal is commonly accompanied by seizures. Estimates vary, but seizures are thought to occur in approximately 10% of patients undergoing alcohol withdrawal. The first seizure typically occurs within 48 hours of the last drink, and the interval from first to last seizure is usually less than 6 hours. A number of studies have addressed the question of immediate- or short-term treatment to prevent recurrent alcohol withdrawal seizures. Many were limited by small sample size, inclusion of patients with a history of seizures unrelated to alcohol, concurrent use of medications that might prevent recurrent seizures, and the use of inadequate dosages of anticonvulsants.

The study by Alldredge and colleagues[19] was not subject to these flaws. These investigators included patients with a recent seizure in the context of acute alcohol withdrawal. Patients with a history of seizures unrelated to alcohol were excluded, as were those who received other medications that might impact on seizure recurrence (including benzodiazepines). Ninety eligible patients were randomized to receive either placebo or 1 g of phenytoin administered intravenously over 20 minutes. Patients were then hospitalized for observation for 12–24 hours. The endpoint of the study was either the recurrence of at least one seizure or a seizure-free period of at least 12 hours from completion of the infusion. There were 45 patients in each group, and seizures occurred in six patients in each group. Clearly, there was no significant difference between the two treatment groups.

More recently, D'Onofrio et al.[20] conducted a prospective double-blind, placebo controlled trial to evaluate the efficacy of a single dose of lorazepam in the prevention of recurrent seizures related to alcohol withdrawal. Patients with a history of alcohol abuse who presented after a witnessed generalized seizure were eligible for inclusion, but patients with an alternative etiology for seizures or who received medications that might alleviate or exacerbate seizures were excluded. Patients were randomly assigned to receive either placebo or a single dose of lorazepam (2 mg) administered intravenously. There were 100 patients in the lorazepam group and 86 who received placebo. Study endpoint was reached with the development of a second generalized seizure or 6 hours after the administration of the study drug. In total, 24 patients developed recurrent seizures: 21 (24%) occurred in the placebo group and three (3%) in the lorazepam group. There were no complications associated with the administration of lorazepam. Notwithstanding the short observation period employed in this study, intravenous lorazepam was found to be safe and effective in preventing seizure recurrence in the context of acute alcohol withdrawal.

Is There Evidence to Support the Use of a Particular Anticonvulsant Regimen in the Treatment of Generalized Convulsive Status Epilepticus?

Shaner et al.[21] conducted a prospective randomized controlled trial comparing the combination of diazepam and phenytoin with phenobarbital as the initial treatment for status epilepticus. *Status epilepticus* was defined as (1) witnessed convulsive seizure activity for at least 5 minutes, (2) history of 30 minutes of continuous or recurrent generalized convulsive activity, or (3) a history of at least three seizures within 1 hour without recovery to baseline mental state. All patients presenting to the emergency room with status epilepticus were eligible for inclusion in the study. Patients were randomized to one of two treatment protocols. In the diazepam/phenytoin protocol, diazepam was infused at 2 mg per minute until seizures were terminated or a total of 20 mg had been administered. Phenytoin was administered simultaneously at a rate of 40 mg per minute. In seizures that were ongoing, a diazepam infusion (8 mg per hour) was continued during the period required to complete the phenytoin load. The patients who were randomized to the phenobarbital protocol received an infusion at a rate of 100 mg per minute until a dose of 10 mg/kg had been administered (a relatively low dose). If seizures continued 10 minutes after initiating treatment, then phenytoin was added. A total of 36 episodes of status (in 35 patients) were treated—18 with the diazepam/phenytoin protocol and 18 with the phenobarbital protocol (five of whom required supplemental phenytoin). The median cumulative convulsion time for patients receiving phenobarbital was 5 minutes compared to 9 minutes for those receiving the combination of diazepam and phenytoin. The median response latency (a measure that includes the time between convulsions when the subject remained obtunded) was also shorter for the phenobarbital group (5.5 minutes vs. 15.0 minutes). These differences were of marginal statistical significance, with largely overlapping confidence intervals. The frequency of complications was similar in the two groups. A conservative interpretation of these results is that phenobarbital is at least as effective as the combination of diazepam and phenytoin.

More recently, Treiman et al.[22] compared four different anticonvulsant regimens for the treatment of status epilepticus in a double-blind, randomized, controlled trial. Two forms of generalized convulsive status epilepticus were recognized: *overt*, in which there were recurrent seizures without complete recovery in between, and *subtle*, in which the subject was continuously comatose with only subtle motor convulsions discernible. Patients were eligible for inclusion irrespective of prior drug treatment as long as there was evidence of overt or subtle status at the time of evaluation. Subjects were randomized to receive intravenous treatment with lorazepam (0.1 mg/kg), phenobarbital (15 mg/kg), phenytoin (18 mg/kg), or the combination of diazepam (0.15 mg/kg) and phenytoin (18 mg/kg). Treatment was considered successful if there was cessation of clinical and electroencephalographic seizure activity within 20 minutes and no recurrence during the period from 20 to 60 minutes after the initiation of treatment. A total of 570 patients were enrolled in the study, 395 with overt status and 175 with subtle status. These are included in the intention-to-treat analysis. In 52 of the 570 patients, the diagnosis of status could not be verified at the time of randomization, leaving a total of 518 for the verified-diagnosis analysis.

In the patients with overt (but not subtle) status, there was a significant difference in the overall frequency of success amongst the four treatments, with lorazepam being more effective than phenytoin ($p = 0.002$). When the patients with overt and subtle status were combined in a post hoc analysis, the success rates between lorazepam (52.2%) and phenytoin (36.8%) remained significant ($p = 0.001$). These differences were not observed in the intention-to-treat analysis. Seizure recurrence rates over the 12-hour study period were not significantly different amongst the four treatment groups. Similarly, there were no significant differences in the frequency of various side effects between the treatment groups. In general, successful treatment was more common amongst those with overt status compared to those with subtle status (55.5% vs. 14.9%), and the 30-day outcome and mortality rates were similarly significantly better amongst those with overt status. The authors concluded that lorazepam was more likely than phenytoin to be successful when used as the initial intravenous treatment for overt generalized convulsive status epilepticus. In evaluating these results and the conclusions drawn, it is instructive to note that the infusion time was only 4.7 minutes for lorazepam and 33 minutes for phenytoin. The implication is that only a limited proportion of the phenytoin loading dose will have been administered within the first 20.0 minutes, during which seizure control was required for the definition of successful treatment. It could, however, be counter-argued that the need to administer phenytoin more slowly provides an additional reason to use a drug like lorazepam that can be administered much more rapidly. It is also worth noting that the differences between the lorazepam and phenytoin groups were not significant in the more conservative intention-to-treat analysis. Finally, this study did not include a treatment arm in which patients were randomized to receive the combination of lorazepam and phenytoin—a regimen currently in common usage.

Therefore, the overall impression from these studies is that there is little difference between the varying anticonvulsant regimens for the treatment of generalized convulsive status epilepticus.

Summary

- The risk of seizure recurrence is difficult to estimate from the available literature, with 1-year risks ranging from 16% to 62% depending on the proportion of patients in the study who received anticonvulsants at the time of the first seizure. Meta-analysis suggests that the 2-year recurrence rate is approximately 42%, although the recurrence rate is strongly determined by etiology.

- Factors that have inconsistently been suggested as predicting a greater risk of recurrence include (1) the presence of an underlying structural brain abnormality (i.e., the index seizure is classified as remote symptomatic); (2) partial (rather than generalized) seizure; (3) the time of seizure onset between 12:00 AM and 9:00 AM; (4) any abnormal finding on neurologic examination; (5) the presence of generalized spike and slow-wave activity on EEG; (6) the presence of any EEG abnormality; and (7) a family history of a sibling with seizures. In a recent meta-analysis, classification of the index seizure as *remote symptomatic* and the presence of any abnormality on EEG are the two features that emerged as most strongly predictive of seizure recurrence.

- There are no placebo-controlled trials that demonstrate the efficacy of the traditional anticonvulsants, and there are only limited data comparing the relative efficacy of these agents. The Veterans Affairs Epilepsy Cooperative Study Group published two trials in 1985 and 1992 that showed carbamazepine to be superior to primidone, phenytoin, valproate, and phenobarbital in the treatment of partial seizures and primidone to be inferior to carbamazepine, phenytoin, and phenobarbital in the treatment of both partial and secondary generalized seizures.

- There is evidence from randomized controlled trials to support the use of gabapentin, lamotrigine, topiramate, oxcarbazepine, vigabatrin, and levetiracetam as monotherapy in the treatment of patients with partial onset seizures with or without secondary generalization.

- The available literature supports the use of magnesium sulfate rather than diazepam or phenytoin in the prevention and treatment of eclampsia.

- The incidence of fetal malformations is increased amongst pregnancies characterized by exposure to anticonvulsants. This increased risk appears to be caused by the anticonvulsants themselves and not simply a result of the mother having epilepsy. Although most often reported with valproate and carbamazepine, there are no good data to indicate that the risk of teratogenicity is greatest with these agents.

- A prospective placebo-controlled trial did not demonstrate the efficacy of early phenytoin therapy in preventing the late occurrence of seizures after traumatic head injury; this study, however, did show the benefit of phenytoin in reducing the occurrence of early seizures.

- Lorazepam, but not phenytoin, is effective in the very short-term or immediate prevention of recurrent alcohol withdrawal seizures. Whether maintenance phenytoin or any other anticonvulsant is effective in preventing alcohol withdrawal seizures in the long term is unknown, as this has not yet been the focus of a controlled trial.

- There are data from a prospective double-blind, controlled trial suggesting that lorazepam is the most effective anticonvulsant in the early treatment of generalized convulsive status epilepticus.

References

1. Hauser WA, Anderson VE, Loewenson RB, McRoberts SM. Seizure recurrence after a first unprovoked seizure. *N Engl J Med* 1982;307:522–528.
2. Annegers JF, Shirts SB, Hauser WA, Kurland LT. Risk of recurrence after an initial unprovoked seizure. *Epilepsia* 1986;27:43–50.
3. Elwes RD, Chesterman P, Reynolds EH. Prognosis after a first untreated tonic-clonic seizure. *Lancet* 1985;2:752–753.
4. Hopkins A, Garman A, Clarke C. The first seizure in adult life. Value of clinical features, electroencephalography, and computerised tomographic scanning in prediction of seizure recurrence. *Lancet* 1988;1:721–726.
5. Berg AT, Shinnar S. The risk of seizure recurrence following a first unprovoked seizure: a quantitative review. *Neurology* 1991;41:965–972.
6. Mattson RH, Cramer JA, Collins JF, et al. Comparison of carbamazepine, phenobarbital, phenytoin and primidone in partial and secondarily generalized tonic-clonic seizures. *N Engl J Med* 1985;313:145–151.
7. Mattson RH, Cramer JA, Collins JF. A comparison of valproate with carbamazepine for the treatment of complex partial seizures and secondarily generalized tonic-clonic seizures in adults. The Department of Veterans Affairs Epilepsy Cooperative Study No. 264 Group. *N Engl J Med* 1992;327:765–771.
8. Chadwick DW, Anhut H, Greiner MJ, et al. A double-blind trial of gabapentin monotherapy for newly diagnosed partial seizures. The International Gabapentin Monotherapy Study Group 945-77. *Neurology* 1998;51:1282–1288.
9. Brodie MJ, Richens A, Yuen AW. Double-blind comparison of lamotrigine and carbamazepine in newly diagnosed epilepsy. The UK Lamotrigine/Carbamazepine Monotherapy Trial Group. *Lancet* 1995;345:476–479.
10. Sachdeo RC, Reife RA, Lim P, Pledger G. Topiramate monotherapy for partial onset seizures. *Epilepsia* 1997;38:294–300.
11. Kälviäinen R, Äikiä M, Saukkonen AM, et al. Vigabatrin vs carbamazepine monotherapy in patients with newly diagnosed epilepsy. A randomized controlled study. *Arch Neurol* 1995;52:989–996.
12. Schachter SC, Vazquez B, Fisher RS, et al. Oxcarbazepine. Double-blind, randomized, placebo-control, monotherapy trial for partial seizures. *Neurology* 1999;52:732–737.
13. Cereghino JJ, Biton V, Abou-Khalil B, et al. Levetiracetam for partial seizures: results of a double-blind, randomized clinical trial. *Neurology* 2000;55:236–242.

14. Crowther C. Magnesium sulphate versus diazepam in the management of eclampsia: a randomized controlled trial. *Br J Obstet Gynaecol* 1990;97:110–117.

15. Which anticonvulsant for women with eclampsia? Evidence from the Collaborative Eclampsia Group. *Lancet* 1995;345:1455–1463.

16. Lucas MJ, Leveno KJ, Cunningham FG. A comparison of magnesium sulfate with phenytoin for the prevention of eclampsia. *N Engl J Med* 1995;333:201–205.

17. Holmes LB, Harvey EA, Coull BA, et al. The teratogenicity of anticonvulsant drugs. *N Engl J Med* 2001;344:1132–1138.

18. Temkin NR, Dikmen SS, Wilensky AJ, et al. A randomized, double-blind study of phenytoin for the prevention of post-traumatic seizures *N Engl J Med* 1990;323:497–502.

19. Alldredge BK, Lowenstein DH, Simon RP. Placebo-controlled trial of intravenous diphenylhydantoin for short-term treatment of alcohol withdrawal seizures. *Am J Med* 1989;87:645–648.

20. D'Onofrio G, Rathlev NK, Ulrich AS, et al. Lorazepam for the prevention of recurrent seizures related to alcohol. *N Engl J Med* 1999;340:915–919.

21. Shaner DM, McCurdy SA, Herring MO, Gabor AJ. Treatment of status epilepticus: a prospective comparison of diazepam and phenytoin versus phenobarbital and optional phenytoin. *Neurology* 1988;38:202–207.

22. Treiman DM, Meyers PD, Walton NY, et al. A comparison of four treatments for generalized convulsive status epilepticus. The Veterans Affairs Status Epileptics Cooperative Study Group. *N Engl J Med* 1998;339:792–798.

APPENDIX 1

Alzheimer's Disease Assessment Scale[1]

The word recognition task is administered first. The next 10 minutes are spent in open-ended conversation to assess various aspects of expressive and receptive speech. Then the remaining cognitive tasks are administered. The noncognitive behaviors are evaluated from report of the patient or reliable informant or observed during the interview. If the patient has more than a mild memory impairment, ratings on behavioral items are based on the informant's report.

Cognitive Behavior

1. *Spoken language ability.* This item is a global rating of the quality of speech (i.e., clarity, difficulty in making oneself understood). Quantity is not rated on this item.
   1 = very mild; one instance of lack of understandability
   2 = mild
   3 = moderate; subject has difficulty 25–50% of the time
   4 = moderately severe; subject has difficulty 50% of the time
   5 = severe; one- or two-word utterances; fluent but empty speech; mute

2. *Comprehension of spoken language.* This item evaluates the patient's ability to understand speech. Do not include responses to commands.
   1 = very mild; one instance of misunderstanding
   2 = mild
   3 = moderate
   4 = moderately severe; requires several repetitions and rephrasing
   5 = severe; patient rarely responds to questions appropriately; not due to poverty of speech

3. *Recall of test instruction.* The patient's ability to remember the requirements of the recognition task is evaluated. On each recognition trial, the patient is asked before presentation of the first two words, "Did you see this word before, or is this a new word?" For the third word, the patient is asked "How about this one?" If the patient responds appropriately (i.e., "yes" or "no"), then recall of instructions is accurate. If the

253

patient does not respond, this signifies that the instructions have been forgotten. Then instruction is repeated for words 4–24. Each instance of recall failure is noted.

4.   *Word-finding difficulty in spontaneous speech.* The patient has difficulty in finding the desired word in spontaneous speech. The problem may be overcome by circumlocution (i.e., giving explanatory phrases or nearly satisfactory synonyms). Do not include finger and object naming in this rating.
>   1 = very mild; one or two instances, not clinically significant
>   2 = mild; noticeable circumlocution or synonym substitution
>   3 = moderate; loss of words without compensation on occasion
>   4 = moderately severe; frequent loss of words without compensation
>   5 = severe; nearly total loss of content words; speech sounds empty;
>   one- or two-word utterances

5.   *Following commands.* Receptive speech is assessed also on the patient's ability to carry out one- to five-step commands.
>   1.   Make a fist.
>   2.   Point to the ceiling, then to the floor.

Line up a pencil, watch, and card (in that order) on a table in front of the patient.
>   3.   Put the pencil on top of the card, then put it back.
>   4.   Put the watch on the other side of the pencil and turn over the card.
>   5.   Tap each shoulder twice with two fingers, keeping your eyes shut.

Each numbered element represents a single step. The command may be repeated once in its entirety. Each command scored is as a whole. Ratings correspond to the highest level of command correctly performed.
>   0 = five steps correct
>   1 = four steps correct
>   2 = three steps correct
>   3 = two steps correct
>   4 = one step correct
>   5 = cannot do one step correctly

6.   *Naming objects and fingers.* The patient names the fingers of his or her dominant hand. The patient also names 12 randomly presented real objects, whose frequency values are high, medium, or low. Objects and their frequency are
High—flower, bed, whistle, pencil
Medium—rattle, mask, scissors, comb
Low—wallet, harmonica, stethoscope, tongs
>   0 = all correct; one finger incorrect and/or one object incorrect
>   1 = two to three fingers and/or two objects incorrect
>   2 = two or more fingers and three to five objects incorrect

3 = three or more fingers and six to seven objects incorrect
4 = three or more fingers and eight to nine objects incorrect

7. *Constructional praxis.* The ability to copy four geometric forms is assessed. These forms, in the order of presentation, are

Circle, approximately 20 cm in diameter

Two overlapping rectangles
   The vertical rectangle is 20 cm × 25 cm.
   The horizontal rectangle is 10 cm × 35 cm.

Rhombus
   Each side is 20 cm.
   Acute angle is 50 degrees.
   Obtuse angle is 130 degrees.

Cube
   Each side is 20 cm.
   Internal lines are present.

Each form is located in the upper middle of a 5.5 × 8.5–in. sheet of white paper. The patient is instructed, "Do you see this figure? Make one that looks like this anywhere on the paper." Two attempts are permitted.
   0 = all four drawings correct
   1 = one form incorrect
   2 = two forms incorrect
   3 = three forms incorrect
   4 = closing in (draws over or around model or uses parts of model); four drawings incorrect
   5 = no figures drawn; scribbles parts of forms; words instead of forms

Scoring criteria for each form (examples show below):
   1. *Circle.* A closed curved figure.
   2. *Two overlapping rectangles.* Forms must be four-sided, and overlap must be similar to presented form. Changes in size are not scored.

Correct   Incorrect

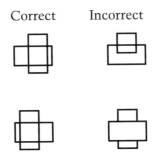

3.   *Rhombus (diamond).* Figure must be four-sided, obliquely oriented, and the sides approximately equal in length. Four measurements are taken (see figure below). These are ac, a'c, bc, and b'c. The ratio of ac/a'c or a'c/ac ranges from 0.75 to 1.00. The ratio of bc/b'c or b'c/bc ranges from 0.60 to 1.00. The ratio of bb'/aa' ranges from 3.00 to 0.75. Figure is incorrect if any ratio is outside these ranges.

Model

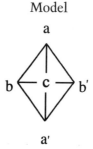

4.   *Cube.* The form is three-dimensional, with front face in the correct orientation, internal lines drawn correctly between corners. If opposite sides of face are not parallel by more than 20 degrees, it is incorrect.

Incorrect

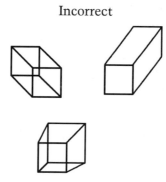

8.   *Ideational praxis.* The patient is given an 8.5 × 11.0–in. sheet of paper and a long envelope. The patient is instructed to send the letter to himself. The patient is told to put the paper into the envelope, seal it, address it to herself, and stamp it. If the patient forgets part of the task, instruction is given again. Impairment of this item should reflect dysfunction in executing an overlearned task only and not recall difficulty. The five components to this task are (1) fold the letter, (2) put letter in the envelope, (3) seal the envelope, (4) address the envelope, and (5) put a stamp on the envelope.

   1 = difficulty with and/or failure to perform one component
   2 = difficulty with and/or failure to perform two components
   3 = difficulty with and/or failure to perform three components
   4 = difficulty with and/or failure to perform four components
   5 = difficulty with and/or failure to perform five components

9. *Orientation.* The components of orientation are date, month, year, day of week, season, time of day, place, and person. One point is given for each incorrect response (maximum = 8). Acceptable answers include ±1 for the date, within 1 hour for the hour, partial name for place, naming of upcoming season within 1 week before its onset, and name of previous season for 2 weeks after its termination.

10. *Word recall task.* The patient reads 10 high-imagery words exposed for 2 seconds each. The patient then recalls the words aloud. Three trials of reading and recall are given. The score equals the mean number of words not recalled on three trials (maximum = 10).

11. *Word recognition task.* The patient reads aloud 12 high-imagery words. These words are then randomly mixed with 12 words the patient has not seen. The patient indicates whether the word was shown previously. Then two more trials of reading the original words and recognition are given. The score equals the mean number of incorrect responses for three trials (maximum = 12).

Noncognitive Behavior

The time period for evaluation includes the entire week before the interview for the following items:
1. Appears or reports feeling sad, down, hopeless, discouraged
2. Is tearful
3. Is delusional
4. Hallucinates
5. Paces
6. Has increased motor activity
7. Has an increase/decrease in appetite

12. *Tearful.* Patient or informant is asked about the frequency of occurrence of tearfulness.
    1 = very mild; occurs one time during week or during test session only
    2 = mild; occurs two to three times during the week
    3 = moderate
    4 = moderately severe; frequent crying spells nearly every day
    5 = severe; frequent and prolonged crying spells every day

13. *Depression.* The patient or informant is asked if the patient has been sad, discouraged, or down. If a positive response is given, further inquiry into the severity and pervasiveness of the mood, loss of interest or pleasure in activities, and reactivity to environmental events is made. The interviewer also assesses the patient for depressed facies and the ability to respond to encouragement and jokes.

1 = feels slightly dysphoric; clinically significant
2 = mild; appears and reports mild dysphoric mood, reactivity present, some loss of interest
3 = moderate; often feels moderately dysphoric
4 = moderately severe; feels dysphoric almost all the time with considerable loss of reactivity and interest
5 = severe; pervasive and severe degree of dysphoric mood; total lack of reactivity; pervasive loss of interest or pleasure

14.   *Concentration/distractibility.* This item rates the frequency with which the patient is distracted by irrelevant stimuli and/or must be reoriented to the ongoing task because of loss of train of thought or the frequency with which the patient appears to be caught up in his or her own thoughts.

1 = very mild; one instance of poor concentration
2 = mild; two to three instances of poor concentration or distractibility
3 = moderate
4 = moderately severe; poor concentration throughout much of the interview and/or frequent instances of distractibility
5 = severe; extreme difficulty in concentration and numerous instances of distractibility

15.   *Uncooperative to testing.* This item rates the degree to which the patient objects to some aspect of the interview.

1 = very mild; one instance of lack of cooperation
2 = mild
3 = moderate
4 = moderately severe; needs frequent cajoling to complete the interview
5 = severe; refuses to continue the interview

16.   *Delusions.* The item rates the extent and conviction of the patient's belief in ideas that are almost certainly not true. In rating severity, consider conviction in delusions, preoccupation, and the effect they have on the patient's actions.

1 = very mild; one transient delusional belief
2 = mild; delusion definitely present but subject questions his or her belief
3 = moderate; patient convinced of delusion but it does not affect behavior
4 = moderately severe; delusion has effect on behavior
5 = severe; significant actions based on delusions

17.   *Hallucinations.* Inquiry about visual, auditory, and tactile hallucinations is made. The frequency and degree of disruptiveness of hallucinations are rated.

1 = very mild; hears voice saying one word; visual hallucination once
2 = mild

3 = moderate; hallucinates numerous times during day, which interferes with normal functioning
4 = moderately severe
5 = severe; nearly constant hallucinating, which totally disrupts normal functioning

18. *Pacing*. Rating on this item must distinguish between normal physical activity and excessive walking back and forth.
1 = very mild; very rare occurrence
2 = mild
3 = moderate; paces frequently each day
4 = moderately severe
5 = severe; cannot sit still and must pace excessively

19. *Increased motor activity*. This item is rated relative to the person's
normal activity level or previously obtained baseline.
1 = very mild; very slight increase
2 = mild
3 = moderate; significant increase in amount of movement
4 = moderately severe
5 = severe; must be moving constantly; rarely sits still

20. *Tremors*. Patient extends both hands in front of body and spreads the
fingers, holding this position for approximately 10 seconds.
1 = very mild; very slight tremor, barely noticeable
2 = mild; noticeable tremor
3 = moderate
4 = moderately severe
5 = severe; very rapid movements with sizable displacements

21. *Increased/decreased appetite*. The item is included because appetite
change may be associated with depression and because clinical observations of some Alzheimer's patients reveal both increases and decreases in
appetite. This item is rated relative to the person's normal appetite or previously obtained baseline.
1 = very mild; slight change, probably clinically significant
2 = mild; noticeable change, patient still eats without encouragement
3 = moderate; marked change, patient needs encouragement to eat, or
patient asks for more food
4 = moderately severe
5 = severe; patient will not eat and needs to be force-fed; patient com-
plains of constant hunger despite consumption of sufficient quan-
tities

APPENDIX 2

Average Muscle Score[2]

Manual muscle strength testing is performed on 32 muscle groups, and results are graded on a modified Medical Research Council (MRC) scale expanded to a 10-point system as outlined below.

MRC Grade	Ten-Point System
0	0
1	1
2	2
3–	3
3	4
3+	5
4–	6
4	7
4+	8
5–	9
5	10

The muscles tested include the neck flexors, neck extensors, shoulder abductors, elbow extensors, elbow flexors, wrist flexors, wrist extensors, thumb abductors, hip flexors, hip extensors, hip abductors, knee extensors, knee flexors, ankle dorsi-flexors, ankle evertors, and ankle plantar-flexors on each side. The scores for all 32 muscle groups are then summated to give an average muscle score (AMS).

APPENDIX 3

Barthel Index[3]

Feeding

Independent (10 points). The patient can feed himself a meal from a tray or table when someone puts the food within his reach. He must put on an assistive device if this is needed, cut up the food, use salt and pepper, spread butter, and so forth. The patient must accomplish this in a reasonable time.

With help (5 points). Some help is necessary (e.g., with cutting up food, as listed above).

Moving from Wheelchair to Bed and Return (Includes Sitting in Bed)

Independent (15 points). Independent in all phases of this activity. Patient can safely approach the bed in her wheelchair, lock brakes, lift footrests, move safely to bed, lie down, come to a sitting position on the side of the bed, change the position of the wheelchair (if necessary, to transfer back into it safely), and return to the wheelchair.

With help (10 points). Either some or minimal help is needed in some step of this activity or the patient needs to be reminded or supervised for safety of one or more parts of this activity.

With help (5 points). Patient can come to a sitting position without the help of a second person but needs to be lifted out of bed, or she transfers with a great deal of help.

Personal Toilet (Wash Face, Comb Hair, Shave, Clean Teeth)

Independent (5 points). Patient can wash hands and face, comb hair, clean teeth, and shave. Male patients may use any kind of razor but must put in blade or plug in razor without help as well as get it from the drawer or cabinet. Female patients must put on own makeup, if used, but need not braid or style hair.

Getting On and Off Toilet (Handling Clothes, Wipe, Flush)

Independent (10 points). Patient is able to get on and off toilet, fasten and unfasten clothes, prevent soiling of clothes, and use toilet paper without help. He may use a wall bar or other stable object for support, if needed. If it is necessary to use a bedpan instead of a toilet, he must be able to place it on a chair, empty it, and clean it.

Some help (5 points). Patient needs help because of imbalance or in handling clothes or in using toilet paper.

Bathing

Independent (5 points). Patient may use a bathtub or a shower or take a complete sponge bath. She must be able to do all the steps involved in whichever method is employed without another person being present.

Walking on Level Surface

Independent (15 points). Patient can walk at least 50 yards without help or supervision. He may wear braces or prostheses and use crutches, canes, or a walkerette but not a rolling walker. Patient must be able to lock and unlock braces if used, assume the standing position and sit down, get the necessary mechanical aids into position for use, and dispose of them when he sits.

With help (5 points). Patient needs help or supervision in any of the above but can walk at least 50 yards with a little help.

Propelling a Wheelchair (Score Only If Unable to Walk)

Independent (5 points). If a patient cannot ambulate but can propel a wheelchair independently. She must be able to go around corners, turn around, maneuver the chair to a table, bed, toilet, and so forth. Patient must be able to push a chair at least 50 yards. Do not score this item if the patient gets score for walking.

Ascending and Descending Stairs

Independent (10 points). Patient is able to go up and down a flight of stairs safely without help or supervision. He may and should use handrails, canes, or crutches when needed. Patient must be able to carry canes or crutches while ascending or descending stairs.

With help (5 points). Patient needs help with or supervision of any one of the above items.

Dressing and Undressing

Independent (10 points). Patient is able to put on, remove, and fasten all clothing and tie shoelaces (unless it is necessary to use adaptations for this). The activity includes putting on, removing, and fastening corset or braces when these are prescribed. Special clothing such as suspenders, loafer shoes, or dresses that open down the front may be used when necessary.

With help (5 points). Patient needs help in putting on, removing, or fastening any clothing. She must do at least half the work alone. Patient must accomplish this in a reasonable time. Women need not be scored on use of a brassiere or girdle unless these are prescribed garments.

Continence of Bowels

Independent (10 points). Patient is able to control his or her bowels and have no accidents. He can use a suppository or take an enema when necessary (as for spinal cord injury patients who have had bowel training).

With help (5 points). Patient needs help in using a suppository or taking an enema or has occasional accidents.

Controlling Bladder

Independent (10 points). Patient is able to control her bladder day and night. Spinal cord injury patients who wear an external device and leg bag must put them on independently, clean and empty the bag, and stay dry day and night.

With help (5 points). Patient has occasional accidents, cannot wait for the bedpan, cannot get to the toilet in time, or needs help with an external device.

A score of 0 is given in all of the above activities when the patient cannot meet the criteria as defined.

APPENDIX 4

Clinical Dementia Rating[4]

Healthy (Clinical Dementia Rating 0)

Memory. No memory loss or slight inconsistent forgetfulness.
Orientation. Fully oriented.
Judgment and problem solving. Solves everyday problems well; judgment good in relation to past performance.
Community affairs. Independent function at usual level in job, shopping, business and financial affairs, and volunteer and social groups.
Home and hobbies. Life at home, hobbies, and intellectual interests well maintained.
Personal care. Fully capable of self care.

Questionable Dementia (Clinical Dementia Rating 0.5)

Memory. Mild consistent forgetfulness; partial recollection of events; "benign" forgetfulness.
Orientation. Fully oriented.
Judgment and problem solving. Only doubtful impairment in solving problems, similarities, differences.
Community affairs. Only doubtful or mild impairment, if any, in these activities.
Home and hobbies. Life at home, hobbies, intellectual interests well maintained or only slightly impaired.
Personal care. Fully capable of self care.

Mild Dementia (Clinical Dementia Rating 1)

Memory. Moderate memory loss, more marked for recent events; defect interferes with everyday activities.
Orientation. Some difficulty with time relationships; oriented for place and person at examination but may have geographic disorientation.

Judgment and problem solving. Moderate difficulty in handling complex problems; social judgment usually maintained.

Community affairs. Unable to function independently at these activities though may still be engaged in some; may still appear normal to casual inspection.

Home and hobbies. Mild but definite impairment of function at home; more difficult chores abandoned; more complicated hobbies and interests abandoned.

Personal care. Needs occasional prompting.

Moderate Dementia (Clinical Dementia Rating 2)

Memory. Severe memory loss; only highly learned material retained; new material rapidly lost.

Orientation. Usually disoriented in time, often to place.

Judgment and problem solving. Severely impaired in handling problems, similarities, differences; social judgment usually impaired.

Community affairs. No pretense of independent function outside home.

Home and hobbies. Only simple chores preserved; very restricted interests; poorly sustained.

Personal care. Requires assistance in dressing, hygiene, and keeping of personal effects.

Severe Dementia (Clinical Dementia Rating 3)

Memory. Severe memory loss; only fragments remain.

Orientation. Orientation to person only.

Judgment and problem solving. Unable to make judgments or solve problems.

Community affairs. No pretense of independent function outside home.

Home and hobbies. No significant function in home outside of own room.

Personal care. Requires much help with personal care; often incontinent.

APPENDIX 5

Clinician's Interview-Based Impression[5] and Clinical Global Impression of Change[6]

Clinician's Interview-Based Impression (CIBI) and Clinical Global Impression of Change (CGIC) are seven-point scales intended to assess change from baseline. The scale intervals range from 1 (very much improved) to 7 (very much worse), with 4 indicating no change since baseline. No guidelines or descriptors are provided to further define the individual ratings; the difference between *minimally improved* and *much improved* is left to the individual rater's clinical judgment.

1 = marked improvement
2 = moderate improvement
3 = minimal improvement
4 = no change
5 = minimal worsening
6 = moderate worsening
7 = marked worsening

APPENDIX 6

Facial Paralysis Recovery Profile[7]

	Points Assigned to Each Unit of Recovery			
Site	0–25%	25–50%	50–75%	75–100%
Forehead	0	+1	+2	+2
Eye	+1	+2	+3	+4
Mouth	+1	+2	+3	+4

This scale is based on the idea that the return of facial function can be measured in units of 25%. The authors assigned plus points to each 25% of return in each of three facial regions (forehead, eye, and mouth). The number of points assigned to the degree of motion of each muscle group was determined on the basis of the functional and cosmetic importance of that group. Profile scores range from +2 to +10.

APPENDIX 7

French Cooperative Guillain-Barré Syndrome Study: Functional Testing Scale[8]

The functional testing evaluates the ability to complete 28 items using a binary outcome: yes or no. All items are given the same weight. A functional score is subsequently derived, ranging from 0 (no items completed) to 100 (all completed).

Function testing of upper limbs*
- Move fingers
- Hold a pen between thumb and forefinger
- Flex forearm over arm in the pronation position
- Flex forearm over arm in the supination position
- Lift elbow above bed plane
- Maintain arms stretched

Function testing of lower limbs*
- Move toes
- Ankle dorsiflexion
- Ankle plantar flexion
- Knee flexion above bed plane
- Raise lower limb above bed plane, knee extended
- Maintain lower limbs above bed plane, knee flexed

Stand up
Walk with assistance
Walk without assistance
Stand up from a squatting position

---

*Tested on both the left and right sides.

APPENDIX 8

Functional Independence Measure[9]

Self Care

Feeding. Includes all aspects of eating and drinking, such as opening containers, pouring liquids, cutting meat, buttering bread, chewing, and swallowing.

Grooming. Includes oral care, hair grooming, washing hands and face, shaving, and applying makeup.

Bathing. Includes bathing the entire body from the neck down.

Dressing—upper body. Includes dressing above the waist as well as donning and removing prosthesis or orthosis when applicable.

Dressing—lower body. Includes dressing from the waist down as well as donning or removing orthosis when applicable.

Toileting. Includes maintaining perineal hygiene and adjusting clothing after toileting.

Sphincter Control

Bladder management. Includes complete intentional control of urinary bladder and management of equipment necessary for emptying.

Bowel management. Includes complete intentional control of bowel movements and use of laxatives, suppositories, and manual evacuation.

Mobility

Transfer—bed, chair, wheelchair. Includes management of all aspects of transferring to and from bed, chair, or wheelchair, or coming to a standing position, if walking is the typical mode of locomotion.

Transfer—toilet. Includes getting on and off toilet.

Transfer—bathtub or shower. Includes getting into and out of a bathtub or shower stall.

Locomotion

Walking or using wheelchair. Includes walking or using a wheelchair, once in a seated position, indoors.
Stairs. Includes going up and down 12–14 stairs (one flight).

Communication

Comprehension. Includes clear comprehension of either auditory or visual communication.
Expression. Includes clear expression of either verbal or nonverbal language.

Social Cognition

Social interaction. Includes skills related to getting along and participating with others in therapeutic and social situations.
Problem solving. Includes skills related to using previously learned information to solve problems of daily living.
Memory. Includes skills related to awareness in performing daily activities in an institutional or community setting.

Functional Independence Measure Description of General Levels of Function

Independence. Another person is not required for the activity.
   (NO HELPER)

   4. *Complete independence.* All of the tasks described as making up the activity are typically performed safely without modification, assistive devices, or aids and within a reasonable time.
   3. *Modified independence.* Activity requires any one or more than one of the following: an assistive device, more than reasonable time, or safety (risk) considerations.

Dependence. Another person is required for either supervision or physical assistance for the activity to be performed or it is not performed. (REQUIRES HELPER)

   2. *Modified dependence.* The subject expends half (50%) or more of the effort. The levels of assistance required are
      a. *Supervision.* Subject requires no more help than cueing or coaxing, without physical contact.

b. *Minimal assistance.* Subject requires no more help than touching, or subject expends 75% or more of the effort.

c. *Moderate assistance.* Subject requires more help than touching, or expends half (50%) or more (up to 75%) of the effort.

1. *Complete dependence.* Subject expends less than half (less than 50%) of the effort. Maximal or total assistance is required, or the activity is not performed. The levels of assistance required are

a. *Maximal assistance.* Subject expends less than 50% of the effort but at least 25% of the effort.

b. *Total assistance.* Subjects expends less than 25% of the effort.

APPENDIX 9

Glasgow Coma Scale[10]

Eye opening	Spontaneous	4
	To speech	3
	To pain	2
	None	1
Best verbal response	Oriented	5
	Confused	4
	Inappropriate	3
	Incomprehensible	2
	None	1
Best motor response	Obeying	6
	Localizing	5
	Withdrawing	4
	Flexing	3
	Extending	2
	None	1

APPENDIX 10

Glasgow Outcome Scale[11]

Grade I   *Good recovery*. Implies resumption of normal life even though there may be minor neurologic and psychological deficits.

Grade II   *Moderate disability (disabled but independent)*. Patients are able to travel by public transport and can work in a sheltered environment and are, therefore, independent in so far as daily life is concerned. The disabilities found include varying degrees of dysphasia, hemiparesis, or ataxia as well as intellectual and memory deficits and personality change.

Grade III   *Severe disability (conscious but disabled)*. These patients are dependent for daily support by reason of mental or physical disability.

Grade IV   *Persistent vegetative state*.

Grade V   *Death*.

APPENDIX 11

Guillain-Barré Syndrome Six-Point Scale[12]

0 = healthy
1 = minor symptoms or signs and capable of running
2 = able to walk 5 m across an open space without assistance, walking frame, or stick but unable to run
3 = able to walk 5 m across an open space with the help of one person and waist-level walking frame or stick(s)
4 = chair-bound or bed-bound, unable to walk as in (3)
5 = assisted ventilation required (for at least part of the day)

APPENDIX 12

Hoehn and Yahr Parkinson's Disease Disability Scale[13]

Stage I   Unilateral involvement only, usually with minimal or no functional impairment.

Stage II   Bilateral or midline involvement, without impairment of balance.

Stage III First sign of impaired righting reflexes. This is evident by unsteadiness as the patient turns or is demonstrated when the patient is pushed from standing equilibrium with the feet together and eyes closed. Functionally, the patient is somewhat restricted in his or her activities but may have some work potential depending on the type of employment. Patient is physically capable of leading an independent life, and the disability is mild to moderate.

Stage IV   Fully developed, severely disabling disease; the patient is still able to walk and stand unassisted but is markedly incapacitated.

Stage V   Confinement to bed or wheelchair unless aided.

APPENDIX 13

House-Brackmann Facial Nerve Grading System[14]

Grade	Definition
I. Normal	Normal facial function in all areas.
II. Mild dysfunction	*Gross*: slight weakness noticeable only on close inspection; may have slight synkinesis. *At rest*: normal symmetry and tone. *Motion*: moderate to good movement of forehead; ability to close eye with minimal effort and slight asymmetry; ability to move corners of mouth with slight asymmetry.
III. Moderate dysfunction	*Gross*: obvious but not disfiguring difference between two sides; noticeable but not severe synkinesis, contracture, and/or hemifacial spasm. *At rest*: normal symmetry and tone. *Motion*: slight to moderate movement of forehead; ability to close eye with maximal effort; mouth slightly weak with maximal effort.
IV. Moderately severe dysfunction	*Gross*: obvious weakness and/or disfiguring asymmetry. *At rest*: normal symmetry and tone. *Motion*: no movement of forehead; inability to close eye completely with maximal effort; asymmetric movement of corners of mouth with maximal effort.
V. Severe dysfunction	*Gross*: only barely perceptible motion. *At rest*: asymmetry. *Motion*: no movement of forehead; incomplete closure of eye and only slight movement of mouth.
VI. Total paralysis	No movement.

APPENDIX 14

Hughes Functional Disability Scale[15]

0 = healthy
1 = minor signs or symptoms
2 = able to walk 5 m without a walker or equivalent support
3 = able to walk 5 m with a walker or support
4 = chair-bound or bed-bound (unable to walk 5 m with a walker or support)
5 = requires assisted ventilation (for at least part of the day)
6 = dead

APPENDIX 15

Hunt and Hess Scale[16]

Grade I   Asymptomatic, or minimal headache and slight nuchal rigidity

Grade II   Moderate to severe headache, nuchal rigidity, no neurologic deficit other than cranial nerve palsy

Grade III   Drowsiness, confusion, or mild focal deficit

Grade IV   Stupor, moderate to severe hemiparesis, possibly carly decerebrate rigidity and vegetative disturbances

Grade V   Deep coma, decerebrate rigidity, moribund appearance

APPENDIX 16

Modified Japanese Orthopedic Association Scale[17]

Score	Definition
Score	*Definition*
Motor dysfunction score of the upper extremities	
0	Inability to move hands
1	Inability to eat with a spoon but able to move hands
2	Inability to button shirt but able to eat with a spoon
3	Able to button shirt with great difficulty
4	Able to button shirt with slight difficulty
5	No dysfunction
Motor dysfunction score of the lower extremities	
0	Complete loss of motor and sensory function
1	Sensory preservation without ability to move legs
2	Able to move legs but unable to walk
3	Able to walk on flat floor with a walking aid (e.g., cane or crutch)
4	Able to walk up and/or down stairs with handrail
5	Moderate to significant lack of stability but able to walk up and/or down stairs without handrail
6	Mild lack of stability but walks with smooth reciprocation unaided
7	No dysfunction
Sensory dysfunction score of the upper extremities	
0	Complete loss of hand sensation
1	Severe sensory loss or pain
2	Mild sensory loss
3	No sensory loss

Score	Definition
Sphincter dysfunction score	
0	Inability to micturate voluntarily
1	Marked difficulty with micturition
2	Mild to moderate difficulty with micturition
3	Normal micturition

APPENDIX 17

Kurtzke Expanded Disability Score[18]

Functional Systems

Pyramidal Functions

    0 = normal
    1 = abnormal signs without disability
    2 = minimal disability
    3 = mild or moderate paraparesis or hemiparesis; severe monoparesis
    4 = marked paraparesis or hemiparesis, moderate quadriparesis, or
        monoplegia
    5 = paraplegia, hemiplegia, or marked quadriparesis
    6 = quadriplegia
    V = unknown

Cerebellar Functions

    0 = normal
    1 = abnormal signs without disability
    2 = mild ataxia
    3 = moderate truncal or limb ataxia
    4 = severe ataxia, all limbs
    5 = unable to perform coordinated movements due to ataxia
    V = unknown
    X = used throughout after each number when weakness (grade 3 or more
        in Pyramidal Functions) interferes with testing

Brainstem Functions

    0 = normal
    1 = signs only
    2 = moderate nystagmus or other mild disability
    3 = severe nystagmus, marked extraocular weakness, or moderate dis-
        ability of other cranial nerves
    4 = marked dysarthria or other marked disability
    5 = inability to swallow or speak
    V = unknown

Sensory Functions (Revised 1982)

0 = normal

1 = vibration or figure writing decrease only, in one or two limbs

2 = mild decrease in touch or pain or position sense and/or moderate decrease in vibration in one or two limbs; or vibratory decrease alone in three or four limbs

3 = moderate decrease in touch or pain or position sense and/or essentially lost vibration in one or two limbs; or mild decrease in touch or pain and/or moderate decrease in all proprioceptive tests in three or four limbs

4 = marked decrease in touch or pain or loss of proprioception, alone or combined, in one or two limbs; or moderate decrease in touch or pain and/or severe proprioceptive decrease in more than two limbs

5 = loss (essentially) of sensation in one or two limbs or moderate decrease in touch or pain and/or loss of proprioception for most of the body below the head

6 = sensation essentially lost below the head

V = unknown

Bowel and Bladder Functions (Revised 1982)

0 = normal

1 = mild urinary hesitancy, urgency, or retention

2 = moderate hesitancy, urgency, retention of bowel or bladder, or rare urinary incontinence

3 = frequent urinary incontinence

4 = in need of almost constant catheterization

5 = loss of bladder function

6 = loss of bowel and bladder function

V = unknown

Visual (or Optic) Functions

0 = normal

1 = scotoma with visual acuity (corrected) better than 20/30

2 = worse eye with scotoma with maximal visual acuity (corrected) of 20/30 to 20/59

3 = worse eye with large scotoma or moderate decrease in fields but with maximal visual acuity (corrected) of 20/60 to 20/99

4 = worse eye with marked decrease of fields and maximal visual acuity (corrected) of 20/100 to 20/200; grade 3 plus maximal visual acuity of better eye of 20/60 or less

5 = worse eye with maximal visual acuity (corrected) less than 20/200; grade 4 plus maximal visual acuity of better eye of 20/60 or less

6 = grade 5 plus maximal visual acuity of better eye of 20/60 or less

V = unknown
X = added to grades 0–6 for presence of temporal pallor

Cerebral (or Mental) Functions

0 = normal
1 = mood alteration only
2 = mild decrease in mentation
3 = moderate decrease in mentation
4 = marked decrease in mentation (chronic brain syndrome–moderate)
5 = dementia or chronic brain syndrome–severe or incompetent
V = unknown

Other Functions

0 = none
1 = any other neurologic findings attributed to multiple sclerosis (specify)
V = unknown

Expanded Disability Status Scale

0 = normal neurologic exam (all grade 0 in Functional Systems [FS]; cerebral grade 1 acceptable)
1.0 = no disability, minimal signs in one FS (i.e., grade 1 excluding cerebral grade 1)
1.5 = no disability minimal signs in more than one FS (more than one grade 1 excluding cerebral grade 1)
2.0 = minimal disability in one FS (one FS grade 2; others 0 or 1)
2.5 = minimal disability in two FS (two FS grade 2; others 0 or 1)
3.0 = moderate disability in one FS (one FS grade 3; others 0 or 1) or mild disability in three or four FS (three or four FS grade 2; others 0 or 1) but fully ambulatory
3.5 = fully ambulatory but with moderate disability in one FS (one grade 3) and one or two FS grade 2; or two FS grade 3; or five FS grade 2 (others 0 or 1)
4.0 = fully ambulatory without aid, self-sufficient, up and about 12 hours a day despite relatively severe disability consisting of one FS grade 4 (others 0 or 1), or combinations of lesser grades exceeding limits of previous steps; able to walk without aid or rest for 500 m
4.5 = fully ambulatory without aid, up and about much of the day, able to work a full day, may otherwise have some limitation of full activity or require minimal assistance; characterized by relatively severe disability, usually consisting of one FS grade 4 (others 0 or 1) or combinations of lesser grades exceeding limits of previous steps; able to walk without aid or rest for 300 m

5.0 = ambulatory without aid or rest for about 200 m; disability severe enough to impair full daily activities (e.g., to work full day without special provisions) (usual FS equivalents are one grade 5 alone, others 0 or 1; or combinations of lesser grades usually exceeding specifications for step 4.0)

5.5 = ambulatory without aid or rest for approximately 100 m; disability severe enough to preclude full daily activities (usual FS equivalents are one grade 5 alone, others 0 or 1; or combinations of lesser grades usually exceeding those for step 4.0)

6.0 = intermittent or unilateral constant assistance (cane, crutch, or brace) required to walk approximately 100 m with or without resting (usual FS equivalents are combinations with more than two FS grade 3+)

6.5 = constant bilateral assistance (canes, crutches, or braces) required to walk approximately 20 m without resting (usual FS equivalents are combinations with more than two FS grade 3+)

7.0 = unable to walk beyond approximately 5 m even with aid, essentially restricted to wheelchair; wheels self in standard wheelchair and transfers alone; up and about in wheelchair 12 hours a day (usual FS equivalents are combinations with more than one FS grade 4+; very rarely pyramidal grade 5 alone)

7.5 = unable to take more than a few steps; restricted to wheelchair; may need aid in transfer; wheels self but cannot carry on in standard wheelchair a full day; may require motorized wheelchair (usual FS equivalents are combinations with more than one FS grade 4+)

8.0 = essentially restricted to bed or chair or perambulated in wheelchair, but may be out of bed itself much of the day; retains many self-care functions; generally has effective use of arms (usual FS equivalents are combinations, generally grade 4+ in several systems)

8.5 = essentially restricted to bed much of the day; has some effective use of arm(s); retains some self-care functions (usual FS equivalents are combinations, generally 4+ in several systems)

9.0 = helpless bed patient; can communicate and eat (usual FS equivalents are combinations, mostly grade 4+)

9.5 = totally helpless bed patient; unable to communicate effectively or eat or swallow (usual FS equivalents are combinations, almost all grade 4+)

10.0 = death due to multiple sclerosis

APPENDIX 18

Mann's Grading for Cervical Spondylotic Myelopathy[19]

Grade A   Normal. No difficulty in walking. Some evidence of spinal cord involvement may be present, such as slightly brisk tendon reflexes and slightly increased tone.

Grade B   Obvious difficulty in walking but can run and hop. Can walk more than 1 km at a time and get up from squatting position holding arms above head. Clinically grossly brisk tendon reflexes, increased tone, and extensor plantar responses. Sphincter muscles intact.

Grade C   Gross difficulty in walking but can do so without help for a distance of at least 400 m. Unable to get up from squatting position; may do so by holding on to furniture. Clinically the same as Grade B, but with ankle and knee clonus, which may be unsustained. Sphincter muscles may be involved.

Grade D   Able to walk only with walking aids. In need of considerable help to get up. Clinically the same as Grade C but showing persistent clonus. Sphincter muscles may be involved.

Grade E   Bedridden. Unable to walk or stand. Clinically the same as Grade D with involved sphincter muscles.

APPENDIX 19

Mini-Mental State Examination[20]

Maximum Score	Score	
		Orientation
5	( )	What is the [year] [season] [date] [day] [month]?
5	( )	Where are we: [state] [country] [town] [hospital] [floor]?
		Registration
3	( )	Name three objects: 1 second to say each. Then ask the patient all three after you have said them. Give 1 point for each correct answer. Then repeat them until she learns all three. Count trials and record.
		Attention and calculation
5	( )	Serial 7s. 1 point for each correct. Stop after five answers. Alternatively spell "world" backwards.
		Recall
3	( )	Ask for the three objects repeated above. Give 1 point for each correct.
		Language
9	( )	Name a pencil and watch (2 points). Repeat the following: "No ifs, ands, or buts" (1 point). Follow a three-stage command: "Take a paper in your right hand, fold it in half, and put it on the floor" (3 points). Read and obey the following: Close your eyes (1 point). Write a sentence (1 point). Copy a design (1 point).

APPENDIX 20

Quantified Myasthenia Gravis Strength Score[21]

A myasthenia gravis score of 0–3 is recorded for each item; possible total scores range from 0 to 39.

	Grade of Weakness			
Test Items	None (0)	Mild (1)	Moderate (2)	Severe (3)
Double vision on lateral gaze (secs)	>60	10–60	1–10	Spontaneous heterotropia
Ptosis on upward gaze (secs)	>60	10–60	1–10	Spontaneous
Facial muscles	Normal	Mild weakness on lid closure; snarl	Incomplete lid closure	Unable to mimic expressions
Chewing	Normal	Fatigue after solid food	Only soft food	Gastric tube
Swallowing	Normal	Fatigue after solid food	Incomplete palatal closure; nasal speech	Gastric tube
Head lifting to 45 degrees while supine (secs)	>120	30–120	0–30	0

Test Items	Grade of Weakness			
	None (0)	Mild (1)	Moderate (2)	Severe (3)
Outstretched right arm to 90 degrees while standing (secs)	>240	90–240	10–90	≤10
Outstretched left arm to 90 degrees while standing (secs)	>240	90–240	10–90	≤10
Vital capacity (L)				
Male	>3.5	2.5–3.5	1.5–2.5	<1.5
Female	>2.5	1.8–2.5	1.2–1.8	<1.2
Outstretched right leg to 45 degrees, supine (secs)	>100	30–100	0–30	0
Outstretched left leg to 45 degrees, supine (secs)	>100	30–100	0–30	0
Right grip				
Male (5 kg)	>45	15–45	5–15	<5
Female (4.5 kg)	>31	10–31	5–10	<5
Left grip				
Male (5 kg)	>35	15–35	5–15	<5
Female (4.5 kg)	>25	10–25	5–10	<5

APPENDIX 21

Myasthenia Muscular Score[22]

Maintain upper limbs horizontally outstretched

    1 point per 10 secs   Maximum 15

                                           Minimum 0

Maintain lower limbs above bed plane while lying on back

    1 point per 5 secs   Maximum 15

                                           Minimum 0

Raise head above bed plane while lying on back

Against resistance	10
Without resistance	5
Impossible	0

Sit up from lying position

Without help of hands	10
Impossible	0

Extrinsic ocular musculature

Normal	10
Ptosis	5
Double vision	0

Eyelid occlusion

Complete	10
Incomplete with corneal covering	5
Incomplete without corneal covering	0

Chewing

Normal	10
Weak	5
Impossible	0

Swallowing

    Normal   10

    Impaired without aspiration   5

    Impaired with aspiration   0

Speech

    Normal   10

    Nasal   5

    Slurred   0

APPENDIX 22

National Institutes of Health Stroke Scale[23,24]

Item	Name	Response	Score
1a	LOC*	Alert	0
		Not alert, obtunded	2
		Unresponsive	3
1b	LOC* questions	Answers both correctly	0
		Answers one correctly	1
		Answers neither correctly	2
1c	LOC* commands	Performs both tasks correctly	0
		Performs one task correctly	1
		Performs neither task	2
2	Gaze	Normal	0
		Partial gaze palsy	1
		Total gaze palsy	2
3	Visual fields	No visual loss	0
		Partial hemianopia	1
		Complete hemianopia	2
		Bilateral hemianopia	3
4	Facial palsy	Normal	0
		Minor paralysis	1
		Partial paralysis	2
		Complete paralysis	3

*LOC = level of consciousness.

Item	Name	Response	Score
5	Motor arm	No drift	0
	a. Left	Drift before 10 secs	1
	b. Right	Fall before 10 secs	2
		No effort against gravity	3
		No movement	4
6	Motor leg	No drift	0
	a. Left	Drift before 5 secs	1
	b. Right	Fall before 5 secs	2
		No effort against gravity	3
		No movement	4
7	Ataxia	Absent	0
		One limb	1
		Two limbs	2
8	Sensory	Normal	0
		Mild loss	1
		Severe loss	2
9	Language	Normal	0
		Mild aphasia	1
		Severe aphasia	2
		Mute or global aphasia	3
10	Dysarthria	Normal	0
		Mild	1
		Severe	2
11	Extinction/inattention	Normal	0
		Mild	1
		Severe	2

APPENDIX 23

Nurick's Clinical Grading of Cervical Spondylotic Myelopathy[25]

Grade 0   Signs or symptoms of root involvement but without evidence of spinal cord disease

Grade 1   Signs of spinal cord disease but no difficulty in walking

Grade 2   Slight difficulty in walking that does not prevent full-time employment

Grade 3   Difficulty in walking, which prevents full-time employment or the ability to do all housework but which is not so severe as to require someone else's help to walk

Grade 4   Able to walk only with someone else's help or with the aid of a frame

Grade 5   Chair-bound or bedridden

APPENDIX 24

Neurological Disability Score[26]

Scoring: Enter *0* for no deficit, *1* for mild deficit, *2* for moderate deficit, *3* for severe deficit, and *4* for complete absence of function or most severe deficit. To obtain a raw Neurological Disability Score, both columns are summated and added together.

	Right	Left
Cranial nerves		
Papilledema		
EOM weakness, Cr III		
EOM weakness, Cr VI		
Face weakness		
Palate weakness		
Tongue weakness		
Muscle weakness		
Respiratory		
Shoulder abduction		
Biceps brachii		
Brachioradialis		
Extension at elbow		
Extension at wrist		
Flexion at wrist		
Extension of fingers		
Flexion of fingers		
Intrinsic hand		
Iliopsoas		

	Right	Left
Glutei		
Quadriceps		
Hamstrings		
Dorsiflexors		
Plantar flexors		
Reflexes		
Biceps brachii		
Triceps brachii		
Brachioradialis		
Quadriceps femoris		
Triceps surae		
Sensation		
Index finger (below base of nail)		
Touch-pressure		
Pricking pain		
Vibration		
Position sense		
Great toe (below base of nail)		
Touch-pressure		
Pricking pain		
Vibration		
Position sense		
Total		

Cr = cranial nerve; EOM = extraocular muscle.

APPENDIX 25

The Neuropsychiatric Inventory[27]

The Neuropsychiatric Inventory evaluates 10 behavioral domains. The domains and a sample question from each are as follows:

1. *Delusions.* Does the patient believe that others are stealing from him?
2. *Hallucinations.* Does the patient talk to people who are not there?
3. *Agitation/aggression.* Is the patient uncooperative or resistant to help from others?
4. *Dysphoria.* Does the patient say or act as if she is sad or in low spirits?
5. *Anxiety.* Does the patient say that he is worried about planned events?
6. *Euphoria.* Does the patient find humor in and laugh at things that others do not find funny?
7. *Apathy.* Does the patient seem less spontaneous and less active than usual?
8. *Disinhibition.* Does the patient say crude things or make sexual remarks that she would not usually say?
9. *Irritability/lability.* Does the patient have sudden flashes of anger?
10. *Aberrant motor activity.* Does the patient pace around the house without apparent purpose?

- After the questions are answered, the interviewer is asked to rate the severity (1 = mild; 2 = moderate; 3 = severe) and frequency (1 = occasionally, less than once per week; 2 = often, approximately once per week; 3 = frequently, several times per week but less than every day; 4 = very frequently, once or more per day or continuously).
- The questions are read aloud by the examiner; defined anchor points for severity and frequency allow caregivers to provide a ratable answer.
- Using this approach, domains with a negative response to the screening question are not explored while data regarding the characteristics, severity, and frequency are garnered for each domain with a positive response to the screening question.

APPENDIX 26

Norris Scale for Amyotrophic Lateral Sclerosis[28]

Item	3 (Normal)	2 (Impaired)	1 (Trace)	0 (Unable)
1. Hold up head				
2. Swallow				
3. Speak				
4. Turn in bed				
5. Sit up				
6. Breathe				
7. Cough				
8. Write name				
9. Use buttons, zippers				
10. Put on shirt, blouse				
11. Put on skirt, trousers				
12. Feed self				
13. Lift glass and drink				
14. Grip and lift				
15. Comb hair				
16. Clean teeth				
17. Lift book or tray				
18. Lift fork, pencil				
19. Change arm position				
20. Climb stairs, one flight				

Item	3 (Normal)	2 (Impaired)	1 (Trace)	0 (Unable)
21. Walk one block				
22. Walk in room				
23. Walk with assistance				
24. Stand up				
25. Change leg position				
Stretch reflexes		Hyper-hypo	Absent	Clonic
26. Arms				
27. Legs				
28. Jaw jerk	Absent	Present	Hyper	Clonic
Plantar responses	**Flexor**	**Mute**	**Equivocal**	**Extensor**
29. Right				
30. Left				
31. Fasciculation	None	Slight	Moderate	Severe
Wasting				
32. Face, tongue				
33. Arms, shoulder				
34. Legs, hips				
35. Labile emotions				
36. Fatigability				
37. Leg rigidity				
38. Arm rigidity				
39. Cramps				
40. Pain				
Totals in case				
Theoretical totals (120)				

APPENDIX 27

Oxford Handicap Scale[29]

Grade	Description
0	No symptoms
1	Minor symptoms that do not interfere with lifestyle
2	Minor handicap, symptoms that lead to some restriction in lifestyle but do not interfere with the patient's capacity to look after herself
3	Moderate handicap, symptoms that significantly restrict lifestyle and prevent totally independent existence
4	Moderately severe handicap, symptoms that clearly prevent independent existence but not needing constant attention
5	Severe handicap, totally dependent patient requiring constant attention night and day

APPENDIX 28

Modified Rankin Scale[30]

Grade	Description
0	No symptoms at all
1	No significant disability despite symptoms; able to carry out all usual duties and activities
2	Slight disability; unable to carry out all previous activities but able to look after own affairs without assistance
3	Moderate disability; requiring some help but able to walk without assistance
4	Moderately severe disability; unable to walk without assistance, and unable to attend to own bodily needs without assistance
5	Severe disability; bedridden, incontinent, and requiring constant nursing care and attention

APPENDIX 29

Scandinavian Stroke Scale[31]

Consciousness	Fully conscious	6
	Somnolent, can be awakened to full consciousness	4
	Reacts to verbal command, but is not fully conscious	2
Eye movements	No gaze palsy	4
	Gaze palsy present	2
	Conjugate eye deviation	0
Arm, motor power*	Raises arm with normal strength	6
	Raises arm with reduced strength	5
	Raises arm with flexion in elbow	4
	Can move but not against gravity	2
	Paralysis	0
Hand, motor power*	Normal strength	6
	Reduced strength in full range	4
	Some movement, fingertips do not reach palm	2
	Paralysis	0
Leg, motor power*	Normal strength	6
	Raises straight leg with reduced strength	5
	Raises leg with flexion of knee	4
	Can move, but not against gravity	2
	Paralysis	0

*Motor power is assessed only on the affected side.

Orientation	Correct for time, place and person	6
	Two of these	4
	One of these	2
	Completely disoriented	0
Speech	No aphasia	10
	Limited vocabulary or incoherent speech	6
	More than yes/no, but no longer sentences	3
	Only yes/no or less	0
Facial palsy	None/dubious	2
	Present	0
Gait	Walks 5 m without aids	12
	Walks with aids	9
	Walks with help of another person	6
	Sits without support	3
	Bedridden/wheelchair	0

APPENDIX 30

Unified Parkinson's Disease Rating Scale

I. Mentation, behavior, and mood

1. Intellectual impairment
   0 = none
   1 = mild; consistent forgetfulness with partial recollection of events and no other difficulties
   2 = moderate memory loss, with disorientation and moderate difficulty handling complex problems; mild but definite impairment of function at home with need of occasional prompting
   3 = severe memory loss with disorientation for time and often to place; severe impairment in handling problems
   4 = severe memory loss with orientation preserved to person only; unable to make judgments or solve problems; requires much help with personal care; cannot be left alone at all

2. Thought disorder (due to dementia or drug intoxication)
   0 = none
   1 = vivid dreaming
   2 = "benign" hallucinations with insight retained
   3 = occasional to frequent hallucinations or delusions; without insight; could interfere with daily activities
   4 = persistent hallucinations, delusions, or florid psychosis; not able to care for self

3. Depression
   1 = periods of sadness or guilt greater than normal, never sustained for days or weeks
   2 = sustained depression (1 week or more)
   3 = sustained depression with vegetative symptoms (insomnia, anorexia, weight loss, loss of interest)
   4 = sustained depression with vegetative symptoms and suicidal thoughts or intent

4. Motivation/initiative
   0 = normal
   1 = less assertive than usual; more passive
   2 = loss of initiative or disinterest in elective (nonroutine) activities
   3 = loss of initiative or disinterest in day to day (routine) activities
   4 = withdrawn, complete loss of motivation

II. Activities of daily living (for both "on" and "off")

5. Speech
   0 = normal
   1 = mildly affected; no difficulty being understood
   2 = moderately affected; sometimes asked to repeat statements
   3 = severely affected; frequently asked to repeat statements
   4 = unintelligible most of the time

6. Salivation
   0 = normal
   1 = slight but definite excess of saliva in mouth; may have nighttime
       drooling
   2 = moderately excessive saliva; may have minimal drooling
   3 = marked excess of saliva with some drooling
   4 = marked drooling, requires constant tissue or handkerchief

7. Swallowing
   0 = normal
   1 = rare choking
   2 = occasional choking
   3 = requires soft food
   4 = requires nasogastric tube or gastrostomy feeding

8. Handwriting
   0 = normal
   1 = slightly slow or small
   2 = moderately slow or small; all words are legible
   3 = severely affected; not all words are legible
   4 = the majority of words are not legible

9. Cutting food and handling utensils
   0 = normal
   1 = somewhat slow and clumsy but no help needed
   2 = can cut most foods, although clumsy and slow; some help needed
   3 = food must be cut by someone but can still feed slowly
   4 = needs to be fed

10. Dressing
    0 = normal
    1 = somewhat slow but no help needed
    2 = occasional assistance with buttoning, getting arms in sleeves
    3 = considerable help required but can do some things alone
    4 = helpless

11. Hygiene
    0 = normal
    1 = somewhat slow but no help needed
    2 = needs help to shower or bathe or very slow in hygienic care
    3 = requires assistance for washing, brushing teeth, combing hair, going
       to bathroom
    4 = Foley catheter or other mechanical aids

12. Turning in bed and adjusting bed clothes
    0 = normal
    1 = somewhat slow and clumsy but no help needed
    2 = can turn alone or adjust sheets but with great difficulty
    3 = can initiate but not turn or adjust sheets alone
    4 = helpless

13. Falling (unrelated to freezing)
    0 = none
    1 = rarely falls
    2 = occasionally falls, less than once per day
    3 = falls an average of once daily
    4 = falls more than once daily

14. Freezing when walking
    0 = none
    1 = rare freezing when walking; may have start hesitation
    2 = occasional freezing when walking
    3 = frequent freezing; occasionally falls from freezing
    4 = frequently falls from freezing

15. Walking
    0 = normal
    1 = mild difficulty; may not swing arms or may tend to drag leg
    2 = moderate difficulty, but requires little or no assistance
    3 = severe disturbance of walking, requiring assistance
    4 = cannot walk at all, even with assistance

16. Tremor (symptomatic complaint of tremor in any part of body)
    0 = absent
    1 = slight and infrequently present
    2 = moderate; bothersome to patient
    3 = severe; interferes with many activities
    4 = marked; interferes with most activities

17. Sensory complaints related to parkinsonism
    0 = none
    1 = occasionally has numbness, tingling, or mild aching
    2 = frequently has numbness, tingling, or aching; not distressing
    3 = frequent painful sensations
    4 = excruciating pain

III. Motor examination

18. Speech
    0 = normal
    1 = slight loss of expression, diction, or volume
    2 = monotone, slurred but understandable; moderately impaired
    3 = marked impairment, difficult to understand
    4 = unintelligible

19. Facial expression
    0 = normal
    1 = minimal hypomimia, could be normal "poker face"
    2 = slight but definitely abnormal diminution of facial expression
    3 = moderate hypomimia; lips parted some of the time
    4 = masked or fixed facies with severe or complete loss of facial expression; lips parted 0.25 in. or more

20. Tremor at rest (head, upper and lower extremities)
    0 = absent
    1 = slight and infrequently present
    2 = mild in amplitude and persistent, or moderate in amplitude but only intermittently present
    3 = moderate in amplitude and present most of the time
    4 = marked in amplitude and present most of the time

21. Action or postural tremor of hands
    0 = absent
    1 = slight; present with action
    2 = moderate in amplitude, present with action
    3 = moderate in amplitude with posture holding as well as action
    4 = marked in amplitude; interferes with feeding

22. Rigidity
    Rigidity is judged on passive movement of major joints with patient relaxed in sitting position. (Cogwheeling is to be ignored.)
    0 = absent
    1 = slight or detectable only when activated by mirror or other movements
    2 = mild to moderate
    3 = marked but full range of motion easily achieved
    4 = severe; range of motion achieved with difficulty

23. Finger taps
    Patient taps thumb with index finger in rapid succession.
    0 = normal
    1 = mild slowing and/or reduction in amplitude
    2 = moderately impaired; definite and early fatiguing; may have occasional arrests in movement
    3 = severely impaired; frequent hesitation in initiating movements or arrests in ongoing movement
    4 = can barely perform the task

24. Hand movements
    Patient opens and closes hands in rapid succession.
    0 = normal
    1 = mild slowing or reduction in amplitude
    2 = moderately impaired; definite and early fatiguing; may have occasional arrests in movement
    3 = severely impaired; frequent hesitation in initiating movements or arrests in ongoing movement
    4 = can barely perform the task

25. Rapid alternating movements of hands
    Rapid alternating movements of hands involve pronation-supination movements of hands, vertically and horizontally, with as large an amplitude as possible, both hands simultaneously.
    0 = normal
    1 = mild slowing or reduction in amplitude
    2 = moderately impaired; definite and early fatiguing; may have occasional arrests in movement
    3 = severely impaired; frequent hesitation in initiating movements or arrests in ongoing movement
    4 = can barely perform the task

26. Leg agility
   Patient taps heel on the ground in rapid succession, picking up entire leg. Amplitude should be at least 3 in.
   0 = normal
   1 = mild slowing or reduction in amplitude
   2 = moderately impaired; definite and early fatiguing; may have occasional arrests in movement
   3 = severely impaired; frequent hesitation in initiating movements or arrests in ongoing movement
   4 = can barely perform the task

27. Arising from chair
   Patient attempts to rise from a straight-backed chair with arms folded across chest.
   0 = normal
   1 = slow; may need more than one attempt
   2 = pushes self up from arms of seat
   3 = tends to fall back and may have to try more than one time but can get up without help
   4 = unable to arise without help

28. Posture
   0 = normal erect
   1 = not quite erect, slightly stooped posture; could be normal for older person
   2 = moderately stooped posture, definitely abnormal; can be slightly leaning to one side
   3 = severely stooped posture with kyphosis; can be moderately leaning to one side
   4 = marked flexion with extreme abnormality of posture

29. Gait
   0 = normal
   1 = walks slowly, may shuffle with short steps but no festination (hastening steps) or propulsion
   2 = walks with difficulty but requires little or no assistance; may have some festination, short steps, or propulsion
   3 = severe disturbance of gait, requiring assistance
   4 = cannot walk at all, even with assistance

30. Postural stability
    Postural stability involves response to sudden, strong posterior displacement produced by pull on shoulders while patient erect with eyes open and feet slightly apart. Patient is prepared.
    0 = normal
    1 = retropulsion but recovers unaided
    2 = absence of postural response; would fall if not caught by examiner
    3 = very unstable, tends to lose balance spontaneously
    4 = unable to stand without assistance

31. Body bradykinesia and hypokinesia
    Assessment of body bradykinesia and hypokinesia combines slowness, hesitancy, decreased arm swing, small amplitude, and poverty of movement in general.
    0 = none
    1 = minimal slowness, giving movement a deliberate character; could be normal for some persons; possibly reduced amplitude
    2 = mild degree of slowness and poverty of movement that is definitely abnormal; alternatively, some reduced amplitude
    3 = moderate slowness, poverty, or small amplitude of movement
    4 = marked slowness, poverty, or small amplitude of movement

IV. Complications of therapy (in the past week)

A. *Dyskinesias*

32. Duration
    What proportion of the waking day are dyskinesias present? (Historical information.)
    0 = none
    1 = 1–25% of day
    2 = 26–50% of day
    3 = 51–75% of day
    4 = 76–100% of day

33. Disability
    How disabling are the dyskinesias? (Historical information; may be modified by office examination.)
    0 = not disabling
    1 = mildly disabling
    2 = moderately disabling
    3 = severely disabling
    4 = completely disabled

34. Painful dyskinesias
     How painful are the dyskinesias?
     0 = no painful dyskinesias
     1 = slight
     2 = moderate
     3 = severe
     4 = marked

35. Presence of early morning dystonia (historical information)
     0 = no
     1 = yes

  B. *Clinical fluctuations*

36. Are "off" periods predictable?
     0 = no
     1 = yes

37. Are "off" periods unpredictable?
     0 = no
     1 = yes

38. Do "off" periods come on suddenly (within a few seconds)?
     0 = no
     1 = yes

39. What proportion of the waking day is the patient "off" on average?
     0 = none
     1 = 1–25% of day
     2 = 26–50% of day
     3 = 51–75% of day
     4 = 76–100% of day

  C. *Other complications*

40. Does the patient have anorexia, nausea, or vomiting?
     0 = no
     1 = yes

41. Does the patient have any sleep disturbances (e.g., insomnia or hyper-
     somnolence)?
     0 = no
     1 = yes

42. Does the patient have symptomatic orthostasis?
     Record the patient's blood pressure, height, and weight on the scoring
     form.
     0 = no
     1 = yes

V. Modified Hoehn and Yahr Staging

Stage 0 = no signs of disease
Stage 1 = unilateral disease
Stage 1.5 = unilateral plus axial involvement
Stage 2 = bilateral disease, without impairment of balance
Stage 2.5 = mild bilateral disease, with recovery on pull test
Stage 3 = mild to moderate bilateral disease; some postural instability; physically independent
Stage 4 = severe disability; still able to walk or stand unassisted
Stage 5 = wheelchair bound or bedridden unless aided

VI. Schwab and England Activities of Daily Living Scale

100% = completely independent; able to do all chores without slowness, difficulty, or impairment; essentially normal; unaware of any difficulty
90% = completely independent; able to do all chores with some degree of slowness, difficulty, and impairment; might take twice as long; beginning to be aware of difficulty
80% = completely independent in most chores; takes twice as long; conscious of difficulty and slowness
70% = not completely independent; more difficulty with some chores; may take three to four times as long in some; must spend a large part of the day with chores
60% = some dependency; can do most chores but exceedingly slowly and with much effort; errors; some chores impossible
50% = more dependent; can help with half of the chores; slower; difficulty with everything
40% = very dependent; can assist with all chores but few alone
30% = with effort, now and then does a few chores alone or begins alone; much help needed
20% = nothing alone; can be a slight help with some chores; severe invalid
10% = totally dependent, helpless; complete invalid
0% = vegetative functions such as swallowing, bladder, and bowel functions are not functioning; bedridden

REFERENCES

1. Rosen WG, Mohs RC, Davis KL. A new rating scale for Alzheimer's disease. *Am J Psychiatry* 1984;141:1356–1364.
2. Barohn RJ, Sahenk Z, Warmolts JR , Mendell JR. The Bruns-Garland Syndrome (diabetic amyotrophy). Revisited 100 years later. *Arch Neurol* 1991;48:1130–1135.
3. Mahoney FI, Barthel DW. Functional evaluation: the Barthel Index. A simple index of independence useful in scoring improvement in the rehabilitation of the chronically ill. *Md State Med J* 1965;14:61–65.
4. Hughes CP, Berg L, Danziger WL, et al. A new clinical scale for the staging of dementia. *Br J Psychiatry* 1982;140:566–572.
5. Knapp MJ, Knopman DS, Solomon PR, et al. A 30-week randomized controlled trial of high-dose tacrine in patients with Alzheimer's disease. *JAMA* 1994;271:985–991.
6. Schneider LS, Olin JT, Doody RS, et al. Validity and reliability of the Alzheimer's Disease Cooperative Study—Clinical Global Impression of Change. *Alzheimer Dis Assoc Disord* 1997;11(Suppl 2):S22–S32.
7. Adour KK, Swanson PJ. Facial paralysis in 403 consecutive patients: emphasis on treatment response in patients with Bell's palsy. *Trans Am Acad Ophthalmol Otolaryngol* 1971;75:1284–1301.
8. Efficiency of plasma exchange in Guillain-Barré Syndrome: role of replacement fluids. French Cooperative Group on Plasma Exchange in Guillain-Barré Syndrome. *Ann Neurol* 1987;22:753–761.
9. Hamilton BB, Granger CV, Sherwin FS, et al. A Uniform National Data System for Medical Rehabilitation. In MJ Fuhrer (ed), Rehabilitation Outcomes—Analysis and Measurement. Baltimore: Paul H Brookes Publishing Co., 1987.
10. Teasdale G, Jennett B. Assessment of coma and impaired consciousness. A practical scale. *Lancet* 1974;2:81–84.
11. Jennett B, Bond M. Assessment of outcome after severe brain damage. *Lancet* 1975;1:480–484.
12. Double-blind trial of intravenous methylprednisolone in Guillain-Barré syndrome. Guillain-Barré Syndrome Steroid Trial Group. *Lancet* 1993;341:586–590.
13. Hoehn MM, Yahr MD. Parkinsonism: onset, progression, and mortality. *Neurology* 1967;17:427–442.
14. House JW, Brackmann DE. Facial nerve grading system. *Otolaryngol Head Neck Surg* 1985;93:146–147.

15. Plasmapheresis and acute Guillain-Barré syndrome. Guillain-Barré Syndrome Study Group. *Neurology* 1985;35:1096–1104.

16. Hunt WE, Hess RM. Surgical risk as related to time of intervention in the repair of intracranial aneurysms. *J Neurosurg* 1968;28:14–20.

17. Benzel EC, Lancon J, Kesterson L, Hadden T. Cervical laminectomy and dentate ligament section for cervical spondylotic myelopathy. *J Spinal Disord* 1991;4:286–295.

18. Kurtzke JF. Rating neurologic impairment in multiple sclerosis: an expanded disability status scale (EDSS). *Neurology* 1983;33:1444–1452.

19. Mann KS, Khosla VK, Gulati DR. Cervical spondylotic myelopathy treated by single-stage multilevel anterior decompression. *J Neurosurg* 1984;60:81–87.

20. Folstein MG, Folstein SE, McHugh PR. "Mini-mental state"—a practical method for grading the cognitive state of patients for the clinician. *J Psychiatr Res* 1975;12:189–198.

21. Tindall RS, Rollins JA, Phillips JT, et al. Preliminary results of a double-blind, randomized, placebo-controlled trial of cyclosporin in myasthenia gravis. *N Engl J Med* 1987;316:719–724.

22. Gajdos P, Chevret S, Clair B, et al. Clinical trial of plasma exchange and high-dose intravenous immunoglobulin in myasthenia gravis. Myasthenia Gravis Clinical Study Group. *Ann Neurol* 1997;41:789–796.

23. Brott T, Adams JP, Olinger CP, et al. Measurements of acute cerebral infarction: a clinical examination scale. *Stroke* 1989;20:864–870.

24. Lyden P, Brott T, Tilley B, et al. Improved reliability of the NIH Stroke Scale using video training. NINDS TPA Stroke Study Group. *Stroke* 1994;25:2220–2226.

25. Nurick S. The pathogenesis of spinal cord disorder associated with cervical spondylosis. *Brain* 1972;95:87–100.

26. Dyck PJ, Sherman WR, Hallcher LM, et al. Human diabetic endoneurial sorbitol, fructose, and myo-inositol related to sural nerve morphometry. *Ann Neurol* 1980;8:590–596.

27. Cummings JL, Mega M, Gray K, et al. The Neuropsychiatric Inventory: comprehensive assessment of psychopathology in dementia. *Neurology* 1994;44:2308–2314.

28. Lacomblez L, Bouche P, Bensimon G, Meininger V. A double-blind, placebo-controlled trial of high doses of gangliosides in amyotrophic lateral sclerosis. *Neurology* 1989;39:1635–1637.

29. Bamford JM, Sandercock PA, Warlow CP, Slattery J. Interobserver agreement for the assessment of handicap in stroke patients. *Stroke* 1989;20:828.

30. van Swieten JC, Koudstaal PJ, Visser MC, et al. Inter-observer agreement for the assessment of handicap in stroke patients. *Stroke* 1988;19:604–607.

31. Lindenstrøm E, Boysen G, Christiansen LW, et al. Reliability of Scandinavian Neurological Stroke Scale. *Cerebrovasc Dis* 1991;1:103–107.

Index

Page numbers followed by *f* indicate figures; numbers followed by *t* indicate tables.